PHANTOM LIMB

BIOPOLITICS: MEDICINE, TECHNOSCIENCE,
AND HEALTH IN THE 21ST CENTURY
General Editors: Monica J. Casper and Lisa Jean Moore

Missing Bodies: The Politics of Visibility
Monica J. Casper and Lisa Jean Moore

*Against Health: How Health
Became the New Morality*
Edited by Jonathan M. Metzl
and Anna Kirkland

*Is Breast Best? Taking on the
Breastfeeding Experts and the New
High Stakes of Motherhood*
Joan B. Wolf

Biopolitics: An Advanced Introduction
Thomas Lemke

*The Material Gene: Gender, Race, and
Heredity after the Human Genome Project*
Kelly E. Happe

*Cloning Wild Life: Zoos, Captivity, and
the Future of Endangered Animals*
Carrie Friese

*Eating Drugs: Psychopharmaceutical
Pluralism in India*
Stefan Ecks

*Phantom Limb: Amputation, Embodiment,
and Prosthetic Technology*
Cassandra S. Crawford

Phantom Limb

Amputation, Embodiment, and Prosthetic Technology

Cassandra S. Crawford

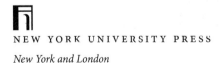

NEW YORK UNIVERSITY PRESS

New York and London

Library Resource Center
Renton Technical College
3000 N.E. 4th Street
Renton, WA 98056

617.9 CRAWFOR 2014

Crawford, Cassandra.

Phantom limb

NEW YORK UNIVERSITY PRESS
New York and London
www.nyupress.org

© 2014 by New York University
All rights reserved

References to Internet websites (URLs) were accurate at the time of writing.
Neither the author nor New York University Press is responsible for URLs that
may have expired or changed since the manuscript was prepared.

LIBRARY OF CONGRESS CATALOGING-IN-PUBLICATION DATA
Crawford, Cassandra S.,
Phantom limb : amputation, embodiment, and prosthetic technology /
Cassandra S. Crawford.
    pages cm
Includes bibliographical references and index.
ISBN 978-0-8147-8928-5 (hardback) — ISBN 978-0-8147-6012-3 (pb)
1. Prosthesis. 2. Phantom limb. I. Title.
RD553.C88 2014
617.9—dc23   2013029822

New York University Press books are printed on acid-free paper,
and their binding materials are chosen for strength and durability.
We strive to use environmentally responsible suppliers and materials
to the greatest extent possible in publishing our books.

Manufactured in the United States of America
10 9 8 7 6 5 4 3 2 1
Also available as an ebook

CONTENTS

Acknowledgments   vii

1. Introduction: Ghost in the Machine   1

2. Characterizing Phantoms: Features of Phantom Limb Syndrome   30

3. From Pleasure to Pain: Accounting for the Rise and Fall in Phantom Pain   73

4. Phantoms in the Mind: The Psychogenic Origins of Ethereal Appendages   107

5. Phantoms in the Brain: The Holy Grail of Neuroscience   149

6. Phantom-Prosthetic Relations: The Modernization of Amputation   193

7. Conclusion: Authenticity and Extinction   223

Notes   251

References   267

Index   301

About the Auhor   307

ACKNOWLEDGMENTS

I want to thank Adele Clark, Lucy Suchman, Virginia Olesen, and Steve Kurzman for their efforts and creative inspiration during the early stages this project. In particular, I am grateful to Adele Clarke for her careful reading and generous commentary. Friends and colleagues have also been invaluable in terms of feedback, critique, and encouragement, including Stephanie Basko, Renee Beard, Gay Becker, Monica Casper, Alexandra Crawford, Emerson Crawford, Alan Czaplicki, Sean Farrell, Chris Ganchoff, Michael Hentschel, Kristin Huffine, Ilene Kalish, Lisa Jean Moore, Diane Rodgers, Dale Rose, and Rachael Washburn. I am especially thankful to the brilliant visual artist Alexa Wright, who generously allowed me to include her beautiful and provocotive photos. The National Institute of General Medical Sciences, the National Science Foundation, the University of California, and Northern Illinois University also provided generous funding and other resources integral to the completion of the book. I have also included previously published material and would like to thank the publishers for giving me permission to reprint those articles here. Chapter 4 includes material from the article "From Pleasure to Pain: The Role of the MPQ in the Language of Phantom Limb Pain" published in *Social Science and Medicine*, 69(5):655-661 in 2009. Chapter 6 includes material from the article "'You Don't Need a Body to Feel a Body': Phantom Limb Syndrome and Corporeal Transgression" published in *Sociology of Health and Illness*, 35(3):1-15 in 2013.

1

Introduction

Ghost in the Machine

In many ways, the conference was like all others. Hundreds of us had taken over the lobby, the hallways, the dining spaces, and many of the meeting rooms in the Fairmont Dallas on an oppressively sultry August weekend. We were all signing in, orienting, mingling—all of those registration day musts. I was given a "first-timer" sticker. But, unlike most of the other first-timers, I was one of a very few at the conference who was not an amputee. The Amputee Coalition of America's (ACA) Annual Education Conference and Exposition was officially devoted to changing direction, and to the technology, prevention, information, and support needed to make that happen. However, another theme was more conspicuous. I found it in the sessions, the workshops, the informal gatherings, and most prominently in the exhibit hall where attendees spent the majority of their time watching presentations, having their gaits analyzed by prosthetists other than their own, and collecting generous amounts of swag. Prosthetization, it seemed, was tantamount to rebirth.

The schedule included two days of technology sessions with presentations on issues such as phantom pain reduction, cutting-edge advances that will change the way amputees live and work, or choosing a microprocessor knee; workshops on issues such as fitness and state advocacy; networking rooms; panels addressing psychological health and finding community resources; a gait analysis clinic; and a very large exhibit hall that included hundreds of exhibited products as well as exhibitor product-theater presentations such as Freedom Innovation's "Join the Revolution." Manufacturers of prostheses and prosthetic paraphernalia were all vying for our attention. Össur, whose slogan was "life without limitations," had world-class amputee athlete Sarah Reinertsen center stage. She and her biking-leg were a seamless extension of the stationary show-bike that she dutifully rode for hours on end. Sarah was a principle member of Team Össur whose mission was public awareness; their message was that "with the help of modern technology, amputees can lead the kind of lives they want, achieving things that were almost unimaginable in previous generations" (Össur 2005, 2). Össur's prosthetic line included the Mauch, a hydraulic knee that presumably transformed its user into a force to be reckoned with. Like anything or anyone capable of mach speeds, Össur's (2010, 1) knee promised to move amputees with the kind of "advanced performance functions" that mocked—perhaps with a hint of contempt—those knees that only permitted basic performance, those made of soft tissue and bone.

Freedom Innovations showcased the Revolution Series, including the Renegade, which apparently enabled its wearer to "reject tradition . . . [and] break away from the pack" (FI 2005, 2) to join another, more worthy cause, one that repudiated prerevolutionary embodiment, espoused radical change, and avowed technologically mediated corporeal transcendence. Freedom Innovations also offered attendees the chance to meet Chad Crittenden, the first amputee to appear on the television show *Survivor*. They made photo opportunities available with Chad, but more importantly, they offered freedom—the kind of freedom that allowed Chad to survive in Vanuatu—freedom from disability, freedom from the limitations of dismemberment.

"Technology for the human race" (CPI 2004, 2), assertedly for all of humanity as well as for the intraspecies evolutionary "race to the top," was College Park Industries' slogan. They presented, among others, their Venture, which as the moniker implied implored its user to embrace an undertaking that was neither trivial nor certain. But, College Park Industries assured transition with ease. The often debilitating phantom pain, the performativity, the abandonment and adoption of embodied technique, the many problems associated with and the work involved in techno-corporeal seaming or coupling were each and all hidden behind shiny prostheses, slogans, and salespeople.

These manufacturers and some forty others inundated attendees with messages about the possibilities of rebirth through prosthetization. In fact, the state of the science was touted as extraordinary, cutting-edge, awe-inspiring, and decidedly futuristic, and we were without exception identified as potential beneficiaries; we were all enthusiastically invited to join the revolution and to embrace technologically achieved corporeal enhancement, self-actualization, aesthetic individuation, moral transcendence, and much more. It was this discourse on the transformative nature and power of prostheses that inspired my work. It was conspicuously apparent at the ACA conference where I observed[1] and conducted both formal and informal interviews, as well as in the 805 prosthetic science, psychiatric/psychological, and (bio)medical articles and texts from circa 1870 to 2011 that I analyzed utilizing a grounded-theory-inspired[2] interpretive content analysis;[3] among the clinicians and researchers whom I interviewed[4] from across the United States and Canada working on various aspects of phantom limb syndrome; and in the often techno-philic or at least techno-friendly arguments of academics and other pundits that I referenced.

Prosthetized Rebirth

Rooted in a form of hegemonic ableism, the discourse on prosthetized rebirth assumes an impoverished body amenable to liberatory enhancement and existential transcendence because it is "in need of" technologic quickening while also assuming its antithesis: the natural, "normal," biologic/biomedical body. As Shildrick (2008, 32; original emphasis) cautioned, "We must constantly remind ourselves that what is called normal is always *normative*, and at the very least devolves on some form of unstated value judgment that may well require intervention and manipulation to achieve." Like the impoverished body, the normal body is a moral, conceptual, technologic, and practical accomplishment, and its often unremarkable and unexamined naturalness is held in place by way of such practices as "achieved" prosthetization and "acquired" physical deficiency or defect. Although outwardly liberatory, the discourse on prosthetized rebirth asserts and reaffirms the distinction between the normal and the hybridized, it secures a form of exclusive biomedical authority as researchers and practitioners assume the role of the legitimate arbitrators of normality, and it reinforces a particular biopolitical order that places some bodies and not others at the center of emerging forms of life and living. When imbricated with a vision of the impending "progressive" cyborgian revolution, this discourse confirms that body modification by way of techno-corporeal conjoin-ment is incontrovertibly desirable and eminently advantageous—augmenting body, mind, and spirit—and by extension, that biomedicine and technoscience are the only or at least the most obvious means of achieving physical, functional, aesthetic, and moral preeminence.

As a core feature of the twenty-first century biopolitical order, the discourse on prosthetized rebirth or transcendent hybridization has enormous implications for the bodies that zealously pursue, migrate towards, or are unwittingly thrust into the center of biomedical and technoscientific projects inspired by the belief in revolutionary and emancipatory techno-corporeality. Casper and Moore (2009, 1) argue that in the age of "proliferating human bodies," it has become imperative that we document precisely which bodies have gone missing or have been made invisible in an effort to confront the processes of erasure-as-social-control. However, it is also crucial in this context to ask, Which bodies do we regularly catch sight of? Which bodies capture our attention? Which bodies do we peek, leer, stare, and gaze at? Which bodies are seen and which bodies are shown? Which bodies are made clearly visible or, in Casper and Moore's (2009, 179) terms, "hypervisible"? In this way, we can also confront the processes of exposure-as-social-control. Taken together, these types of inquiries help to define the emerging biopolitical order or the means through which power is exercised on, over, and though the body in order to regulate ever more aspects of the biophysical (what is fundamentally "organic" or indicative and derivative of the organism and assertedly distinct from the cultural, the artificial, and the inorganic), the corporeal (what constitutes the physical or tangible attributes of the body when overdetermined), the embodied (what makes up, classifies, and is produced by living through the body), the visceral (what makes up and originates in the interior but manifests outside of bodies becoming collective), and the flesh (what composes the body's exterior or surface that is both amenable and resistant to attempts at "inscription").

As an exemplar of what Foucault (1978, 141) referred to as "anatomo-politics" or the purposive surveillance, categorization, regimentation, and manipulation of the human body with the intention of optimizing its capacities, extorting its forces, and rendering it docile, the discourse on prosthetized rebirth establishes the historicity of technologic quickening—a narrative of authenticity about techno-corporeality and its properties; it reinforces internalized self-order and control—by way of identification with species cyborg and the mandates that citizenship entails; and it individuates the responsibility for "successful" actualization—after all, biomedicine can show you the way, but you have to want it first.

I engage the discourse on prosthetic transcendence or rebirth critically, interested in deconstructing the naturalized, purportedly "unmediated" relationship between prosthetization and corporeal transformation. This kind of critical approach allows for the conditions under which the discourse surfaced, matured, and elaborated to be made apparent. It also exposes the past, present, and potential future effects of its dissemination, while opening up the possibilities for and the implications of its disruption. In Rose's (2007, 4, 5) terms, discourses are dissected and denatured in order to "destabilize a present that has forgotten its contingency . . . [and] destabilize the future by recognizing its openness." It also destabilizes a reified past by denaturing an origin story and a developmental or evolutionary history that has been a source of definitiveness rather than contingency and completion rather than openness.

Thus, I ask precisely *how* and in *what ways* has prosthetization transformed the bodies, selves, and identities of the men, women, and children who have survived amputation? How does historicizing and contextualizing these transformations give us insight into the ways in which bodies and corporeal technologies relate as well as into the ways in which past bodies and future bodies are inflected within present technologies of the body? What part has the evolution of prostheses played in the modernization of amputation? Furthermore, what are the implications of such transformations for all of us, for how we collectively envision what prosthetization does to bodies? How do the promises and realizations of revolutionary forms of techno-corporeality alter what we expect from these technologies and from bodies, especially the "disfigured" or "functionally impaired"?

Ghost in the Machine

I have taken pains not to celebrate or fetishize prosthetic technologies, not to be eagerly or even cautiously seduced by the arguably imminent or actualized revolution, not to be mesmerized by the transformative power of prostheses because prosthetization is not simply or straightforwardly done to bodies. Instead, it is always a relational process of technologization-in-the-making. Transcendent prosthetization, for example, has only been realized for amputees, prosthetists, clinicians, and others as a consequence of the relationship forged between artificial limbs and phantom limbs or those ghostly appendages that can persist sometimes with uncanny realness long after fleshy limbs have been traumatically, surgically, congenitally, or electively amputated. For instance, Simmel (1966b, 346) described how convincingly haunted limbs could present themselves to amputees; she wrote,

> The first meeting between a phantom limb and its owner is, typically, a rather dramatic affair. As the patient wakes up from surgery he feels his leg present, he seems to be able to wiggle his toes quite normally—and then someone steps up to him and tells him that the operation went very well and he will be able to walk on an artificial limb in no time at all. No matter how well and how long before the operation he was prepared for the loss of the leg, the patient typically cannot believe that it is really gone . . . [because] he continues to feel the absent limb as if it were still present.

Phantom limbs have often been conceptualized as thoroughly mimetic, all but faultless copies of the genuine thing, or even as possessing more

awareness than the preamputated limbs they emulated and consequently, as exceptionally pleasant or pleasurable. One of Simmel's (1956,
641) patients reported, "The leg felt good . . . real good." For other amputees, phantoms have been sensed as paralyzed and functionally dead
to the world, as if submerged in mercury, weighed down by plaster, or
imbedded in a block of ice. And quite disturbingly, these bodily apparitions have also subjected some amputees to a lifetime of one of the most
intractable and merciless pains ever known.

Phantom limbs are curious to be sure because they often move in the
world like fleshy limbs—waving goodbye or gesticulating during conversation—because they possess lovely or disturbing histories—wearing precious engagement rings, favorite lace-lined socks, or blood-filled
boots; because they can exist tenaciously and sometimes audaciously—
penetrating solids, objects, and even the very viscera of others; and
because they "physically" detach from the body—leaving gaping holes as
the hovering bit follows the body with reverence and in perfect harmony.
Embodied ghosts are curious for these and many other reasons, and it
is their curiousness—their many eccentricities—that make phantom
limbs a uniquely productive ingress into epistemological and ontological
questions about the body,[5] techno-corporeality, and embodiment, questions that have surfaced over the last few decades as the dismembered
body has become an increasingly fruitful object and site of biomedical intervention, and as phantoms have become ever more productive
technologies-of-the-body. To be sure, shadowy limbs are "technologies";
they are the practical application of biomedical and scientific knowledge
intended to accomplish a task, the creation and use of technical means
to serve a purpose, even if that purpose goes unrealized, is converted,
is intentionally subverted, or is deliberately (or naively) appropriated.

Deeply Embodied Technologies

Without question, prostheses are invested in and become vital via
human labor and inventiveness —by designers—but they are also vitalized by those who embody them—by users (Oudshoorn and Pinch

2005). Technologies are imagined and constructed with "user represen-tatives" in mind (Akrich 1995; Woolgar 1991), but they are also always negotiated in-use both deliberately and as a consequence of the recalci-trant nature of the body. *Deeply embodied technologies* leave transitory and lasting traces on physical bodies, just as "body-based traces" (Hocky and Draper 2005, 47) of various kinds are left on those same technolo-gies. Prostheses bruise, rub, lacerate, and fatigue, while also being "worn in" and lived-as-flesh. And, it is because of the profound intimacy had with phantom limbs—the tendency for prostheses to rouse and civilize unruly phantoms and for phantoms to animate lifeless prostheses—that prostheses have become invested with therapeutic, transcendent, evoca-tive, and other qualities.

In other words, the corporeality (in addition to the subjectivity) of users will always have an effect on technologies just as those same tech-nologies function to shape the bodies of users precisely because they are of-the-body, because they are *embodied*. I use the term "embodiment" to signal the engaged process of both having and being a body, of pos-sessing a body while also being possessed by it, of simultaneously being both object and subject to oneself (Mead and Morris 1934). The body-as-object is shaped by normative understandings of private and public behavior, techniques, acts, practices, and the like, all of which are gov-erned by those individuals, collectives, institutions, and knowledges that colonize bodies, define the body-collective, and regulate, delimit, and normalize populations. The body-as-subject is purposefully individu-ated, reflexively managed, and intentionally inhabited (Adler and Adler 2011). It is used, shaped, ornamented, performed, and done. Undeni-ably, "The body is alive, which means that it is as capable of influencing and transforming social languages as they are capable of influencing and transforming it" (Siebers 2008, 68). Thus, we intentionally and uninten-tionally *take on* both material and ideational features of the social world such that we *come to* embody (to express, personify, or exemplify), pro-vide a body for (to make incarnate by living), and comprise (to make up while embracing, rejecting, or modifying) that very world. As opposed to pure object—the body objectified and treated as "thing"—as opposed to the pure subject—the "deciding force" and foundational impulse—we are of-our-bodies, and it is through them that the world itself comes into being.

Foregrounding the concept of embodiment circumvents the trappings of technological determinism that threatens projects like these. It also exposes not only the ways in which amputation surgery and prosthetic science have related as disciplines or the ways in which amputees and their prosthetists have related interpersonally, but also the ways in which amputated bodies and prostheses themselves have related. In other words, focusing the analytic lens on amputated bodies (rather than selves, identities, psyches, etc.) with their undeniably uncanny phantomed limbs and their deeply embodied artificial limbs takes seriously the role that haunted limbs have played in the representation of technologic appendages as transformative while simultaneously acknowledging the role that prostheses have played in phantom limbs becoming productive technologies-of-the-body, becoming socially and materially substantive. Inquiry into how phantom limbs and prosthetic limbs relate, into *phantom-prosthetic relations*, tells us as much about what is "known" and knowable about these curious and illusive ghosts as it does about how prostheses transform or precisely what prosthetized rebirth entails, for whom, and why. Indeed, whether intended for functional restoration or for radical enhancement, whether relatively crude or comparatively sophisticated, whether mimetic or revolutionary, modern prostheses have transformed; they have transformed the bodies, the minds, and the brains of amputees while also transforming the prosthetic imaginary.

Transforming Bodies

In the early history of American prosthetic science, the aim of designers and manufacturers was to return the male body to a functional state, enabling the amputee to regain his role as productive citizen and to fend off accusations of dependency, emasculation, and radical impairment. At times this entailed prioritizing the functionality of the artificial limb at the expense of its "look." For the mid-twentieth-century skilled laborer, for example, upper limb prostheses were sometimes adapted through work-specific attachments to interface with industrial machinery, making the amputee a living extension of industry (Meier 2004). These prostheses, intended for functional *restoration*, were far from mimetic of fleshy limbs. That is not to say that the aesthetic of artificial limbs was inconsequential. In fact, from the postbellum context onward, imitation has been a guiding principle of prosthetic design even when efficiency and operability needed to be sacrificed (Ott 2002). Underlying both of these impulses, nevertheless, has been a desire to reestablish mobility and restore productivity, especially to the boys and men who had sacrificed limbs in the service of their country.

In the contemporary context, prosthetization has been guided by functional and, for some amputees, aesthetic *enhancement*. Enhancement innovations have included the use of novel materials, including acrylics, epoxies, fiberglass, and Kevlar; the addition of microprocessor knees with hydraulic systems; dynamic response feet that store and release energy; the harnessing of remaining nerves and musculature; novel and more efficient power sources; the renewal of sensation; direct neural interfacing with the brain;[6] osseointegration or direct attachment to bone; bionic ankles that imitate muscles and tendons; and the application of biomechanical and animal models, among many others.

Since the turn of the twenty-first century, bodies have been mediated by prosthetization in ways that are profoundly different from past transformations. Though the coupling of bodies and technologies has been an elemental aspect of social life throughout modern history, contemporary prostheses are unique in terms of the degree to which they are intimately integrated with and into the tissues of the body. In fact, some scholars have argued that current hybridization is dissimilar from that of the past in that today's technologies have come to degrade our essential human-ness; we are less of ourselves for having developed such indelible intimacies with machines. Others, such as Luke (1996, 7), proposed that we consider the "dehuman . . . cyborg-anized quasi-object/quasi-subject . . . [as the] ontological constant rather than a technological aberration." In a similar vein, Rabinow (1996, 108) suggested that "nature's malleability offers an 'invitation' to the artificial. . . . Once understood in this way, the only natural thing for man to do would be to facilitate, encourage, accelerate its unfurling." Ironically, artificiality is an inevitable expression of all things natural. And, challenging the argument that the flesh is endangered by technologies-of-the-body like these, Balsamo (1996, 40) asserted that the cyborg actually reasserts the materiality of the body because "cyborgs never leave the meat behind" (Balsamo 1996, 40). In fact, bodies may be considered hypermaterial at the same time that they are understood to be patently nonnatural.[7]

Unquestionably in the late-modern context, we are pressed to ask, How transcendent are techno-corporeal con-joinments of this kind, or, more to the point, how transcendent should they be? What can be said with certainty is that the material and symbolic effects of past, present, and imagined future iterations of prostheses on embodiment and corporeality cannot be differentiated by the extent of functional replacement alone. Late-modern prostheses have developed a lived "taken-for-grantedness" (Olesen 1992, 210) because they increasingly interface deeply and indelibly with remaining nerves and musculature, with skeletal systems, with cortices, and the like; they have become of-the-body in novel ways as our morphology, physiology, neurology, and our very humanity have been reimagined. Not inconsequentially, this level of intimacy has only been possible in the case of amputees because of the relations had between phantoms and prostheses. Embodied ghosts have engendered prosthetic taken-for-grantedness because they have inhabited and vitalized artificial limbs with evident ease and because they are devoted to the practice of technologic quickening. Phantoms and prostheses have long had a tendency to affiliate, have long been "companion technologies" that clinicians, researchers, and amputees alike have wanted and, at times, needed to exploit.

Transforming Minds and Brains

Artificial limbs have also historically been designed with the intent of transforming individual and societal psyches. Dismemberment can

Library Resource Center
Renton Technical College
3000 N.E. 4th Street
Renton, WA 98056

impart physical and functional as well as psychological and social losses, and accordingly, artificial limbs have been envisioned as therapeutic. For example, turn-of-the-twentieth-century prostheses were thought to reestablish productivity, returning the masculine body to industriousness, while also staving off problematic adjustment to limb loss (Herschbach 1997). Despite this expectation, however, amputees were often regarded as evincing the kinds of physical and psychical characteristics that typified the fragility and instability of femininity. The emasculating effects of amputation have long been a concern of clinicians, and one of the most obvious indicators of poor adaptation was the manifestation of a phantom limb. Those amputees who reported ethereal appendages that felt, "looked," and moved like intact limbs, particularly those amputees who reported cruel and debilitating pain, were, during the late 1800s, for example, equated with the female hysteric (Long 2004). Because the integrity of the mind was thought to be dependent on the integrity of the body, dismemberment undermined the self and made the amputee a literal and figurative "fraction" of a man (Mitchell 1871; O'Connor 2000); phantoms were proof that dismemberment altered the psyches of even the toughest, most commanding, and proudest of men, and were proof that maladjustment could be found in the healthiest and most vigorous of communities.

The assumption that amputation emasculated men and that phantoms were the "material" expression of psychical troubles remained relatively unchallenged until the post–World War II years. Postwar renormalization efforts involved the intensive rehabilitation of demobilized wounded, significant and unparalleled state investment in prosthetic technologies, and the strategic conflation of the prosthetized amputee with military technological prowess (Serlin 2004). Together these came to constitute a national program that was incommensurate with the association of dismemberment with emasculation and mental instability, and consequently, phantoms were reconceptualized as fundamentally neurophysiologic in origin. This shift from the psychologization to the medicalization of phantom limb syndrome, from phantoms originating in disturbed minds to phantoms originating in reorganized brains,

had many implications, not the least of which was that it altered the kinds of stories that were or could be told by researchers, practitioners, and amputees themselves about how phantoms felt, about their size and shape, about when they materialized, and about what they did or how they could be used.

Over the next few decades, the brain became an increasingly viable site for locating the origins of phantoms in large part because of the emergence, proliferation, and advance of medical imaging technologies during the 1970s and 1980s and because the then-nascent field of neuroscience was gaining legitimacy. Americans became fascinated with the brain, and neuroscience surfaced as the predominant means through which we understood everything from memory and emotion to perception and the development of a sense of self. By the early 1990s and consonant with the trend in neuroscientific research of challenging the relative stability of neuronal connections in the adult human brain (the hardwired paradigm), phantom phenomena began to be attributed to neuronal malleability (the plasticity paradigm). Relocated in the brains rather than the minds of amputees, the phantom was rendered biomedically "real," factual, and authentic rather than fictitious, fraudulent, and fanciful. Equally notable, however, was the reconceptualization of prostheses. Because of the neuroscientific research on phantom limb syndrome, artificial limbs became key to appreciating, preventing, and/or harnessing the capacity of the human cortex to reorganize itself. The phantom functioned as an unexpected window enabling researchers to see that prostheses fundamentally transformed the structure and function not only of bodies but of brains as well.

Transforming the Prosthetic Imaginary

Innovations in prosthetic science have also transformed the prosthetic imaginary or the shared ideas that both establish and reflect what we envision that prosthetization does to bodies, and the circulated symbols and stories that encapsulate how we make visible and visualize prosthetic embodiment. Fixated on the "miracles" of biomedicine and technoscience, Americans readily consume the stories and images regularly circulated in the media and beyond. Indeed, Friedman (2004, 2) argued, "The intricate web spun jointly by medicine and the media results from a collaborative process that resembles a mating ritual as much as a professional relationship." What is so powerful about these representations is that they carry both authority and appeal (Friedman 2004); they are lovely, evocative, compelling, and outwardly ingenuous. And, we believe in the promise of biomedical and technoscientific "fixes" to fundamentally alter bodies and, maybe more importantly, selves. The rhetoric of personal transformation (Featherstone 1999), expressive individualism (Hewitt 1997; Sweetman 1999), self-actualization (Haiken 1997), or spiritual cure (Gilman 1998) is intoxicating, and many of us want our fix; we want to be "some body new" (Glassner 1995, 175). There is something unmistakably paradoxical about our anxious desire to realize individual authenticity through (sometimes) radical and dramatic change. Yet, even as we are torn between desire and loathing, awe and skepticism, exhilaration and fear, we still want to be some body new. In fact, those who are born again seem to be exceptional, exceptionally "health[y], enhance[d] and fully functional—more real than real" (Balsamo 1995, 216). They seem to have been resurrected with all the concomitant advantages that rebirth entails. Like the discarnate ghost who no longer bleeds, the technologically mediated body loses its "pathetic vulnerability" (Blum 2003, 49) and a life-affirming spirit rises from the ashes of the sacrificial flesh. Sara Reinertsen on *The Amazing Race*, Chad Chittenden on *Survivor: Vanuatu*, Kelly Bruno on *Survivor: Redemption Island*, Steve Gill on *Big Brother 11*, and Heather Mills on *Dancing with the Stars* are just a very few of the extraordinary prosthetized amputees who appear to demonstrate that through the wonders of prosthetization and an achieved indomitable spirit, amputees can be reborn and accomplish the truly miraculous.

As the hype suggests, rebirth entails rupture, a radical departure that leads ultimately to consummate rapture. Rebirth entails disassociation from the fragility of the flesh that leads ultimately to a resolute devotion to revolutionary ideals and, finally, to an enduring fidelity to species cyborg. What receives little exposure is the fact that rebirth also entails pain, the pain of "passing" as well as the "growing pains" involved in becoming some body new. And as Shildrick (2008, 35) pointed out, "Given the acceptability and sometimes quite considerable pain in the pursuit of reconstruction, we might see that what is treated is a pathology in the cultural imaginary, rather than in the individual body." Pain is an acceptable if unfortunate side effect of treating the pathologized prosthetic imaginary, one that the public can tolerate even if the amputee cannot.

In many respects our fascination with techno-miracles is an outgrowth of and testifies to the contemporary biomedical trend toward technological fetishism and highly technologically mediated transformations (Clarke 2003). This has played out in the prosthetic sciences in a number of ways over the last few decades. Design is no longer inspired by the desire to return bodies to "normal" states but rather by the desire to transcend the inadequacies of the human body, its pathetic vulnerability, and the weaknesses of its problematical architecture. Prosthetists consequently began looking toward animal and mechanical models with the intention of expanding on human biomechanics. As Ott (2002, 24–25) explained, "The design trajectory of a technology—from mimicry to modification and then to dissociation with the original—has happened many times in history. . . . Many prosthetic makers in the late twentieth century took a turn into visionary engineering, where parts replicated neither form nor function of the human body." Visionaries often commune with and find their muse in hybrids, those that reside between worlds. And sometimes, they quite simply engineer them.

The image of Aimee Mullins, the professional athlete, actress, and model featured on the cover of *Dazed and Confused,* shows us that prosthetization enables the amputee to be beautiful not only on the inside—with an otherworldly spirit that seems to glow—but on the outside as well. One of *People Magazine's* fifty most beautiful people in 1999 (Toepter 1999), Aimee became "fashion-able" through technologically mediated conjoin-ment with the cheetah. Össur's Cheetah feet allowed her to move off the paralympic racing track and onto the sleek catwalk

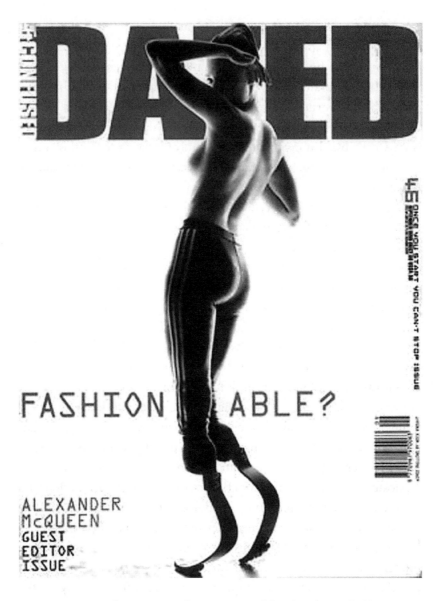

Figure 1.1. Aimee Mullins. Aimee Mullins, actress, model, and professional athlete, featured on the September 1998 cover of *Dazed and Confused Magazine*. (Reprinted with permission from Dazedgroup.)

with the commanding power, the breathtaking agility, and the enchanting grace of bodies that are not just able, but remark-able. Hers is the kind of spectacular body that might just leave an observer a bit dazed and confused.

Unquestionably, prosthetization has been a project in the aesthetics of corporeality and today there is beauty in the convergence of the "natural" with futuristic technologies of the body that both enable and "exoticize." With visible fuchsia and aqua-tinted tibia and fibula equivalents, for example, prostheses at the ACA conference were quite stunning to be sure. Most were worn without the "skin," exposing both the internal mechanics of their legs and arms as well as their membership in species cyborg. Counter to Hughes's (2007) claim that the disabled are not objects of desire in part because they evoke fears of physical frailty, the contemporary prosthetized amputee with seemingly invulnerable and unquestionably exotic limbs represents not fragility but imperviousness. And, as one of "the people's" most beautiful, Aimee is far from undesirable.

With intent and unwittingly, amputees have come to dwell at the border of present and future techno-corporeality, to embody the liberatory promises of medicine, science, and technology, to exemplify human/animal/mechanic hybridization, and to occupy a position of primacy in our prosthetic imaginary. Amputees are central to our understanding of how prosthetization in all of its guises is done, to what revolutionary techno-corporeality purportedly entails or might someday entail, and to the ways in which aesthetics and morality, beauty and spirit, are understood to be incontrovertibly transformed by prosthetic technologies.

Phantom-Prosthetic Relations

Prostheses are and have been pregnant with so much power and significance because they affiliate. Throughout their history, prostheses and phantoms have affiliated conceptually as well as in practice, and consequently, the researchers and practitioners working on the myriad "problems of dismemberment" and technologic augmentation have always had to grapple with this relationship in one way or another. For example, in order to aid in facile prosthesis use, in order to treat phantom limb pain, in order to rehabilitate the bodies, minds, and brains of amputees, in order to restore physical, economic, and social productivity to the disabled, diseased, and, perhaps most notably, to those who sacrificed limbs in defense of their country, clinicians have needed to understand, to exploit, and, often, to cultivate friendly phantom-prosthetic relations. This has meant that both of these technologies-of-the-body have been conceived, constructed, and deployed with the intent of perfecting techno-corporeal conjoin-ment and as such, they represent notable facets of biomedical "body-building."

Ethereal limbs and artificial appendages have long had an asserted natural proclivity for one another. Indeed, the phantoms that have animated inert prostheses have been offered up as proof of the effortless synergism had between embodied ghosts and machines. Amputated *bodies* and "adjusting" *minds* or psyches have for the most part welcomed affiliations with prostheses; prosthetization has historically restored mobility, independence, and productivity while staving off the feminizing and other "deleterious" effects of limb loss. Moreover, by the end of the twentieth century, the *brains* of amputees were constructed as nothing less than built for these kinds of intimacies, wired for techno-corporeal synergism.

Exploring techno-corporeality through phantom-prosthetic relations demands that *synergy* be thrust to the center of analysis, and perhaps somewhat ironically, it demands the same of *absence*. On the one hand, centering synergy exposes the reciprocity inherent in what Knorr-Cetina (1997, 23) termed "object-centered socialities," or those social relations (with scientific objects of knowledge in particular) that are characterized by openness and insufficiencies and are "sources of the self, of relational intimacy, of shared subjectivity and social integration." These objects come to define us as much as we define those same objects. In fact, it is careless to think of prostheses simply as man-made tools, appliances, machines, or commodities that we try on or use and discard at will, or to think of them as imposing themselves on individuals, bodies, or populations without resistance or negotiation. Prostheses-as-objects do have (negotiable) intent, a (dynamic) purpose, a (working) agenda, and as such are meaningfully socialized with. However, technologies are never simply self-evident (Suchman et al., 1999), often not even user friendly (Suchman 2005), and are frequently used for unintended purposes or in unintended ways. They are characterized by openness so that despite their "intent," prostheses are negotiated-in-use by the agential self as well as by the agential body. Consonant with an appreciation of the body as leaky (Shildrick 1997; Shildrick 1999), unruly resistant (Mitchell 2002), recalcitrant (Williams and Bendelow 2000), naturally subversive (Scheper-Hughes 1994; Scheper-Hughes and Lock 1991), seepy (Lawton 1998), or transgressive (Falk 1994; Monaghan 2001; Williams 1998), this line of argumentation assumes that physical bodies often join sociocultural and political projects both extraordinary and mundane, and may contravene or transgress in unplanned or unimaginable ways.

On the other hand, centering absence allows moments of sociality *between objects*, between ghosts and machines, to be taken seriously even if these seem inconsequential, abhorrently abstract, or perhaps, entirely incomprehensible. Phantoms have undeniably been at times ethereal, embodied traces characterized by inauthenticity and devoid of an essential ontology. But, they have also unequivocally been objects invested with social substance and with material integrity. Throughout their history, ethereal limbs have been for some researchers and practitioners the Holy Grail of neuroscience, sacred objects with miraculous powers. For others, they have been pure vacuousness, mere vestiges, or worthless psychic baggage. Given their tumultuous history, one might ask, How can such wildly disparate representations characterize the same phenomenon? The ambiguity that characterizes the biography of phantoms is in some measure a consequent of the ambivalence of clinicians, researchers, and others rooted in changing norms regarding the legitimation of scientific and medical knowledge claims, as well as the desire to distance contemporary work in the field from its disreputable past and to elevate the import of phantom phenomena for neuroscience and beyond. It is also a result of the phantom's protean nature and, as such, demonstrative of the tendency for haunted limbs to resist biomedical, technoscientific, and other institutionalized attempts at rationalization. The most notable consequent, however, is the extraordinary proliferation of phantoms over the twentieth and into the twenty-first centuries.

Phantom Proliferation

With substantial advances in amputation surgery, with "quantum leaps" in biomedical knowledge concerning the origins and features of phantoms, with dramatic increases in treatment and prevention modalities, one might expect the biomedical discourse on phantom limb syndrome to contract and for phantoms themselves to become increasingly "managed" or disciplined through biomedical intervention and prevention efforts. In fact by about 1980, painful phantoms were normative, distortion became more and more commonplace, and phantoms of all kinds had proliferated with utter abandon.

What was known about phantoms during the late nineteenth century when the phrase was coined was predominantly derived from the work of Silas Weir Mitchell (1829–1914), who depicted phantoms as alienating, as intrusive, and as capable of profound betrayal. Mitchell (1871, 365–366) wrote,

> There is something almost tragical, something ghastly, in the notion of these thousands of spirit limbs haunting as many good soldiers, and every now and then tormenting them with the disappointments which arise when, the memory being off guard for a moment, the keen sense of the limb's presence betrays the man into some effort, the failure of which of a sudden reminds him of his loss.

Deceit or trickery was a common game that phantoms played. For instance, they might shorten or lengthen, disappear or reappear, and they caused forgetting. "'Indeed,' says one sufferer, writing of this point,

Table 1.1. Late-Nineteenth Century Typology: A Late-Nineteenth
Century Typology of Phantom Limbs and Digits

Phanom Type	Description
	Sensorial
The Sensory Ghost	Phantoms that are more definite and intrusive than the living member
Spirit Limbs	Phantoms that are so real that they betray a man into some effort
The Painful Phantom	Exceptionally rare phantoms that are sensed as painful
	Kinesthetic
The Indelibly Fixed Phantom	Phantoms that represent the last scene which it reflected during life
Automatic Shadows	Phantoms that are in a perpetual state of automatic activity
Exact Exertions	Phantoms that are moved at will
Automatic Gymnastics	Phantoms that cause painless thrashing about of the stump
Rigid for Life	Phantoms that have never stirred
	Temporal
The Summoned Phantom	Phantoms called forth by weather, a blow on the stump or reamputation
The Forgotten Phantom	Phantoms that are forgotten over time
	Morphologic
The Incomplete Spirit	Phantoms that include parts that are indistinct or absent
Gradual Shortening	Phantoms that gradually shorten over time
Re-lengthening	Phantoms that return to normal length after shortening

'Every morning I have to learn anew that my leg is enriching a Virginia wheat crop or ornamenting some horrible museum" (Mitchell 1871, 566–67). They were also characterized by spite and were marked by *automatic shadows* or spasms such that the residual limb moved perpetually, never able to be quieted. These spasms testified to the phantom's wild and meaningless ways:

> The spasms of stumps are very interesting and too often incurable, but they involve no pain, and only such annoyance as may come from the part thrashing about in a wild and meaningless fashion, so as to excite for its owner attention wherever he goes. . . . The sufferer . . . engaged in politics, he has only to uncover his jerky arm in order, as he says, to make

the greatest kind of a stump speech, and to carry with him the sympathies of the audience. (Mitchell 1871, 565)

As the early-twenty-first century typology shows, one could easily claim an affinity between *the sensory ghost* of the past and *the vial phantom* of the present felt as possessing more awareness than the intact limb. *The incomplete spirit* with absent pieces or bits may have been a precursor to *phantom gaps* or those phantoms that seemed to float mysteriously in space. *Spirit limbs* that so viciously betrayed men many decades ago may very well be equatable to *phantom forgetting* when, for example, men fall hard to the floor upon "rising" from sleep. *Phantom gymnastics* that caused such violent thrashing that it eternally excited its possessor may be the antecedent of *phantom jactitation* marked by involuntary spasms the likes of which could drive a man to tie down or lie upon his disobliging stump. Or, *phantom paralysis*, the fixed or frozen phantom, may be a later version of those phantoms that had never stirred, those that were cursed with *rigidity for life*.

All of these continuities are interesting and hugely significant, but what is arguably more conspicuous and ultimately more curious is the extraordinary proliferation of phantoms of all kinds, including distorted and painful phantoms—no doubt, important moments in their biography. Most notably, however, is the emergence of a qualitatively distinct type or class of phantom, those that were intelligible only in relation to prostheses. As the field of prosthetic science matured and prostheses grew increasingly sophisticated, a new class of phantoms surfaced that were defined not by what they did or did not do, when they manifested, how they felt, or what they "looked like" but rather by how they related to artificial limbs. *Phantom occupation*—or those phantoms that occupied or penetrated things and people with audacity—and *phantom animation*—or those phantoms that inhabited and animated the materiality of prostheses—were nonexistent during the late nineteenth century. Likewise, the phenomenon of *phantom fusion* or the experience of absolute synchronicity between phantoms and prostheses was simply

Table 1.2. Early-Twenty-First Century Typology: An Early-Twenty-First Century Typology of Phantom Parts

Phantom Type	Description
Sensorial	
The Natural Phantom	Phantoms that are not painful or distorted
Limb Facsimile	Phantoms that are mimetic and are exact replicas of intact limbs
Phantom Limb Awareness	Consciousness of a phantom limited to a general impression of a limb
Phantom Limb Sensation	Phantom sensations equivalent to those of intact limbs
The Pleasant Phantom	Phantoms that feel exceptionally pleasing
The Vital Phantom	Phantoms that possess more awareness than the intact limb
Phantom Mislocation	Phantom sensations felt as far removed from the site of amputation
The Painful Phantom	Transiently, temporarily, or permanently painful sensations
Phantom Pain Memories	Phantom pain that emulates pain experienced prior to amputation
Endless Regression	The multiplication of phantoms after successive re-amputations
The Disposal Phantom	Phantom pain that emulates the experience of the part after disposal
Kinesthetic	
The Willed Phantom	Phantoms that move at will
Phantom Forgetting	Phantoms that are unconsciously used, for example in balancing
The Conjunctive Phantom	Phantoms that move in synchronicity with other body parts
The Reflexive Phantom	Phantoms that move autonomously
The Spontaneous Phantom	Phantom movement that is outside of volitional control
Phantom Jactitation	Phantoms that cause often painful involuntary spasms of the stump
Phantom Paralysis	Phantoms that feel fixed or frozen
Temporal	
Phantom Provocation	Phantom sensation or pain exacerbated by stimuli
Phantoms Reawakening	Phantoms that reappear after having disappeared
The Exposure Phantom	Phantoms that appear after having been "exposed" to another amputee
The Experimental Phantom	Phantoms induced in non-amputees
Phantom Fading	Phantoms that become increasingly vague and disappear over time
Morphologic	
The Last Moment of Life	Phantoms that mimic the posture of the limb just prior to amputation
Superadded Sensations	Phantoms that are sensed as wearing a ring, watch, shoe, etc.
Phantom Regrowth	Phantoms that regrow to normal length after having shrunken
Dream Morphology	Phantoms that appear in the dreams of amputees in various states

Table 1.2. (continued) Early-Twenty-First Century Typology: An Early Twenty-First Century Typology of Phantom Parts

Phantom Type	Description
	Morphological
The Distorted Phantom	Phantoms that are not mimetic of fleshy limbs
Supernumerary Phantoms	Multiple phantoms growing from numerous sites
The Telescoped Phantom	Phantoms that shrink toward or into the stump
Phantom Gaps	Phantoms that are sensed as gapped such that they float in space
Phantom Shrinking	Phantoms that shrink often to the size of a child's hand
Disturbances of Continuity	The dropping out of pieces or the development of holes
	Relational
Phantom Animation	Phantoms that occupy or inhabit the materiality of the prosthesis
Phantom Occupation	Phantoms that occupy the same space as things or people
Phantom Shunning	Phantoms that disappear, move within the stump, or bend to the side
Phantom Fusion	Phantoms that become fussed to or synchronized with prostheses
Phantom Utility	The innate utility that phantoms possess

incomprehensible. And consequently, *phantom utility* or the assertion that ethereal limbs had an innate utility that could and should be harnessed in the service of facile prosthesis use was utterly unimaginable. Phantom occupation, phantom animation, phantom fusion, and phantom utility are exemplars of phantom-prosthetic relations. As we shall see, this relationship between ghosts and machines has at times been pleasant, accommodating, and mutually beneficial. At other times, it has been fraught with discord, competition, betrayal, coercion, and even the brutal threat of extinction.

Overview of the Book

Chapter 2, "Characterizing Phantoms: Features of Phantom Limb Syndrome," explores how corporeal ideology informed understandings of phantom peculiarities and influenced efforts to legitimate the work being done on phantom limb syndrome whether in the form of (1) the modern "culture of the copy" (Schwartz 1996), which was motivated by the tendency for replication to cause both confusion and distrust; (2) the mechanistic body, which was envisioned as a system of perfectly interchangeable parts; (3) American Taylorism, which emphasized efficiency and the rationalization of motion; (4) the elaboration of the human kinesthetic, which associated purposeful movement with the soundness of the body and spirit; (5) the theory of the phylogenic recapitulation of ontology, which conceived of human development as a reenactment of the "evolution of man"; (6) or the principle of object relations, which presupposed an embodied reverence for the material world and, perhaps more importantly, the incarnate.

As researchers and clinicians debated what counted as valid or reliable research and data, past work was reimagined as illegitimate and modern-day phantoms as more "real" than those of the past, which were considered fanciful and flawed because they were mired in material acquisition, measurement, operationalization, detection, ego, and truthtelling problems, among others. Uncoupled from poor science, capricious stories, and painful stumps, the very morphology of phantoms was rethought, altering what phantoms "looked" like, what they did, and how they felt; mimetic phantoms—those that were faithful facsimiles—became increasingly uncommon while distorted phantoms— those that were fundamentally restructured and divorced from the laws that had always governed fleshy limbs—became more and more commonplace.

One of the most significant impulses for revisioning the field was a need to explain the grossly discrepant and ephemeral knowledge that characterized the literature particularly with regard to phantom pain incidence (the number of new cases) and prevalence (the total number of cases). As the exceptionally rare symptom of "shadowy" pain became epidemic by the late 1970s, researchers were pressured to clarify, to justify, and to account for the dramatic change in the biomedical narrative about rates of phantom limb pain among amputees and others. Chapter 3, "From Pleasure to Pain: Accounting for the Rise and Fall in Phantom Pain," investigates the extraordinary increase and subsequent decrease of phantom limb pain within the American context. Consonant with the invention of pain medicine, the instantiation of the pain clinic, the institutionalization of pain therapeutics, the clinical management of the pained patient, and the American "plague" of pain around 1975, phantom pain became pervasive. Through the introduction of a specific language of phantom limb pain by way of the widespread adoption of the McGill Pain Questionnaire (MPQ), the pleasurable phantom lapsed into rarity, and the painful phantom proliferated. The MPQ provided a linguistic structure that has shaped the qualitative dimensions of phantom pain unto this day—a trend that is antithetical to the widely accepted presupposition that pain is unshared/able and, thus, inherently indescribable. Further, virtually mirroring the increase in pain reporting was the incredible swell of available treatments for this particularly virulent form of neuropathic pain; a biomedical industry devoted to and dependent on painful and distorted phantoms burgeoned as pain became a common sequela of phantom limb syndrome.

Nonetheless, throughout the 2000s, pain prevalence began to decline despite the inadequacy of the myriad treatments available to amputees suffering from "inexplicable," often intractable, torturous, and, in some cases, life-long pain. If practitioners and their interventions were not responsible for the decline, what was? The answer lies in the multifarious and convoluted history of the syndrome's etiology or cause. The next two chapters show how the shift from the psychologization to the medicalization of phantoms (from phantoms originating in the disturbed mind to phantoms originating in the reorganized brain) led to the intelligibility of distortion and the elaboration of pain. Chapter 4, "Phantoms in the Mind: The Psychogenic Origins of Ethereal Appendages," begins the survey of the phantom origin story, detailing how the major psychogenic theories of phantom phenomena exposed the obvious anxiety that dismemberment evoked throughout the late-nineteenth and the first half of the twentieth centuries, while also demonstrating how particular features of the phenomena were foregrounded and engaged as proof of theory. Specifically, the central concept of the body scheme is dissected in order to trace its evolution and to show how proponents enlisted peculiar phantoms in an effort to buttress claims about the primordial nature of the body scheme, including congenital phantoms, or those that were reported in cases of congenitally lost or malformed limbs; paralyzed phantoms, or those that were permanently frozen or fixed, often in the position in which the limb was last "felt"; exposure phantoms, or those that materialized as a consequence of seeing another amputee; penetrating phantoms, or those that pierced through objects, including bodies (both the self and others); dreamt phantoms, or those that were similar to or profoundly different from waking phantoms; and disposal phantoms, or those that remained connected to the lost part capable, in some cases, of "feeling" how the remainder was handled after amputation.

Dispute about the nature of the body scheme in its various incarnations and consequently what could be hypothesized with respect to body-traces with often vibrant corporeal histories caused the further proliferation of phantoms. In fact, as the body scheme fractured and split, phantoms spread to newly theorized "vulnerable" or at-risk populations and multiplied in kind, enlisting more and more of the sensorial body in the "phantom problem."

By the latter half of the twentieth century, psychogenic theories were overtly maligned. They were purposively undermined and—as it was forcefully asserted—systematically debunked. Phantoms were no longer found in the troubled minds of amputees with adjustment problems of one kind or another, but rather could be found—by way of imaging technologies—in the pink, viscous tissue of the cerebral cortex. Phantom limbs became brain based, and so too did fleshy limbs. In fact, the human body was relegated to the realm of the epiphenomenal and, ironically, phantom limbs became more "real" than the intact limbs they emulated with, at times, such exactitude.

Chapter 5, "Phantoms in the Brain: The Holy Grail of Neuroscience," shows how phantoms have not simply been "passive"—sensitive to changes in corporeal ideology, the advent of the pain clinic, or the revisioning of neuroscientific knowledge—but have also been agents in their own right, causing transformations within the field of neuroscience, within the bodies, minds, and brains of amputees, and between bodies and prosthetic technologies. Today, the phantom is considered a precious window into the most historically elusive questions about the mind-body connection, the self, consciousness, and many others, and because amputees have been identified as conduits of valuable "research material," they have become pioneers at the edge of experimentation exploring the implications of the prosthetized and haunted "body-in-the-brain." The hard-wired dogma of cortical organization is now juxtaposed to the discourse on cortical plasticity (whether in the form of redundancy or the growth of new connections), and amputees have become both a means of adjudicating between the two hypotheses and among the many beneficiaries of this "functional" tendency for the human brain to reorganize itself. References to the causal role of cortical plasticity in phantom manifestation after major limb amputation began to emerge around 1990, and in fact, this tendency, it was asserted, could and should be exploited in an effort to facilitate the successful embodiment of artificial limbs and effectively stave off phantom pain and distortion.

Because ethereal limbs had the capacity to pathologize, prostheses, with their ability to tame or civilize unruly phantoms, were touted as therapeutic. Prostheses both provoked phantoms into productive relations with machines and cured phantom limb pain, contributing to their increasing remarkability. Still, phantoms retained their long-recognized utility. Chapter 6, "Phantom-Prosthetic Relations: The Modernization of Amputation," details how phantom-prosthetic relations unfolded in the context of the modernization of amputation, including the rapid state-sponsored expansion and maturation of the prosthetic industry and the development of a collaborative relationship between amputation surgery and prosthetic science. These and other events engendered a shift in phantom-prosthetic relations over the twentieth and into the twenty-first centuries from (1) the *prosthetization of phantoms* to (2) the *phantomization of prostheses,* and finally to (3) *phantom-prosthetic reciprocity.*

The remarkability of the prosthesis ceded to the extraordinariness of the phantom. Ultimately, however, phantom-prosthetic relations would be characterized by reciprocity, by the vital phantom animating the inert prosthesis, while the prosthesis provided the structure necessary for disciplining the restless phantom. Nevertheless, despite the friendly intimacy had with prostheses and despite their essential utility, contemporary phantoms became endangered, at risk for being theorized into extinction, for being displaced by the very machines they had always had such an affinity with.

The final chapter, "Conclusion: Authenticity and Extinction," employs the concept of authenticity as a rhetorical frame and asks, What is at stake in how the future of phantom-prosthetic relations unfolds and what has this particular history revealed about prostheses, amputation, the body-in-the-brain, the prosthetic imaginary, techno-corporeality, neuroscientific authority, and more? First, the case of phantom penis is used to demystify claims of *scientific authenticity*, showing that biomedical knowledge systems are always a reflection of the social milieu in which they are engendered. Second, through the struggle to secure *phantom authenticity*, to find the real McCoy, embodied fraudulence in the form of the feminized mind and emasculated body gave way to the epiphenomenal man-made body, a conceptual move that has enormous implications for our understanding of *authentic embodiment*, for how prostheses transform human bodies, and for phantom-prosthetic relations. Third, as transsexuals and apotemnophiles—or those who desire amputation of "healthy" limbs—have been enlisted in the debate over the experientially based versus hard-wired body-in-the-brain, what counts as *authentic amputation*, as well as embodied wholeness and *authentic disability*, has been thrown into doubt. Fourth, reengaging with the concept of prosthetized rebirth or transcendence, I explore *authentic corporeal transformations* and ask what implications this discourse has for amputees, as well as the social or communal body. Lastly, I confront the idea of the impending displacement or theoretical extinction of phantoms addressing *authentic death*. In the end, I suggest that phantom endangerment tells us as much about biomedicine and biopolitics in the second decade of the twenty-first century as it does about how ghosts haunt machines.

2

Characterizing Phantoms

Features of Phantom Limb Syndrome

Official medical accounts of a disease, illness, disorder, or syndrome communicate as much about corporeal ideology, as much about what is normative and what is moral, as it does about what has "gone terribly wrong" with the body's structures or processes. Biomedical knowledge links specific characterizations of the pathological and the natural/normal/normative body with what Foucault (1978, 139) called "anatamo-politics," or a politics intended to render human corporeality useful and the physical body docile. As biomedical and techno-scientific knowledge systems elaborate, we are increasingly immersed within an ever more expansive and complex set of discourses and practices that engender the internalization of both the biomedical gaze—or the ideas, techniques, and practices used to objectify, scrutinize, and dehumanize the ill and "the disabled" as well as the "at risk"—and corporeal ideology—or the set of ideas used to justify and legitimate the subordination of some bodies over others.

Corporeal ideology encompasses what we know about the body, its nature, its capacities, its potentialities, its weaknesses. It comprises the ideas, values, and beliefs that determine and justify "knowledge" concerning various aspects of corporeality and embodiment, including ontology, or what human bodies are and can be; aesthetics, or what constitutes achieved and ascribed beauty; morality, or how bodies should be managed, regulated, and governed; sociality, or who and what bodies should develop relations and the nature of those relations; structure, or how bodies should be composed, including ideas about reorganization, replacement, and interior/exterior; function, or what constitutes health, wellness, healing, illness, dying, death, and disability, as well as the distinction between physical and mental processes; symbolism, or what the body and body parts connote and invoke, in addition to how the body is used as a metaphoric source; and economy, or what defines the worth or value of bodies in part or in toto including the body's status as a commodity. In short, corporeal ideology determines what "makes up" the body, defines its facticity, its purpose, and its value, and establishes how it can, should, and often will be used; it gives the human body material integrity and social significance even when the body materializes and becomes meaningful in opposition to such forces.

As a "classical" form of what Lemke (2011, 6) termed the "mode of politics" —or how representations of the body and biopolitical articulations arise and are employed within the context of medical and scientific dominance—corporeal ideology has operated as a means through which the amputated body has been strategically mobilized for political purposes, not the least of which has been biomedical legitimation. Corporeal ideology has certainly shaped constructions of the temporal (phantoms in time), kinesthetic (phantom movement), sensorial (phantom sensation), and morphologic (phantom size and shape) aspects of embodied ghosts. But, it has also been enlisted at various times in an effort to revise and "re-vision" (Clarke and Olesen 1999, 5) the work being done on phantom limb syndrome and to reevaluate what should and should not be counted as valid or reliable and why. In recent decades, this has meant that past data, research, and researchers have been brought under the microscope so that poor research and "pure speculation" could give way to rigorous science and systematic knowing. Consequently, the long-held dogma of phantom mimesis relented to the spread of phantom distortion, and the all but faultless replicas of the past became capable of grotesque reorganization.

Ambiguity and the Phantom Complex

The medical literature on phantom limb syndrome is replete with contradictory and often ephemeral knowledge. Scholars of the recent past have attempted to explain the many drifts and discontinuities in what is known and knowable about these embodied ghosts, to explain why phantoms have so persistently eluded characterization even by history's best, brightest, and most curious minds. Some of these scholars advanced arguments accounting for the discrepant state of the knowledge and others put forward reviews as well as provided fresh data intended to parse the valid and reliable from the mythical and the messy. For example, Ribbers, Mulder, and Rijken (1989) attributed the astonishing degree of ambiguity found in the literature to terminological confusion, sloppy sample selection, differences in patient reporting, and observer misinterpretation. In other words, some studies were reread as suffering from the insufficiencies of poorly practiced science and others from the inadequacies of unreliable respondents.

At the close of the twentieth century, researchers and clinicians suggested that past studies and amputees themselves had confounded the distinct elements of what Jensen and Nikolajsen (2000) termed "the phantom complex," a tripartite concept that included (1) *phantom limb pain*, or pain that is "referred" to or felt as if it originates in the phantom; (2) *phantom limb sensations*, or nonpainful sensations that are referred to the phantom; (3) and *stump pain*, or pain that originates in and is localized to the stump. A few years later, researchers added a fourth element that further convoluted phantom phenomena; *phantom limb awareness* was defined as the general consciousness of a limb often limited to a vague impression (see for example Hunter, Katz, and Davis 2003). Dr. Joseph M. Czerniecki, professor in the Department of Rehabilitation Medicine at the University of Washington and associate director for the Veterans Administration (VA) Rehabilitation Research and Development Center in Seattle, elaborated on the differentiation problem:

> You may have a condition where there is a pathophysiologic process in the residual limb that causes pain in the stump and pain in the phantom. So, there is a kind of overlapping process that can cause some confusion in discerning phantom only, stump only, or stump and phantom pain. It

can be complicated. I often hear people say, "My phantom pain is driving me nuts." I say, "Okay, point to where it is," and they point right to their stump. That is stump pain, not phantom pain. Sometimes, they just think that if there is pain after amputation, then it's phantom pain. (Czerniecki 2005)

Whether attributable to bemused clinicians or undiscerning amputees, at least some of the ambiguity that has characterized the work on phantoms was attributed to the failure of researchers and amputees alike to systematically discriminate between the flesh and its ghosts. The debate about analytic messiness ultimately led researchers to distinguish between phantoms of the past and those of the present; past phantoms were reworked as problematic, as poor copies of the genuine thing. They were problematical conflations of specter and soma, while contemporary phantoms were depicted as more "real," genuine, and valid than their historical equivalents because they were analytically clean and clear. Consequently, past phantoms were measured against present phantoms in an effort to sort the authentic from the chimerical, to rationalize phantoms, and to distance more current scientific work in the field from its fanciful and flawed history.

Long imagined as faithful copies of fleshy limbs, phantoms are today conceived as parts not accountable to gravity, symmetry, time, or the principles of human morphology, not answerable to the laws that had always governed the physiology of human bodies. That is not to say that past phantoms were faithful copies. In fact, they often were not, but distortions were ultimately deemed explicable. As Roth (2005, 30, 32) argued, researchers often co-construct shared knowledge in order to establish some kind of certainty and the unclassified/able cases, the "'crosses,' 'mongrels,' or even 'monsters' that are inherently out of bounds," become part of a disturbing "pea-soup." However, pea-soup in the sciences is invariably managed just as it is in all fields of work; outliers, crosses, anomalies are often attributed to flawed technique, to faulty assumptions, or to genuine discovery (Star and Gerson 1987). Indeed, there is "an enormous amount of work needed to stabilize knowledge, freeze action, [and] delete outliers" (Lampland and Star 2009, 13). In the case of embodied ghosts, the anomalous, distorted phantom at the turn of the twentieth century was pure mongrel or monster, while at the turn of the twenty-first century, the protean nature of the phantom was its quintessence.

Limb Facsimile

Mitchell (1871, 566), in his seminal article on "the strange and even startling" spirit member, observed, "Many persons feel the lost limb as existing the moment they awaken from the merciful stupor of the ether given to destroy the torments of the knife." Since the late nineteenth century, amputees have commonly described awakening from surgery to sensations so real that they questioned whether or not the procedure had actually taken place. In fact, the uncanny realness of phantom sensations has provoked some patients to peer under the covers for visual confirmation that the surgeon had truly done his or her job. Simmel (1966b, 346; emphasis added) wrote of the tendency in the mid-1960s:

> The first meeting between a phantom limb and its owner is, typically, a rather dramatic affair. As the patient wakes up from surgery he feels his leg present, he seems to be able to wiggle his toes quite normally—and then someone steps up to him and tells him that the operation went very well and he will be able to walk on an artificial limb in no time at all. No matter how well and how long before the operation he was prepared for the loss of the leg, the patient typically cannot believe that it is really gone, until he can convince himself by looking under the covers. And though he thus verifies the true state of affairs, he continues to feel the absent limb as if it were still present. . . . Needless to say, this is a very puzzling experience for the amputee, so much so that many have commented "I thought I must be out of my mind."

Even after seeing with his own eyes that the limb was no longer present, not infrequently an amputee might still refuse to acknowledge the surgery because of how convincingly the phantom could be sensed. Vivid sensation seemed to originate in a limb that was rationally understood as gone, and it was the phantom's persuasiveness, its ability to imitate the preamputated limb in compelling detail, that made the apparition at times undeniable. Gallinek (1939, 416; emphasis added) wrote of case number three, "Thirteen years before the examination the patient had had amputations through the left calf and the upper third of the right thigh. Phantom limbs had appeared on both sides immediately after the amputation. When the patient was told about the operation *he would not believe it.*"

As skillful imitators, phantom limbs were long thought of as replicas of the original, copies in terms of size, shape, posture, and movement. In fact, phantoms were frequently described as emulating the preamputated limb in very precise ways. Mitchell (1871, 568) wrote,

> Many readers will recall a bit of newspaper science which described the retina of the eye as having indelibly fixed upon it the last scene which it reflected during life. This fable is realized in the case of many lost limbs. . . . There are some cases of hands which have been crushed or burned, and the fingers remained painfully rigid in life or bound on a splint. . . . The latest and most overpowering sensation is thus for all time engraved upon the brain.

Until about 1980, most clinicians, researchers, and amputees described them as thoroughly mimetic. It was not that phantom "replicas" disappeared from the literature after the 1970s—in fact, examples can still be found—but rather, phantom distortion elaborated and became normative while flawless mimesis grew increasingly rare and replication became one of many tricks that phantoms performed. Prior to this, the phantom was in most cases an authentic facsimile, an all but faultless copy of its physical complement, and as such, it was often described as mimicking the preamputated limb with precision.

In terms of posture, phantoms often maintained the fixed, relaxed, flexed, or twisted posture of preamputated limbs, particularly the position of the limb *just prior* to loss—what Simmel (1956, 641) termed the "last moment of life." For instance, an amputee who had tried to protect himself from flying shrapnel on the battlefield permanently sensed his splayed phantom hand in the same position it had occupied at the moment of traumatic amputation; when he was asked to describe it, the soldier replied, "the hand is right in front of my face. I'm looking at it" (Harber 1958, 20). In another example, Henderson and Smyth (1948, 103) detailed the case of a soldier who, after first having a toe removed, underwent amputation of the leg just below the knee, resulting in a phantom that imitated the unique characteristics of his preamputation foot:

> Another example is that of a soldier whose second toe was removed together with the distal part of the metatarsal a few days after being wounded; this left a "V-shaped gap" which he had seen during dressings. Several weeks later it was necessary to amputate through the leg. The usual phantom appeared in which he could feel all the toes except the second and the V-shaped gap was [present].

Sacks (1987) presented the case of a sailor who had accidentally amputated his right index finger, a finger that had been rigidly extended prior to its removal. Over the course of forty years, the sailor lived with the unyielding fear that his pointed phantom finger might poke his eye out while he was eating. These "dangerously life-like and real phantoms," as Sacks (1987, 66) called them, were at times constructed as untrustworthy and mean-spirited tricksters. Indeed, in our early-modern "culture of the copy," we became confused about the quality of the replica; we became confused about the role of "impostors, 'evil' twins, puppets, 'apes,' tricksters, fakes" (Schwartz 1996, 17), and it was because of our anxiety about the possibility that the dangerously life-like could actually endanger the "real" that facsimiles of limbs—like all copies—acquired a reputation for malicious disregard.

Because these sensations were so realistic, some amputees reported that their phantoms were seriously disquieting impediments causing them to alter the manner in which they moved in or through the world. For instance, amputees might purposively move in ways intended to protect the protruding phantom for fear of hurting it or others or to accommodate the ghost's sometimes atypical angle.

> We observed a patient who felt his flexed and immovable phantom arm pressed upon his chest, just in the same way in which he had carried his arm in a sling for months . . . [or] the case of a patient who *had to sleep on his belly because his phantom hand remained inconveniently situated on his back*. (Frederiks 1963, 77; emphasis added)

Fredericks (1963) was also one of many researchers who argued that the mimetic phantom was best understood as a consequent of the integrated, "mechanistic" quality of the human body, particularly of the peripheral and central nervous systems. He theorized that when a part of the body is amputated, it is not experienced as a "lack" but rather as "unpatterning" and, accordingly, "organically-induced illusions and hallucinations" would necessarily be sensed as characteristically life-like (Frederiks 1963, 73). His hypothesis was consistent with a facet of corporeal ideology that predominated during the post–World War years.

To be sure, corporeal ideology often originates from within the social worlds of biomedicine and techno-science, but prevailing "knowledge" about the body's functionality, aesthetics, morality, symbolism, economy, and the like also originates within other realms or spheres of social life informing scientific "discovery" and medical "advance." Ideas about the functionality of the body in the postwar years borrowed from the organic-machine metaphor that dominated popular culture, especially during the 1950s and 1960s, and continued to be influential long afterward (Bowring 2003; Featherstone 1991; Gray 2002; Gray and Mentor 1995; Gray, Mentor, and Figueroa-Sarriera 1995 Grenville 2001; Martin 1999) whether in the form of the human-motor (Gleyse 1998; Kimbrell 1993; Rabinbach 1990), the human-computer (Gleyse 1998; Lynch and Collins 1998), or the cyborg (Gray and Mentor 1995; Gray, Mentor, and Figueroa-Sarriera 1995; Grenville 2001; Tofts 2002). From this perspective, the body was essentially conceived as a complex machine standardized in terms of its forces, parts, and processes.

> Modern life, with its essentially industrial momentum had processed our world and our bodies into dissociated, fetishized, ultimately empty and machinable elements. . . . [T]his was certainly congruent with a scientific worldview that has tended increasingly to treat human behavior as patterns of stimuli and responses, reducing mind to brain and brain to electrochemical impulses, and treating organs as interchangeable parts. . . . [T]he commanding image is now the machine: the well-oiled machine, the corrupt machine, the broken-down machine, the totalitarian juggernaut, the scrap heap. Our bodies themselves have been configured into machinehood. (Schwartz 1992, 105)

This concept of "machinehood," that the body was reducible to mechanistic qualities and standardized elements, led scholars and practitioners of the day to presume that limbs, even in their shadowy form, would emulate or imitate with the kind of exactness that one would expect from "interchangeable parts."

The Sensorial Peculiarities of Phantoms

In addition to posture, phantoms have also aped the sensorial quality of intact limbs. Nearly everything the body feels has been sensed as originated in or on the phantom, including the lightest touch, the deepest pressure, the most irritating itch, or the softest texture. Phantoms have felt vibration, pressure, heat/warmth, and cold/coolness, as well as itch, tickle, swelling, wetness, numbness, pain, effort, and fatigue. Amputees have provided detailed descriptions of sensing the icy cool rigidity of metal, the subtle warmth of a slight breeze, the unmistakable roughness of stepping on pebbles, the scratchiness of long wet grass, or the cold wet of pants slapping against irritated skin. In Der Beeck (1953, 225) gave the following first-person account of an itchy phantom: "Immediately after the amputation I felt the left leg throughout its whole length. . . . [I]t was a prickling sensation, as though the leg were hanging down with the hollow of the knee on one edge of the bed. It was an itching, furry feeling, a continual to-ing and fro-ing."

Ethereal appendages have also at times been characterized as adept imitators because they responded readily to external stimuli of all kinds. For example, when walking through a puddle of water, the phantom foot may feel wet (Sherman, et al. 1997), a sensation that might also be accompanied by a distinct awareness of temperature so that on a dismal rainy day, the soaked phantom is also unmistakably cold. Others have reported sensations that varied with dramatic or even slight changes in the weather, including temperature and humidity. In fact, phantoms have been used by amputees to predict rainfall with astonishing accuracy (see for example Ramachandran and Hirstein 1998). One amputee observed that "the foot was never quite normal. . . . [W]eather conditions affected it, so that the toes might feel crushed if it was frosty or feel immersed in moving water before a rain came" (Buxton 1957, 500). Similarly, In Der Beeck (1953, 225) presented the case of an amputee whose toenails were his barometer:

> Whenever the weather changes, I have the feeling as though the toe-nails are being pulled upwards . . . [and] the toes rise up of themselves, but do not go down again without my will. I always have to push them down again first. If I did not do that they would remain standing up. That gives a feeling of cramp and causes me trouble, and that is why I always have to push them down.

Moreover, reports have long documented the incorporation of what have been termed superadded features such as a bandage, tourniquet, cast, ring, watch, shoe, glove, piece of clothing, cane, hot stick, or blood-filled boot (see for example Giummarra, et al. 2011; Katz 1992b), and contemporary studies suggest that the prevalence rate of this arguably bizarre phenomenon among amputees is 15 percent (Giummarra, et al. 2011). Ramchandran and Hirstein (1998, 1605–6) wrote of a patient who wore a wooden splint in the days before his amputation:

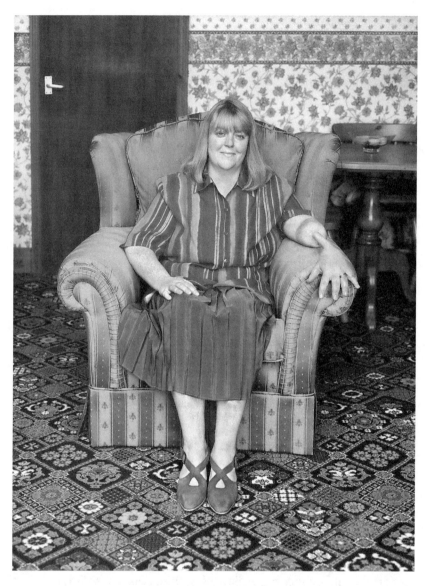

Figure 2.1. Superadded Features. Working in collaboration with neurologist Dr. John Kew and neuropsychologist Dr. Peter Halligan, English visual artist Alexa Wright manipulated photographic portraits enabling the visualization of phantoms as they were described by amputees. J.N.'s phantom hand was often experienced as larger and as heavier than her intact limb. Her wrist was virtually absent, but the joints were large and stiff. Her phantom finger still wore an engagement ring. (Reprinted with permission from Wright, Alexa. 1997. *After Image*. London, England: www.alexawright.com.)

We have seen a patient whose arm was in a vertical wooden splint, flexed at the elbow, with the fingers hooked over the end of the splint, gripping it tightly. Two days later his arm was amputated, and when we saw him several weeks later, his phantom was in exactly the same position that his real arm had occupied, with the fingers hooked over an imaginary splint.

Amputees might carry with them a cumbersome, imaginary, wooden splint, grip a trusted and sturdy cane, clutch a lethal grenade, feel the tight constriction of a tourniquet, or wear beloved and valued jewelry. Jackson (2002, 71) described the sensation of an absent finger wearing a nonexistent ring as "almost holographic." One amputee knew precisely which ring his phantom finger wore because it had been bent in the past and was consequently tight in some places (Harber 1958). Harber (1958) also detailed the case of an amputee who wore two watches at the same time prior to his amputation, and although he was rather irritated by the fact that these had not been returned to him after the surgery, his phantom wrist wore both. One wonders if they kept time in their phantom-ed state.

L.B.'s phantom hand donned two bracelets and ten rings made of gold, leading him to surmise that his "apparent" amputation must have been the work of God:

> He believes that his missing hand is really present, but rendered invisible by God. . . . On the wrist he feels two bracelets and on the first and second joint of each finger he feels rings, so that he wears 10 rings on the phantom hand. (Actually he wore only one ring when he cut off his hand.) God has given him the rings. "Yes sir, absolutely, in fact, all of them." God adorned the phantom hand with these rings about a year after he had cut off his hand and the phantom hand had made its appearance. The rings are made of metal, "they are gold," and because they are metallic he feels them even more strongly than the hand. (Gallinek 1939, 421)

Because they have been so well integrated into and such integral aspects of the phantom experience, in many cases these objects were felt as if they belonged to the body, as if they were a component of the "self." Still, for others these objects were not sensed as embodied and amputees perceived them to be foreign, distinct, or alien. For example, Noritaka and Mita's (2009, 479) patient was restricted by a massive metal bar:

> The patient (A.S.) was a 60-year-old man amputated at the left forearm. A.S. suffered an injury in which his hand was crushed by a machine at his workplace. . . . When A.S. tried to move the wrist joint of his phantom forearm, he said "I cannot move it because the metal bar is preventing wrist flexion." According to him the metal bar was massive, cold, and approximately 10 cm long. He felt the metal bar more as an artificial object than as a part of his body. He also said that the extent of the feeling of the metal bar changed somewhat day by day, but that the bar was continuously grasped in the phantom hand.

Phantoms have also incorporated what have been termed "multimodal superadded sensations" (Harber 1956), such as a "white sock and a black patent leather shoe with straps" (Katz and Melzack 1990, 328). Amputees, in these cases, have been able to relay the quality and features of superadded sensations with astonishing exactitude. In the above example, not only was the type, shape, and texture of the shoe sensed but color was a fundamental aspect of the sensation. Moreover, olfactory cues have been integrated so that the phantom was sensed as possessing "the foul smell of putrid diabetic ulcers and gangrene" (Katz and Melzack 1990, 332). Superadded features demonstrated that lost limbs had corporeal histories. Long after amputation, they continued sensing tepid water, the slippery wet of melting ice, or the pleasure of a friendly tickle. They continued wearing precious engagement rings, favorite pink lace-lined socks, or dreaded blood-filled boots.

Forgetting the Phantom

The vividness and at times eerie reality of phantom-ed mimicry and the accuracy with which ethereal limbs were positioned in and occupied space has long been evidenced by what has been termed "forgetting." Reflexively or "unconsciously," amputees have attempted to step out of bed, answer the phone, rub an eye, or shake hands only to find that the effort was in vain. Not only did phantoms disappoint when a man's efforts went unrealized, but they were also cruel reminders of functional and physical losses. The gross irony of forgetting was that it was ultimately about remembering.

In the first few decades of the twentieth century, as Rabinbach (1990) argued, American Taylorism, with its emphasis on efficiency and rationalization, influenced ideas about how bodies should be used, particularly in terms of the economy of motion. Professionals of all stripes thought that bodies did and should move with underlying purpose and with efficiency. Bodies "naturally" moved efficaciously and competently in ways that were not wasteful or pointless, and when they did not, professionals in all sectors of society moved in to show them how. Within the medical community, phantoms too became governed by a vital purpose; these fictive and wish-fulfilling body parts moved in ways that ultimately made sense and had a point. Forgetting testified to the remarkable capacity of phantoms to emulate the limbs they originated from, but as an inevitable consequent of limb loss, mimesis also attested to the fact that natural phantoms moved with an underlying intent.

> It is *quite natural* that, for a time the missing part *should seek to take its place along with the other limbs* in the performance of more or less automatic every-day actions, as in dressing, using the hand to pick up objects or catch a ball, stepping out of bed on the missing foot, crossing the knees with a thigh stump, or, while in bed moving the stump if anyone is about to sit where the foot appears to be. (Henderson and Smyth 1948, 97; emphasis added)

Taking its place alongside other limbs, the phantom was expectedly used in everyday life to break a fall, catch an object, and fend off a blow or to point, wave, grasp for a falling object, or reach for something desirable. When an aromatic cup of steaming coffee enticed, the phantom might reflexively reach for a warm sip. When leaving the room, the phantom might blow a kiss or wave goodbye. Unfortunately, though, phantoms were not good at these things; they failed to grab, reach, grasp, catch, or gesture to others. Regardless of their inadequacies, however, phantoms as devoted imitators did what they were "supposed to do." And at times, phantoms *were* notably productive. They aided amputees during walking, running, crawling, or stepping, and they "helped" during the act of sitting, getting up, steadying, or standing. Fairley's (2004, 1) patient remarked, "When I play tennis, my phantom will do what it's supposed to do. . . . It will give me balance in hard shots."

Still, by the late twentieth century, amputees began to relay something very unlike forgetting, a decisiveness about phantom "use," something more like intentional exploitation. For instance, Scatena (1990, 1230) provided the story of a young girl's calculated use of her outstretched phantom fingers enabling her to solve problems:

> An 11-yr.-old girl with congenital absence of both forearms and hands . . . said that from the age of six she had felt two phantom hands hanging below her stumps. She claimed to feel these hands clearly and to be able to move them at will. . . . [I]n her first years in school she had learned to solve simple arithmetic problems by counting her fingers . . . on these occasions she would place her phantoms on the table and count the outstretched fingers one by one.

Although researchers and amputees themselves had described forgetting since the late 1900s, accounts of intentional exploitation did not surface until around 1980, including general references to phantom utility, as well as specific reports of their benefit in counting, writing, or shaking hands (with a prosthesis). Increasingly, phantoms were characterized as vitally productive; they were not "natural" agents of the body that at times proved to be beneficial, but rather, they were inherently productive and beneficial phenomena because they were "natural" agents of the body. For instance, Abramson and Fiebel (1981, 103; emphasis added) observed that "natural [phantoms] are known to persist in terms of size, of perception of sensation, of movement, and of *incorporation into function,*" and despite the attention given to dysfunctional or abnormal phantoms most, they argued, were "restorative." And, as Sacks (1987, 67) relayed, "Its value to the amputee is enormous." The misbehaving and deceptive phantom of the past, prone to trickery and betrayal—those that amputees needed to be protected against—came to possess a vital purpose and utility. Because they came to "matter," and it was no longer the amputee but rather the phantom that needed to be safeguarded.

The Kinesthetic Peculiarities of Phantoms

Just as phantoms emulated limbs in terms of posture and sensation, they moved in stereotyped ways indicative of the bodies they mimicked. Phantoms covered mouths during surprise, waved to taxis, spread their toes in sand, kicked balls, and slapped cheeks. They quite literally moved in social contexts just as fleshy limbs did. Ramachandran and Hirstein (1998, 1606) provided the case of D.B.:

> We recently reported the presence of phantom arms in a patient (D.B.), a 20-year-old woman whose arms had both been missing from birth. All she had on each side were the upper ends of the humerus—there were no hand bones, and no radius or ulna. However, she claimed to experience very vivid phantom limbs that often gesticulated during conversation.

Schwartz (1992) argued that throughout the twentieth century, there was an elaboration of the human kinesthetic, which was increasingly regarded as "expressive," as evincing the soundness of body and soul. Character could be read through the body in motion, and yet, movement was also conceived as operative in that both the physical body and the psyche could be treated through proper rhythm. As Schwartz (1992, 77, 95) proposed, apposite movement, gesture, and rhythm became curative and transformative; "if one moved wisely, gesture would be a true reflection of the self. . . . This, of course, was an essential pivot in the semantics of the new kinaesthetic, as it moved from the expressive to the operative, and from the operative to the transformative."

In the case of amputees, the rationalization of natural and authentic movement—certain, earnest, willed movement—was evidenced by the value placed on adequate prosthetic technologies and successful reha- bilitation (Schwartz 1992). However, it was also evidenced by an impulse to catalogue and evaluate the kinesthetic features of phantom-ed limbs. Four types of movement were of particular interest by the mid-twenti- eth century: synkinetic or conjunctive, automatic reflexive, spontane- ous, and willed. Conjunctive movements were described as those that were synchronized with the intact limb or other parts of the physical body. A phantom arm might swing in coordination with the intact arm while walking or a phantom leg may move conjunctively or reflexively as an amputee sat, lay down, bent, stooped, or performed other acts. For instance, Henderson and Smyth (1948, 96) wrote,

> During change of body posture, for example, a knee which is straight when the patient is recumbent may bend to a right angle when he sits on the side of the bed so that the foot appears to hang down, or when he turns on his side in bed with the normal leg flexed so that "the legs are alike."

In some cases, phantoms moved like living, organic extensions coor- dinated with and to the body in both time and space. In other cases, amputees reported that phantoms behaved autonomously, as if they had a will of their own, often with distressing consequences. For example, Melzack (1989, 4) described the pain and fatigue that one of his patients suffered as a consequence of his inability to stop his phantom legs from cycling continuously. These spontaneous movements were most typi- cally described as completely outside of the amputee's volitional control.

> The dystonic spasms of the phantom arm and hand were so real and pow- erful that she avoided close contact with other people and objects because of the fear of hitting them. . . . At times she reached out with their right

hand "to calm" the involuntary movement in the phantom arm. The perception of constant movement of the left arm often awoke her from sleep, resulting in chronic insomnia. (Jankovic and Glass 1985, 433)

And in many cases, spontaneous movements did not seem to serve a purpose, nor did they resemble the kinds of movement that fleshy limbs might engage in. "The involuntary movements of his left fingers were purposeless and consisted of flexion-extension, adduction-abduction and clawing-fanning. He could stop them by an effort of will for a few seconds, and they were so peculiar and clumsy as not to be capable of imitation by his right fingers" (Funakawa, Mano, and Takayanagi 1987, 342). In fact, because his movements were so purposeless, the authors concluded the article with the observation that he could be considered psychologically compromised; they wrote, "It is possible that these patients might be considered to be hysterical or psychotic."

Phantoms have never been typified by one type of movement, nor has one category of movement necessarily exemplified a phantom over its entire lifecycle. Some types have been lost or recovered, and some phantoms have expressed two or more forms of movement. For instance, Katz and Melzack (1987, 54; emphasis added) wrote of a patient whose phantom moved conjunctively, reflexively, and spontaneously, sometimes causing him to fall flat on his back or stir uncontrollably in his sleep:

> His limb consisted solely of the lower arm and hand, with a gap between the stump and the beginning of the phantom elbow. He described the limb as suspended in space. Whenever he walked, it behaved as a real limb would, *swinging naturally back and forth in synchrony with his contralateral leg.* Such automatic movements of the limb are common. He described how, while walking down a flight of stairs, he *instinctively reached out to grab the banister with his phantom arm* to avoid a fall, only to find himself lying on the landing below. In contrast, it required considerable effort for him to willfully move the phantom limb: he reported that he was able to partially open the hand, but this was a slow and frustrating process that required enormous concentration. . . . [O]n his first

visit to the pain center one of his primary complaints was that he had great trouble falling asleep at night, for if he lay on his right side he would experience a sharp increase in pain, and when he turned over, *the phantom arm would rise upward like a helium-filled balloon until it was fully extended over his head*. After several minutes in this posture, his arm would become heavy with fatigue, and an unbearable pain would ensue forcing him to shift position again. (Katz and Melzack 1987, 54; emphasis added)

The import placed on the kinesthetic features of phantoms reflected a desire to keep bodies in motion, a desire indicative of the "healthy" body since the turn of the twentieth century (Schwartz 1992). Since the late 1900s, willed movement of the phantom had been advised because it was considered restorative and crucial to prosthetic animation. In Mitchell's (1871, 567) terms, "an artificial member . . . competently supplies the place of the missing limb" and the phantom's role was to assure that the artificial member gave the right "impression." Similarly, Harber (1958, 625) advised that amputees regularly exercise their phantoms in order to facilitate facile prosthesis use; he wrote, "Phantom sensations can be kept more 'natural' and more vivid if soon after amputation the patient takes daily exercises in 'willing' phantom movements; such exercises are said to make a patient better able to use a mobile (cineplastic) prosthesis."

Involuntary movements, on the other hand, have been represented as out of control, as mongrel or monster, throughout much of the twentieth century. Some of the descriptors used to convey involuntary or spontaneous movements included "squirming" (Falconer 1953), "flapping" (Harber 1958), "swaying" (Melzack, et al. 1997), "tensing" (Harber 1958), "writhing" (Ramachandran and Rogers-Ramachandran 1996), "trembling" (Melzack, et al. 1997), and "stiffened and seem[ing] to fly in all directions" (Ament, et al. 1964, 2908). One of the most frequently mentioned, most aberrant, and most out-of-control involuntary movements has varyingly been referred to as "stump jumping," "stump epilepsy," "phantom spasms," "jactitation," and more recently as "phantom restless leg" (Hanna, Kumar, and Walters 2004). McGrath and Hiller (1992, 50) wrote of the phenomenon, "She experienced an unusual sensation that she referred to as nerves jumping. She described it as: 'you first get a weird tingling that starts in your toes and goes up to your stump and the nerves jump. The stump jumps up and down (1 or 2 inches) for a few seconds.'"

These involuntary spasms were described at times as originating in the stump and at other times as originating in the phantom. Regardless, the stump itself might have "never ceased to fly up and down and in and out" or might "politely show . . . an interest in its owner by ceasing to quiver for the whole day on which he had made an offer of marriage" (Mitchell 1871, 565). Throughout the twentieth century, stump jumping—even in the absence of pain—was most often presented in conjunction with some means of treating the affliction, with some means of silencing the movement such as immobilizing the stump by lying on it or tying it down. Because movement, as Schwartz (1992) argued, was a true reflection of the self and because it revealed the nature or disposition of one's character, orchestrated, decisive movement with a rhythmic aesthetic was celebrated while involuntary, unintentional movement was maligned. What typified laudable, vigorous, authentic bodies and their parts also exemplified healthy, proper, and "natural" specters of limbs. After the turn of the twenty-first century, willed movement remained privileged but not because it was demonstrative of a quality character or because it was physically and psychically curative. It was privileged because phantoms had a fundamental utility that could and should be exploited.

Phantom Paralysis and Object Relations

Ramachandran and Hirstein (1998) have employed the term "learned paralysis" to describe a frozen or fixed phantom that imitates the paralysis of a limb prior to amputation or to describe a phantom that becomes paralyzed through nonuse. The neglected phantom, one that was not exercised and willfully moved, could become frozen, immobile, and hence experienced as passive, empty, a mere object with no vital interiority. As if cast in cement, as if submerged in mercury, as if weighed down by plaster, or as if imbedded in a block of ice, the fixed phantom had a remarkable quality possibly indicative of all phantoms; it was not impeded by interposed objects and was often felt as if it pierced or penetrated solids such as a table, mirror, bureau, couch, wall, or even an amputee's own body. "The phantom seems to go blithely through the object, and the experience seems to be so 'natural' to the patient that it is rarely commented upon spontaneously" (Simmel 1956, 642). In fact, it was thought to happen "without arousing any feeling of obstruction or unpleasant sensation" (Henderson and Smyth 1948, 98). For example, a phantom leg bent at a right angle might pierce a mattress when lying down so that the foot was felt as though it was inside the mattress or poking out below it.

> Upon regaining consciousness after the operation he perceived the presence of a phantom limb. The ghost consisted chiefly of a foot and the lower leg. It seemed bent so that when he was lying on his abdomen, the foot felt as thought it was suspended above him. When he was lying on his back the foot seemed to be protruding through the mattress. (Browder and Gallagher 1948, 460)

At other times, paralyzed phantoms were consciously accommodated for because coming in contact with objects or surfaces (such as glass, metal, stone, or netting), one's own or another person's physical body (including the torso, an appendage, or the head), another phantom (in the case of bilateral amputation or conflict with another person's phantom), or a part of the phantom itself (for example, the finger penetrating the wrist) was unsettling, uncomfortable, and sometimes excruciatingly painful.

> In one person, the phantom arm was felt to extend straight out at the shoulder and at a right angle to the body; the phantom was so vivid that he turned sideways to walk though a doorway so the phantom would not

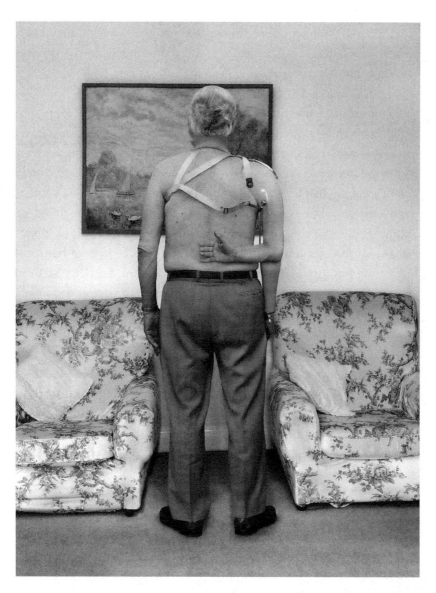

Figure 2.2. Phantom Paralysis. As if encased in plaster, L.N.'s phantom moved laterally, but it was fixed at a right angle and would pass through his body when his stump was angled toward the back. He commented, "It's just there. I can't scratch it, I can't hit it, I can't do anything with it; it's not there except that it feels as though it is there." (Reprinted with permission from Wright, Alexa. 1997. *After Image*. London, England: www.alexawright. com.)

hit the wall. Another person, whose phantom arm was felt behind his back, slept only on his abdomen or a side but could not sleep on his back because his phantom arm was in the way. (Melzack 1989, 3)

Phantoms have had different strategies for "adapting" to the physical world. In the most comprehensive study done on object relations, Jalavisto (1954, 175) suggested that *phantom shunning* (disappearing, moving within the stump, or "bending" to the side), as opposed to *phantom occupation* (moving inside of a wall or another person's body) was demonstrative of the degree to which a person's phantom limb was adaptive. Shunning phantoms were regarded as "adaptable," while "rigid" phantoms were those that did not yield to "real" objects. One of her most interesting findings was that amputees between the ages of seventeen and twenty-four described their phantoms as disappearing or moving when approaching a wall, while amputees over age twenty-five tended to describe their phantoms as passing into the wall. The idea that phantoms either adapt to their environment or rigidly resist the material world communicates as much about the assumed "substance" of phantoms as it does about the author's preconceptions about amputees (particularly with regard to the age-related rigidity). Implicit in her dichotomy is an evaluative judgment about the appropriate ways in which bodies should relate to objects and others. Phantoms that bent or disappeared respected the materiality of the world, while phantoms that "occupied" objects or persons disrespected the integrity of that same world, as well as the sacredness of the subject. Frozen or paralyzed phantoms that confronted the physical world with disrespect were problematized both because of their immobility—their failure to move expressively, curatively, and "naturally" —and because of their irreverence for materiality and the living.

The Temporal Peculiarities of Phantoms

The seemingly idiosyncratic manner in which phantoms have occupied time has consistently been one of the most considered and perplexing aspects of the phenomenon. Why should phantoms have such variability in terms of when they materialize, how long they last, or how frequently they are sensed? Like much of the ambiguity within the literature on phantom phenomena broadly speaking, variability concerning onset, frequency, persistence, and duration has been attributed to poor study design, to methodological flaws, or, most commonly, to deficits in the personalities of amputees. For example Shukla and colleagues (1982, 56) speculated that in cases of delayed onset, "the difference may be because our patients, being educationally backward and rather unsophisticated, were slow to recognize its presence."

Immediately after surgery, phantoms regularly abruptly appeared so that an amputee woke up with a distinct impression of the limb that had been removed. Still, amputees have reported that their phantoms had "grown" (spread, lengthened, or broadened), "materialized" as if they were being brought into the world at a molecular level, "fattened up," "matured" like all limbs, "faded in" before steadying, began as a hollow shell becoming progressively more "dense," "inflated," "swelled" into existence, "dropped in" like a heavy weight or "floated in" like a feather, or increased in intensity, becoming more vivid even after hours, days, months, or years. For example, Jensen and Nikolajsen (2000) reported a case of phantom onset forty-four years after amputation. Often in cases of delayed onset, a precipitating event like puberty (Murphy 1957) or an injury to the stump was attributed to provoking the phantom into existence:

> Another subject, aged 18 years, had a congenital absence of the left arm below the elbow. At the age of 16 years, she had a horse riding accident. Her artificial limb fell off her stump and she landed on the tip of the stump, producing a small haematoma which was eventually resolved. Shortly after the accident, she developed a constant feeling of a full-length phantom arm, hand and full-length fingers. She had never experienced any phantom feelings before this time. (Melzack, et al. 1997, 1604)

Many precipitating factors have been identified that purportedly accounted for the onset, reappearance, or exacerbation of phantom sensation or pain. In addition to stump, knee, hip, wrist, elbow, back, neck, and face pain, general fatigue, illness (such as angina, herpes zoster, prostate cancer, or aneurysm) or injury (especially to the back or stump), stimulation of the stump by means of prosthesis use, or physical exertion have provoked phantom sensations or pain.[1] So too have psychological or emotional events such as stress, anxiety, anger, or fright, everyday behaviors or actions like coughing, yawning, urination, defecation, hemorrhoid irritation, menstruation, orgasm, or sleep, and seemingly benign events like writing, playing ball, smoking, shaving, or seeing another amputee. For instance, a 21-year-old male whose amputation was a result of gangrene experienced the sensation of numbness when thinking or talking about his phantom, when bumping his residual limb, or when coming into contact with anything that resembled a snake (Melzack, et al. 1997).

Phantoms have materialized intermittently, but they have also maintained constancy enduring over the life course, abruptly disappeared, and even reappeared or "reawakened" after having been long gone. Amputees were commonly told that their phantoms would fade and/ or disappear over time despite evidence to the contrary. Weiss's (1956) review of the typical temporal progression of the syndrome was typical of what amputees were told until around 1980; he wrote, "Gradually the

Table 2.1. Provoking Phantom Limb

Author and Year	Precipitant
Weinstein et al. 1969	PL provoked by epileptic attack
Chong-cheng 1986	PL provoked by acupuncture and labor
Dernham 1986	PLP induced/exacerbated by catheterization and prostate exam
Yuh et al. 1992	PL provoked by MRI
Saadah & Melzack 1994	PL provoked by cyst removal and removal of toenails
Knox et al. 1995	PLP provoked by chemotherapy
Melzack et al. 1997	PL induced by anything resembling a snake
Braverman & Root 1997	PLP provoked by carpal tunnel syndrome
Satchithananda et al. 1998	PL lengthening subsequent to heart transplant

tingling becomes weaker and recurs less frequently. For a while it may be present only during changes of weather, just before a patient falls asleep, after he wakens, or at the onset of micturition [urination]. Usually it disappears in two or three years."

By the 1990s, references to phantom fading and disappearance within the literature had doubled. This was not because fading occurred more frequently by the close of the twentieth century but rather because researchers and practitioners became increasingly anxious about the loss of phantoms. The discourse on the "natural" utility of phantoms that had surfaced around 1980 led to greater interest in maintaining healthy and, importantly, mobile phantoms. For example, Abramson and Feibel (1981, 111; emphasis added) warned that "disuse" was the enemy of "restoration":

> Like all . . . processes, it [the phantom] *responds to the adverse affects of disuse* and to the constructive effects of use. This implies that the phantom experience is useful for function, a viewpoint that is the direct antithesis of the attitude of the great American psychologist, William James, who stated that 'The feeling of the lost foot tells us absolutely nothing which can practically be of use to us. It is a superfluous item in our conscious baggage.' . . . The restorative process attempts to prevent or minimize those aspects of disuse that lead to pathological consequences. . . . Function does not flow from the edge of a scalpel, from inactivity. . . . *Only function breeds function.*

Consequently, fading occupied a more prominent place in the literature typically as something that should be cautioned against. Fading, disappearance, and immobility could all lead to potentially long-lasting and harmful effects. Phantom fading and disappearance could leave an amputee impoverished of the naturally occuring productive potential of a mimetic limb, and phantom immobility could lead to paralysis and other "pathological consequences," particularly with respect to phantom pain. Phantom exercise not only aided the amputee in the form of forgetting, but it functioned to stave off some of the most extreme and extraordinary forms of distortion.

The Morphologic Peculiarities of Phantoms

The most distal parts of the limb, the toes or fingers, hands or feet, have been regarded as the sites of the strongest and most persistent sensation and have often been depicted as the sole representation of the phantom despite amputation of, for example, the entire leg or forearm such that the phantom hand or foot is felt as if it essentially floats in midair. R.D.'s entire phantom hand was vividly experienced, but his wrist and forearm were experientially absent so that his phantom hovered almost magically in the position that the intact hand would have occupied. As R.D. moved his prosthesis, the hovering hand followed in perfect synchronization. Simmel (1956, 643) considered floating to be a corollary of phantom fading. She surmised that as the proximal parts of the phantom faded over time, the distal parts would maintain their "proper place":

> When parts of the phantom first begin to fade, the position of the remaining parts is unchanged. The patient may no longer have a phantom thigh, but the remainder of the phantom limb is in its usual and proper place. At this stage the patient is not aware of any holes or empty spaces between the stump and the remaining phantom parts. For some patients there then follows a period during which they experience the emptiness of the interspace, and they describe the persisting phantom as disconnected, as "floating down there."

Areas of a phantom limb may fade, sensed only imperceptibly, or they may "drop out," sensed as missing altogether, as "interspace." For example, Buxton (1957, 500) wrote, "He had always been aware of a phantom right foot, stating that the instep and big toe were most clear and resembled the real foot although the ankle was not part of the phantom." The shaded regions in figure 2.4 show areas or pieces of phantom toes, feet, legs, fingers, hands, and arms that were reported as experientially vivid by Melzack's (1990) patients, and the dotted lines demarcate areas of the missing limbs that did not experience phantom sensation or awareness. For example, the big toe or the sole of the foot might be represented while the other parts of the foot or leg might feel nonexistent. In

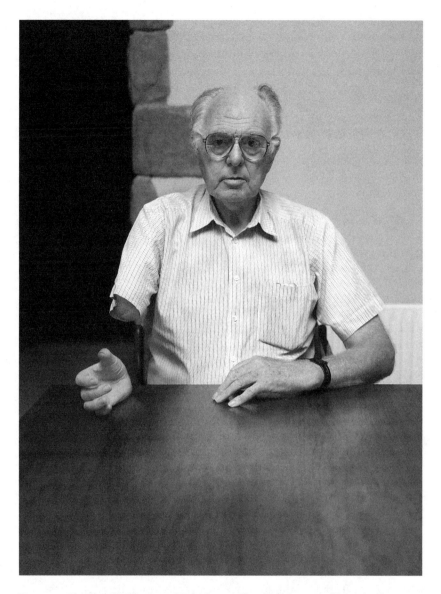

Figure 2.3. The Floating Phantom. R.D.'s phantom hand was heavy and his itchy fingers floated in space. Despite the fact that it was irritating, he admitted that he would "rather keep it as it is than risk losing it." (Reprinted with permission from Wright, Alexa. 1997. *After Image*. London, England: www.alexawright.com.)

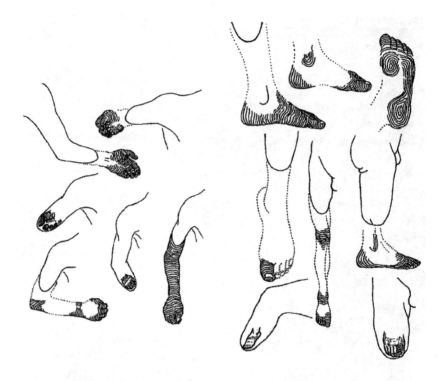

Figure 2.4. Disturbances of Continuity. Based on patient reports, these drawings depict phantom vividness; solid lines indicate the most vivid parts of the phantom while dotted lines illustrate areas where sensation is less vivid or not experienced. Phantoms that have telescoped into the residual limb are also shown. (Reprinted from Melzack, Ronald. 1990. "Phantom limbs and the concept of a neuromatrix." *Trends in Neurosciences* 13:88–92, with permission from Elsevier.)

other cases, these silent sensorial zones were consciously "felt" such that amputees were perceptually aware of zones of absence.

Other phantom pieces have been sensed as if they were not strongly attached, as if one might simply pluck off the dangling bit. These *disturbances of continuity* have been varyingly referred to in the literature as "phantom gaps" or "holes," and are sometimes thought to be similar to (or synonymous with) what has been termed "telescoping" and/or strongly correlated with diminution of size, or "phantom shrinking." Zuk (1956) suggested that the "dropping out of parts" was a subphenomenon of telescoping, while others have argued that diminution in size, disturbances of continuity, and telescoping are distinct phenomena. Consonant with the latter, Simmel (1956, 643) argued that disturbances of continuity produced telescoping; she proposed that when the upper thigh, knee, and calf begin to fade, a "hole or empty space" opens up between the body and the remaining vivid parts—the foot and toes, for instance—and because "phantoms and their owners seem to abhor a vacuum as much as nature is said to do . . . we find the separate parts moving together and approaching the stump." Sobchack (2010, 57) provided the following first-person account, writing,

> Most prominently and clearly defined, I experienced my former foot: even two of the outer toes felt numb just as they had before the surgery. However, I felt little more of the leg itself than a certain ill-defined verticality. . . . That is, I had no formal sense of a knee and only the barest sense of narrowing that might have been an ankle and, of course, did not proprioceptively feel the weight of my thigh or sense some equivalent of my calf against the sofa cushion. The leg's connection to my bandaged stump was also ambiguous; there seemed to be a certain auratic area around my residual limb, a sort of vaguely bounded band of "unfilled" space, a no-man's land separating two different perceptions of my body that would admit no trespass.

These peculiar embodied holes functioned as compelling evidence that some body parts "mattered" more than others: fingers more than wrists, toes more than ankles, knees more than shins, elbows more than forearms. However, the empty spaces between body parts were often considered more revealing than any of the suspended or precariously perched bits or pieces that persisted with tenacity. These gaps testified to the fact that our "connection" to physical parts is meaningfully embodied and that this bond could materialize overtly in terms of how "disconnected" less significant parts could become.

At times, these floating parts were described as unequivocally belonging to the body and sensed as intimate and important aspect of the "self." For example, Melzack (1990, 90) observed,

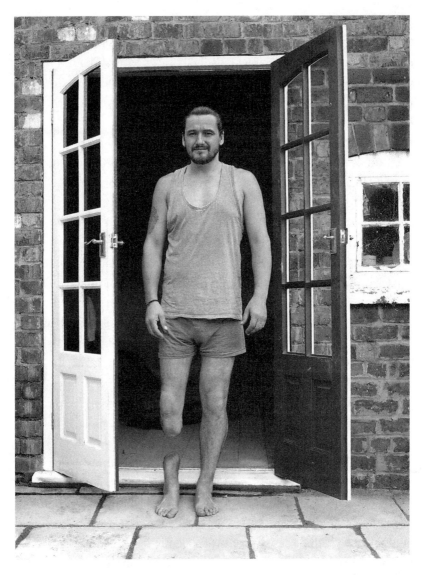

Figure 2.5. Phantom Gapping. A.M.'s phantom allowed him to feel as if his leg was back when walking. He said, "Sometimes the phantom feels like my own leg, but it feels like having a dead piece of meat touching the floor. I can feel a vibration when the leg hits the floor, although I know it's not there. It's basically a part of me which moves normally when I walk or run, although I feel my foot as it was after the accident when it was damaged. Sometimes it feels like there are bits of the foot there and sometimes there are bits missing. It seems real, as if I or someone else can touch it." (Reprinted with permission from Wright, Alexa. 1997. *After Image*. London, England: www.alexawright.com.)

One of the most striking features of the phantom of a limb or any other body part, including half of the body in many paraplegics, is that it is perceived as an integral part of one's self. Even when a phantom foot dangles "in mid-air" (without connecting leg) a few inches below the stump, it still moves appropriately with the other limbs and is unmistakably felt to be part of one's body.

However, amputees have also reported that these suspended parts have a distinctive nature. For example, A.M.'s leg felt like his own, but it was experienced as a "dead piece of meat" with "bits missing."

Telescoping is a curious event that was originally introduced by Gueniot (1861) and has been described as the process of the gradual decrease in the length and/or size of the phantom, such that it shrinks and withdraws toward or into the stump. As Miller (1978) observed, the phantom has also been felt as if it had grown in size in order to "engulf" itself. He wrote, "As time goes on, the phantom dwindles, but it does so in very peculiar ways. The arm part may go, leaving a maddening piece of hand waggling invisibly from the edge of the real shoulders; the hand may enlarge itself to engulf the rest of the limb" (Miller 1978, 20).

Gueniot originally proposed that an amputee's phantom limb *regressed* to that of a child's over time (Katz 1992a), and in fact, phantom hands have been described by amputees and others as child-sized (Spitzer, et al. 1995), as resembling "a 'baby's hand' curled up inside the stump" (Murphy 1957, 474), or as approximating a "doll's hand" (Browder and Gallagher 1948, 459). For some, the tiny hand was felt as if it were attached immediately to the stump's exterior or as if it were barely hanging from the edge of the residual limb. In other cases, the shrunken fingers protruded through the stump "hanging straight down" or they "curl[ed] around the end of the stump as if grasping it" (Henderson and Smyth 1948, 91). Still, haunted limbs were at times felt as if they had been pushed completely inside the residual limb. G.N.'s phantom arm had telescoped almost entirely into his shoulder stump with the exception of his thumb, which protruded through the end, remaining intact and vivid.

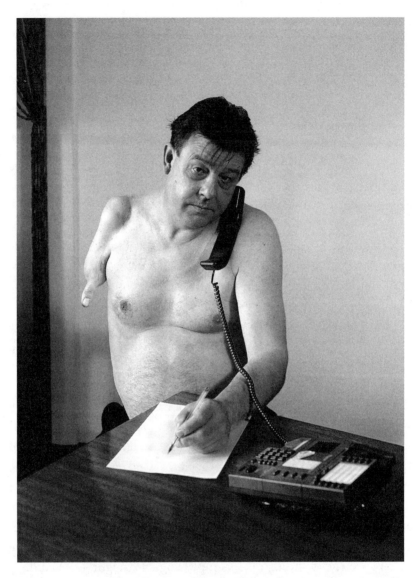

Figure 2.6. The Telescoped Phantom. G.N.'s phantom telescoped into his residual limb so that only the phantom thumb remained. Commenting on the changes in his phantom over time, he said, "The phantom used to float away from where the arm was. I was in a hospital bed and it would float through the bedclothes and get cold, so I developed this habit of sleeping on my right side so the phantom limb drifted into the mattress and stayed warm. At the beginning I used to believe I could get the arm back. Now nearly all of the arm has disappeared." (Reprinted with permission from Wright, Alexa. 1997. *After Image*. London, England: www.alexawright.com.)

This sensation of the phantom foot or hand slipping inside the body, becoming enclosed by or embedded in the stump—what Winston (1950, 299) termed "melting" —has often been described as a kind of lived tension. For example, Scatena (1990, 1230) relayed an account of a congenital amputee whose telescoped phantom was struggling; she said, "If the end of the stump was open, a hand would grow out of it, for I am sure there is something inside which wants to come out. It feels as though a lump inside is struggling."

There is a great deal of ambiguity within the literature about the degree to which telescoping is a common sequela of phantom limb syndrome. The earliest published prevalence report within the American medical literature appeared in 1972, and during the 1970s, reports were as high as 80 percent (see for example Varma, Lal, and Mukherjee 1972). Prevalence was expectedly high because as Pontius (1964, 697) argued, borrowing from the law of biogenetics, telescoping was demonstrative of the atavistic form of the phylogenetic recapitulation of human ontology. Human embryonic development assertedly followed the same path as the evolutionary development of "man" and accordingly, during telescoping "limbs analogous to those of fish are experienced." From this perspective the "natural" phantom shrunk or regressed to a primordial state, and because phylogenetic recapitulation was central to human physiologic development, telescoping was expectedly highly prevalent among amputees. In fact, some shrunken phantoms were described as "like that of an embryo" (Frederiks 1963, 80).

By the 1980s, the prevalence rate had dropped to between 30 and 33 percent (see for example Jensen, et al. 1983), where it remained until the turn of the twenty-first century. Over the next decade, the prevalence rate plummeted; reports were as low as 3.8 percent (Probstner, et al. 2010). The dramatic decline in the telescoping prevalence rate was a corollary of the reconceptualization of phantoms as principally productive phenomena, as having a fundamental utility, and like both fading and disappearance, phantom telescoping precluded the possibility of harnessing the phantom's productive potential. Telescoping increasingly made clinicians, researchers, and others quite anxious because as Sacks (1987, 67) relayed, "Its value to the amputee is enormous."

However, contemporarily, phantoms have also been depicted as having the capacity to return to full length or to regrow. For example, G.N.'s entire phantom had telescoped into his residual limb with the exception of his thumb, but when he donned a prosthesis, his phantom grew to normal length so that his phantom thumb was felt as superimposed on the prosthetic thumb; he described the sensation as that of a hand fitting nicely inside a glove. Similarly, in the case of a lower limb phantom, Melzack (1990, 89) wrote, "The phantom fills the artificial leg when it

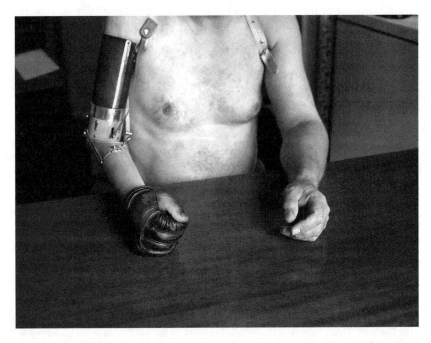

Figure 2.7. Phantom Regrowth. G.N.'s phantom hand was sensed as inside a glove when his prosthesis was donned, and his thumb would come to reside in its former position. However, he could also be "wrong" sometimes. He said, "If I can't see the artificial hand I can be wrong; I could be six inches out as to the location of the hand: the phantom hand can miss the artificial one in terms of spatial placing. There is an intermittent crushing pain, but the phantom is always there. It's part of me; it will never go away completely. I will always be this; I will always have two arms, it's just that one of them is missing." (Reprinted with permission from Wright, Alexa. 1997. *After Image*. London, England: www.alexawright.com.)

is strapped on [so that] the phantom foot now occupies the space of the artificial foot in its shoe." Telescoped phantoms also temporarily "zoomed out" in an effort to reach for objects or greet an outstretched hand. For example, Ramachandran and Blakeslee (1998, 1606) wrote,

> One of our patients, for example, had his right forearm amputated below the elbow, and his hand was usually telescoped into the stump just below the elbow. However, if he attempted to shake hands or reach out to grab a cup, his phantom would extend to normal length. Indeed, in one instance, when we suddenly pulled the cup away he yelped in pain, claiming that we had wrenched the cup away from his phantom fingers, causing his arm to telescope unexpectedly.

Not only did the telescoping prevalence rate decline circa 1980, but telescoping was increasingly understood as potentially transitory and reversible. As embodied ghosts morphed into productive phenomena, the tendency for them to regress or telescope became more and more remote, and those phantoms that did withdraw into the body or curl up inside residual limbs as if to hibernate—not doing "what they should be doing"—could, with the right strategy, be coaxed out again.

Phantom Distortion and the Case of Supernumerary Phantoms

Despite the fact that phantoms were principally imagined as replicas until about 1980, researchers had always wrestled with some phantoms that were not like real limbs in very fundamental ways, anomalies that were part of their disturbing "pea-soup." Throughout most of the twentieth century, the literature classified some of these monsters as explicable while others remained out of bounds, epistemologically sequestered. One of the most fantastical manifestations of phantom "distortion" is what has been termed "supernumerary limb." These surplus or extra phantom limbs have also been referred to as doubled limbs, surplus limbs, spare limbs, or reduplicative limbs, and have been documented in cases of paralysis, traumatic brain injury, multiple sclerosis, brain tumor, epilepsy, stroke, amputation, and others. Bakheit and Roundhill (2005, 1) wrote of one patient's third leg and its fleshless "bone plate":

> The patient repeatedly reported that he had a third leg protruding from his left knee. He consistently maintained that the phantom leg was attached to his knee with a "bone plate" that "had no flesh on it." . . . [T]he phantom limb prevented him from turning over in bed, but did not adversely affect him otherwise. . . . [H]e believed that the phantom belonged to him, although he readily accepted that it was not "normal." . . . [I]nitially he reported that the "leg" was growing from his own knee, but then reasoned that (given its size) he would have noticed it before. . . . At other times he believed the leg was attached to him by the nursing staff, but could not explain why.

Commonly, supernumerary limbs originated from the same joint as the "real" or fleshy limb. However, patients have also reported only a vague sense of how the limb was attached, and sometimes they could not articulate exactly where the connection was made. Surplus limbs have also been documented as growing from an atypical site—from the middle of the chest, for example (Sakagami, Murai, and Sugiyama 2002); as partial in nature—for instance, the presence of three and a half legs (Fredericks 1963); or as replicating immoderately—as in the case of a man who complained of having a nest of hands in his bed. These, he concluded, should rightly be "put in a bag" because that is where hands without arms go.

> A 59 year old right hemisphere stroke patient is described who, according to his doctor, complained of having "a nest of hands in his bed." This patient . . . requested that the "hands" should be amputated and put in a bag. . . . Six days after the stroke . . . he maintained that his old left hand had begun to shrink and that a new hand had emerged, becoming fleshier and more voluminous. Subsequent questioning confirmed that the patient believed in the existence of several hands (without arms), two on the left and one on the right, the former of which were thought to be located in the region of his left knee. (Halligan, Marshall, and Wade 1993, 159)

Melzack and his colleagues were instrumental in chronicling spare limbs in the case of amputation. For example, Lacroix, Melzack, Smith and Mitchell (1992, 504–5) reported on the case of a young girl who "grew" two feet and three sets of toes after amputation of a congenitally malformed limb. The girl described a deformed phantom foot and toes that seemed to replace the amputated foot (a congenitally deformed phantom), which was felt to be ten centimeters higher than the normal foot (her "good" foot). Another set of "baby" toes extended from the end of the stump (a new set that protruded from/through her new residual limb), which she described as at times itchy and at other times constantly wiggling. Her third phantom was perceived as a shell of a leg composed of a calf, foot, and toes that were otherwise "normal" in size and position (a full-length phantom of a limb that, in fact, she never had).

Amputees and others, although psychologically normal, often used bizarre logic to rationalize these inexplicable surplus limbs. When pressed, the inadequacy of their rationalizations typically did not deter patients from insisting on the limb's "reality." For example, L.M. felt confident when she screwed on her surplus or spare arm:

> The spare limb could be moved and controlled by L.M. who was able to screw it on when needed. . . . I concentrated myself on the arm that I did not move in order to try to perceive even the smallest movement, I looked at the arm carefully; all of the sudden I started to have a strange sensation which can't be explained well with words: I had an extra arm, in addition to the one that I couldn't move, a sort of spare arm; so at times I thought that I could unscrew the paralysed one and screw on the good one. . . . It gave me confidence. It was an arm like the other two; sometimes I could feel it so much that I was surprised by not being able to see it. (Grossi, Di Cesare, and Tamburro 2002)

Halligan and his colleagues (1993, 162) presented the case of 65-year-old man whose third arm originated from the upper left side of his chest. They provided the following excerpt from an interview with the patient (P) three days after admission into the hospital:

E: So tell me now at the moment, how many hands do you have?

P: Three.

E: Three! . . . Show me your right hand (raises right arm). Count the
    number of hands you have for me.

P: (Looking down and pointing) . . . One . . . two . . . three.

E: How many actually work?

P: Two.

E: Two of them work? Where are the good working hands?

P: On the right side and the left side and the middle I suppose.

E: So which one does not work?

P: The one in the middle

E: How is the middle one attached to your body?

P: It's not . . . it's attached but detached in the sense of it was taken
    off. . . . I don't know. I really don't know. I'm in a muddle about this.

E: It's quite confusing, isn't it?

P: Yes, it is. . . . I know that the right one is alright.

E: Can you move the left one?

P: Yes, but not very much. . . . I can't do very much with it.

E: Where is the other hand that does not work?

P: In the middle . . . (pointing with right hand).

E: Does it fit under your clothes?

P: No, it does not. . . . No, it is not covered with any clothes.

E: Does it get cold?

P: Yes, it does get cold.

E: Can you feel it?

P: Yes, I do! . . .

E: What do you think of a person having three hands?

P: It's an odd situation! . . . I'm a bit vague about it I must say.

What is most noteworthy about supernumerary limbs is that although
very few references can be found within the literature before the late
1990s, in almost every year between 1997 and 2012 the phenomenon
was documented and with revealing detail, a pattern that attests to the
increased intelligibility of phantom distortion. The mimetic phantom

of the past "seem[ed] to maintain such perfect connexion and harmony with the stump . . . [and] as a rule the phantom seemed to be a replica of the original" (Henderson and Smyth 1948, 99); "show[ed] considerable uniformity, since [it] reflect[ed] constant and generic features" (Harber 1956, 625); "[was] experienced as self-evident and belonging to the normal integrity of the body" (Frederiks 1963, 75); and "[felt] as the original limb did in every respect as to shape, size, consistency, position, sensation and ability to move" (Frazier and Kolb 1970, 487). But, something was happening to these benign copycats, shadows, replicas, these curious tricksters, these devoted and skillful imitators, these relics of man's evolutionary history, these standardized parts of our biophysical "machines."

The Natural Phantom and the Plague of Pain

Given the assumption that phantoms were mimetic of preamputated limbs in form and function, distortion was unintelligible and thus, rare specimens were typically described as incomplete, resized, or strangely postured versions of what was referred to as the "natural phantom." Incomplete phantoms were just "not filled in" or finished, while resized phantoms were nothing more than tiny or large versions of the real McCoy. Phantoms that occupied a strange position or posture did so for the most part within anatomical limits and importantly, in ways that reflected the positioning of the limb just prior to amputation, a tendency that actually testified to their mimetic nature.

By about 1980, the "unnatural" phantom was typical, and strange distortions of the past were recast as among the many forms that phantoms could assume. Phantoms appreciably deviated from normal structure and were reorganized in profoundly perverted ways. They were depicted as out of place, as protean, or as grotesquely disturbed in size and shape. Abramson and Feibel (1981, 105) commented, "There are many reports of images [phantoms] that are deformed in amputees and images that are uncoupled and markedly out of place from where they should be." The phantom was also characterized as "a fluid, frequently changing perceptual experience" (Katz 1992b, 295). And as Sobchack (2010, 54) urged,

"Even the most reported and recurrent structural features of the 'phantom limb' must be taken as provisional rather than essential forms: that is, as inherently dynamic and open to myriad variations of being and meaning." Phantoms also began to be sensed as dis/reorganized in ways that did not reflect normal human morphology, including impossible anatomical configurations (Giummarra et al. 2011) such as a phantom leg with a knee located lower than normal at shin level (Melzack, et al. 1997), a phantom arm irregularly shaped with a thin forearm (Cole, et al. 2009), "unnatural limb contortion" (Zeher, et al. 2011, 730), a clump of fingers of unknown quantity (Melzack, et al. 1997), a phantom foot on backwards (DiMartino 2000), or a pulverized foot that "feels 'confused' and all over the place" (Giummarra, et al. 2011, 696).

Despite attempts by researchers and practitioners to rationalize phantoms, to delimit the parameters of phantom morphology, embodied ghosts morphed or shape-shifted. They twisted, contorted, warped, spread, flattened, and "pathologized" in many other ways. Phantoms increasingly refused to abide by the laws that had always governed bodies, such as gravity (floating like helium-filled balloons), symmetry (growing from the middle of the chest or multiplying immoderately), time (suddenly disappearing or reappearing, popping in and out of sensorial experience), or permanence (telescoping to curl up inside the stump as if hibernating or giving up altogether). In response to medical attempts at "containment," phantoms transgressed; they did not acquiesce to an origin story that defined them as nothing more than copies, replicas, fakes.

Incontrovertibly, the all-but-faultless facsimile of the past was no fake, nor did pleasurable copies come into being by way of inadequate, flawed, or inferior science. Phantom mimesis did not materialize out of errors in judgment, sloppy practices, or ulterior motives—a notion predicated on the idea that with adequate tools, the proper techniques, and a systematic and rigorous approach to inquiry, it is possible to "get it right," to definitively understand the phantom and its qualities, its origin story, and its purpose. Rather than being "matter" revealed to us accurately or with error by way of empiricism, phantom limb syndrome, like all diseases, illnesses, conditions, etc,, becomes "substantive" and, hence, understood, diagnosable, treatable, and made intersubjectively mean-ingful, within political, social-cultural, and historical contexts.

To be clear, it is not my intent to be naively dismissive of the role of biomedicine and technoscience in constructing phantoms. Instead, I want to undermine the sanctity of neuroscientific preeminence, its claims of superiority and rightful authority rooted in the fundamental tenets of objectivity and value neutrality, to expose the fact that phantoms are faith-based. Undoubtedly, biopower entails the elaboration and refine-ment of technical knowledge that functions to enhance the authority of those in positions of expertise through, among many other means, the generation of a set of knowledge-filters that (1) *naturalize* disease in order to distance the biophysical from the sociocultural and safeguard knowl-edge from social-scientific and other sources of scrutiny, (2) *produce* the very objects that are presumably under biomedical and techno-scientific investigation and intervention, and (3) *mediate* the myriad social rela-tions within and outside of the laboratory, the hospital, and the clinic.

However, it is important to note that biomedical and technoscientific "objects" are rarely stable for long (Rosenberg 1992, 2007). Perturbations in the logics and practices constitutive of the biopolitical order come from within—via turf wars, paradigmatic drift or shifts (Kuhn 1962), politicization, and the like—as well as from without—from the broader sociocultural milieu, shifts in corporeal ideology, lived accounts of ill-ness or disability, and the recalcitrant nature of the body. It is because of such perturbations that Klepinger (1980, 481) maintained, "Some diseases change their expression; new diseases arise and some die out." Unequivocally, phantom limb syndrome has "changed its expression." Haunted limbs began to materialize in ways that were quite "unnatural," and they did so despite the widely accepted assumption of their mimetic nature, an assumption that made distortion entirely incomprehensible.

The recharacterization of the phantom from replica to deviant shape-shifter, from fundamentally mimetic and generic to protean and idiosyn-cratic, was at least partly a consequence of the need to rethink phantoms as research on the phenomenon began to produce data that was widely discrepant from past reports. Most notably, researchers had to explain the onset of an epidemic of phantom limb pain that surfaced around 1980. If pain was a widespread sequela of the syndrome, researchers and clinicians were pressed to ask, Why were past studies so erroneous, so fatally flawed? Why had phantom pain of epidemic proportions gone unreported, unrecognized, and untreated for so long? Why had the keepers of truth and the caretakers of the body of evidence on haunted limbs been so remiss?

As pain became normative, distortion became increasingly intelligible and mimesis grew to be atypical, the flawless "natural" copy lapsed into rarity, and the phenomenon of phantom "emulation" (of phantoms mimicking the posture and other qualities of the intact limb *just prior to amputation*) evolved into what was termed "pain memories" by 1990. Emulation was no longer relatively benign with the evident charm of superadded features—phantoms with glittering rings, trusty watches, and scuffed patent leather shoes. In the form of pain memories, emulation was the worst of all nightmares.

Because pain came to be considered widespread and because reports told of the cruelty of such pain, researchers and clinicians surmised that phantoms must be amenable to treatment. Indeed, the underlying nature of phantoms became their ability to adapt and their essential utility. Forgetting—using a phantom hand to steady oneself, for example—regularly assumed the form of intentional exploitation, and phantom exercise or willed movement became associated not just with "helping" the amputee but with staving off phantom pain. Willed movement was characterized as integral to recovery because it was an elemental aspect of phantom utility and because it effectively ameliorated pain. The idle phantom, by contrast, was the devil's plaything. Without willed movement, the phantom could "pathologize," torturing the body and spirit with the most unrelenting, agonizing, and intractable pain ever known—a pain one patient described as like "50 devils . . . [with] stabbing needles" (Nikolajsen, et al. 1997, 398).

3

From Pleasure to Pain

Accounting for the Rise and Fall in Phantom Pain

Consonant with the invention of pain medicine (Baszanger 1992, 1998a), the instantiation of the pain clinic (Baszanger 1992, 1998a; Kugelmann 1997), the institutionalization and codification of pain therapeutics and clinical management (Baszanger 1998a; Rey 1993), and the emerging "epidemic" of pain in the United States around 1975 (Morris 1991; Osterweis, Kleinman, and Mechanic 1987), phantoms became painful, and through the advance of a specific language of pain vis-à-vis the McGill Pain Questionnaire (MPQ), phantoms became cruelly, gruelingly, exhaustingly painful. The terminology advanced by the MPQ became pivotal for understanding and, in fact, expressing phantom pain. In other words, phantom pain became linguistic, standardized, and sharable via an instrument or technology intended to measure neurophysiological processes, scrutinize the peculiarities of enigmatic pain, broaden understanding of the nature of pain itself, give voice to amputees and others suffering from seemingly inexplicable pain, and pin down pain for diagnostic purposes.

As a corollary of a paradigmatic shift in pain theorizing that occurred around 1965, the new language of phantom pain engendered by the MPQ had its origins in attending to the objectification of pain and the creation of a more responsive, more sensitive tool for capturing the newly understood complexity and multidimensionality of pain. Indeed, the purpose of the MPQ was to make the objectification of pain increasingly possible. And, it did. It also caused pre-MPQ pain to be reimagined as poorly measured and pain reporting of the past to be viewed by researchers and practitioners as fraught with inauthenticity.

As the discourse on the quality of phantom sensations elaborated—at least in part provoked by the advent and widespread use of the MPQ—painful phantoms proliferated. The development and implementation of a new technology intended to increase biomedical control over dismembered (and other) bodies had the effect of accentuating and refining pain. Phantom pain became the rule rather than the exception, and when phantoms hurt, they burned, stabbed, and cut. Because pain can enslave and because pain operates as a means through which bodies can be managed and governed, it is always relevant to ask who is in pain, why, and, perhaps disturbingly, to whose benefit. The contemporary plague of pain is a core expression of late-modern biopower, and in the case of phantoms, it has functioned as nothing less than a form of the biopolitical "reinvention of nature" itself (Haraway 1991; Lemke 2011, 93). The body's "absent" parts have become profitable and industrious sites of intervention. As it turns out, what is missing can be biomedically territorialized too.

Increasingly, the discursive practices available to people in pain have been those endemic to pain medicine, which characterized, classified, codified, and institutionalized the properties of pain and the pained subject. With the emergence and entrenchment of pain medicine over the latter half of the twentieth century and into the twenty-first, pain has been dissevered, particularized, deepened, and elaborated, and like many pain syndromes, the prevalence rate of phantom pain reached its peak. Phantom pleasure lapsed into pain, the "natural" phantom became a mere specter of itself, and the quality of phantom sensations became unequivocally painful. The etiology of pain was fractured according to distinct burning, shooting, and lancinating classes, while the treatment, prevention, and management of phantom pain became a clinical problem of vital import. Clinical practice and research became oriented toward not just cure and management but prevention, thus expanding the legitimate jurisdiction of pain medicine. As the role of pain medicine has broadened to include diagnosis, treatment, management, and prevention, the public discourse on pain has expanded, engendering changes in the way pain has been made meaningful, historicized, and given context, the way pain has been accomplished, practiced, and experienced, and the way pain has been communicated, shared, and made relational.

The Pleasurable Phantom

Phantoms were historically conceptualized as morphologically and kinesthetically mimetic of fleshy limbs; they "looked" and "acted" like intact limbs with few exceptions. Until the late 1960s, phantoms were thought of as uncanny imitators that as a rule were replicas of the original except that they possessed a unique vitality, they "possess[ed] *more awareness than the real limb*" (Frederiks 1963, 76; original emphasis).[1] As early as the late 1800s, Mitchell (1871, 564) published on the vividness of the "remainder," which was felt as "more definite and intrusive than is that of its truly living fellow-member." At mid-twentieth century, Cook and Druckemiller (1952, 509–10; emphasis added) wrote of one amputee's experience of feeling his limbs both dead and alive:

> As with many patients with this syndrome he was, at first, unable to reconcile the objective absence of his limb with the fact that it felt as if it were still present. This conflict must have been particularly disturbing since he said, "This one (left lower extremity) is here and dead, but this one (amputated extremity) is gone, yet it *feels alive.*" From his description there was apparently a distinct sensation of *viability* in the phantom, and subsequently, he explained that it felt as if he could kick someone with it.

As somehow *better* than the best fleshy limbs—as more present or "there"—phantoms had a distinct viability or vitality that differentiated them from intact limbs, and an amputee had to "simply learn . . . to live with a phantom limb of which he was more conscious than the one present" (Bailey and Moersch 1941, 41). Henderson and Smyth (1948, 90) observed, "The sensation is always stronger than any vague awareness of the intact limb (which is not consciously felt, at least as a positive sensation)." The vague awareness indicative of the intact limb is a state that is tantamount to what Leder (1990) characterized as the experiential absence of the body in everyday life, its taken-for-granted-ness. "Whilst in one sense the body is the most abiding and inescapable presence in our lives, it is also characterized by absence. That is, one's own body is rarely the thematic object of experience. . . . [T]he body, as a ground . . . tends to recede" (Leder 1990, 1). In contrast, when the body *dys-appears* because of pain, it is brought fully into our conscious awareness, becoming phenomenologically present, and when we are free of pain, we experience the absence of absence.

Just as the "pained" body forces itself into the forefront of our conscious awareness, so too does the "pleasured" body. In the case of phantom limb, the exceptionally vital ghost member was remarkably pleasant and welcomed until around 1980.[2] In fact, it was the characteristic pleasurable tingling of phantoms that made them feel so alive, so remarkable, so distinctive, and so vibrant. For example, Simmel's (1956, 641) patient quite enjoyed the sensation he felt: "The foot of the amputated leg may tingle and itch, and, as the patient reaches down to scratch it, he reaches for an empty space. He may feel the bedsheets on the arm or leg; he may feel a mild, perhaps pleasant tingling. . . . [T]hus one patient told me that 'the leg felt good . . . real good.'"

From around 1980 onward, only a few studies documented pleasurable phantoms, and those accounts generally either referenced the phantom's favorable role in prosthesis use or were associated with body parts that have a natural proclivity for providing pleasure, such as the breast or penis. In terms of the former, Hill (1999, 125) argued that the phantom was "seldom distressing" and was "in fact, welcome[ed, because] . . . it allows them [amputees] to use a prosthesis naturally." And, in terms of the latter Melzack (1989, 3) explained, "The painless phantom breast after a mastectomy, in which the nipple is the most vivid part, is usually a pleasant experience because the phantom breast seems to fill out the padded brassiere and feels extremely real." In both cases, pleasure was understood as a facet of functionality unlike past accounts when pleasure was pleasure for its own sake, when it was simply titillating.

The fact that pleasurable phantoms lapsed into rarity had as much to do with normative expressions of pain as it did with the implications of eerie and often menacing specters of limbs invoking genuinely realized pleasure. Pain and pleasure alike always involve a set of codified social rules, norms, mores "which sets the parameters of allowable overt manifestations ... [that are] defined by society's standards of permissiveness or notions of transgression" (Rey 1993, 4). Prior to pain becoming an object of scientific and biomedical inquiry of distict importance, confessing to pain that originated in a limb, breast, or other body part that no longer existed was outside the parameters of allowable manifestation. Pain was expectedly exceptional, and thus, phantom sensation was characterized by its opposite. We always feel *something* about what we feel. If a sensation is clearly not pain, and cannot by its very definition be *nothing*, it must be pleasure. With the instantiation of the pain clinic and the rise in pain prevalence, pleasure became peculiar and inexplicable; why would the after-effect, the sensorial consequent, of dismemberment feel pleasant, pleasing, welcomed, pleasurable, or "real good"? This was not just a strange supposition. It was ludicrous because it was undeniably disturbing.

As the pleasurable phantom became increasingly rare, the painful phantom proliferated. By the 1980s, 85 percent of phantom limbs were reportedly painful (see for example Sherman and Sherman 1983). Disturbingly, what was once thought to be a relatively infrequent occurrence for a very few amputees became widespread and often described as an unrelenting, unbearable, and exquisite form of torture. A number of researchers and clinicians speculated as to why this incredible discrepancy existed in the literature, principally arguing that "earlier studies grossly underestimated the incidence of this dreaded phenomenon" (Davis 1993, 79). Underestimation was attributed to methodological issues (particularly the choice of study population), terminological confusion or differing operational definitions of pain, the failure to differentiate between phantom sensations and phantom pain, issues related to patient recall, and/or observer misinterpretation (see for example Hazelgrove and Rogers 2002; Mortimer, et al. 2004; Ribbers, Mulder, and Rijken 1989; Weeks, Anderson-Barnes, and Tsao 2010). Czerniecki elaborated on the problem of study population:

I think it [the prevalence rate] depends on how the question is asked. Some of the early data looked at people who presented with phantom pain at their clinical visits. Results will differ if you count the prevalence of phantom limb pain based upon that clinical context, as opposed to asking somebody: "Do you ever have pain in the part of your limb that is missing?" Ever is a very broad statement. Even if you had someone who had a transient electric jolt six years ago, they would have to answer yes to that question. So, now you've got a much more sensitive means of detecting phantom limb pain than waiting for somebody to come to you with problematic, symptomatic, functionally-limiting phantom limb pain. (Czerniecki 2005)

Others have suggested that the discrepancy was a result of changes in patient reticence to report inexplicable pain. However, one recent study demonstrated that 50 percent of amputees who experienced pain did not consult their general practitioner about treatment (Whyte and Carroll 2002). Moreover, White and Niven (2004) showed that general practitioners underestimated the prevalence, intensity, and duration of phantom limb pain, and that when a specialist referral is made, there is significant variation in the preferred approach to pain management; referrals are made to prosthetic clinics, pain clinics, and/or psychological, psychiatric, or other counseling services. In addition, insufficient and inconsistent information is frequently given to patients about phantom limb pain, especially prior to amputation, because some practitioners believe that encouraging the expectation of pain may actually cause it (see for example Mortimer, et al. 2004). Indeed, Deuchar (1981, 117; emphasis added) believed that "most patients are *brainwashed* into accepting pain as inevitable." And, In Der Beeck (1953, 223) suggested that it was only through "close and intensive investigation" that phantoms "were bought to life":

During investigations which were made of 75 cases of persons amputated during the second world war it was noticed that many of the affected persons had never thought of their phantom limb. They only became acquainted with the feeling for their phantom as the result of the close and intensive investigation. Some of them were surprised at the large number of sensory impressions, which were brought to life.

Infrequent pain reporting was also attributed to patients' fears of being labeled mentally compromised. For example, Hsu and Sliwa (2004, 659) wrote, "Poor understanding of how pain could be perceived in an absent body part led many physicians to believe that such pain was psychogenic and led many patients to believe that reporting such pain would make their physician think they were mentally ill." The fear of being thought foolish or insane by family, friends, practitioners, or others is a theme that repeatedly appears in the literature even after the turn of the twenty-first century (see for example Whyte and Niven 2004). In the mid-1960s, Simmel (1967, 64) elaborated on what happened to amputees who were accused of "not playing by the rules" or of disgracing the family:

> The wise patient quickly discovers that he had better not talk about the phantom. While most physicians and surgeons know about phantoms, they seem to have an almost universal antipathy towards them. They too think of sensation in terms of concurrent stimulus input, and when the patient reports sensation in an absent limb they too accuse him of not playing by the accepted rules. For somewhat different reasons, the patient's family and friends often react in much the same way. They are ready to discuss what they regard as the realistic aspects of the situation, and the phantom does not belong among these. The family may be full of sympathy about the loss of a leg but they resent what seems to them the loss of the mind. The former is a misfortune; the latter reflects on the family honor and possibly the genes.

Likewise, in the mid-1990s, Sherman (1994, 96) wrote about amputees' fears of broaching the subject of inexplicable pain in absent limbs with health care providers and others. Such an inquiry could render him or her unreliable and preclude thoughtful consideration of other legitimate concerns. In fact, being labeled "nuts" could seriously interfere with rehabilitation:

> We asked why they did not discuss their phantom pain with health care providers. Most very bluntly said that they were afraid that their providers would think they were crazy and would then ignore other problems involving . . . the residual limb and prosthetic fit. Their view that this would be the reaction was probably accurate because most patients who did report phantom pain to their physicians were either told that they had a psychological reaction, were "nuts," or were ignored. Many were sent for psychiatric evaluations.

The Prevalence of Phantom Pain

> After the surgery, my amputated legs and feet still hurt. . . . [I]t was another item on a long list of things that didn't seem fair. If I have no legs, why should I have to suffer them hurting me? (Goldman and Cagan 2001, 84)

Phantom pain is a particularly mystifying example of neuropathic pain, pain associated with disorders of the central and peripheral nervous system as opposed to being produced by some external physical cause. Most amputees who develop phantom pain are thought to do so within the first few days after amputation, although the onset can be delayed even for decades. Just as with nonpainful phantoms, pain is often most distinct in distal parts, the hands and feet, fingers and toes (Jensen and Nikolajsen 2000),[3] and is correlative with the maintenance of detail (Sherman, et al. 1997). And, just as painless phantoms vary in terms of experiential vibrancy, their painful counterparts have been varyingly described as mild and transient or ceaseless and "exquisite torture" (Ament, et al. 1964, 2907). The hallux or great toe might feel especially "fleshed out" and relentlessly inclined toward soreness, ache, and tenderness. The fingers might pile on top of one another or "crumble . . . together with a cramping pain" (Rosen, et al. 2001, 41). The following is a particularly macabre description of a burning phantom leg being slowly eaten away: "The burning in my phantom limb does not come like the burning that occurs when one comes [briefly] in contact with a live coal; rather, it eats away at my phantom like a corrosive chemical ravages flesh" (Williams and Deaton 1997, 75).

By the 1990s, ambiguity within the literature about phantom pain prevalence was pronounced a problem of the past (see for example Ribbers, Mulder, and Rijken 1989). And still, reported pain prevalence rates[4] continued to vary drastically. Prior to the 1960s—although phantom limb *sensation or awareness* was considered universal (or nearly so)—phantom *pain* was thought to be relatively rare, occurring in less than 1 percent of the amputee population (see for example Henderson and Smyth 1948; Simmel 1959). During the 1960s, reported pain prevalence rates were commonly between 5 and 15 percent (see for example Ament, et al. 1964), and in the 1970s, it was between 35 and 50 percent (see for example Melzack 1973). By the early 1980s, pain became a common sequela of the syndrome, and "phantom limb pain [became] one of the most terrible of all the pain phenomena" (Prasad and Das 1982,

Table 3.1. *Phantom Pain Prevalence: Reports of Phantom Pain Prevalence Rates*

Date	Prevalence	As Low As	As High As
1910–1919	Unknown	Unknown	Unknown
1920–1929	Unknown	Unknown	Unknown
1930–1939	Not Infrequent	Unknown	Unknown
1940–1949	1%	1%	30%
1950–1959	1%	1%	98%
1960–1969	5%–15%	1%	56%
1970–1979	35%–50%	2%	65%
1980–1989	50%–85%	2%	98%
1990–1999	70%–85%	1%	100%
2000–2009	50%–80%	0%	100%

30). Prevalence rates were typically between 50 and 85 percent during the 1980s (see for example Kessel and Worz 1987). This trend continued throughout the 1990s with reports regularly of 85 percent (see for example Jahangiri, et al. 1994) but as high as 97 percent (see for example Stannard 1993). Throughout the 2000s, the vast majority of reports were 80 percent or below (see for example Acerra, Souvlis, and Moseley 2007) with more than thirty reports of 50 percent or below, either as part of a range or alone, and reports were as low as 46.7 percent (see for example Sumitani, et al. 2010). In short, phantom pain became widespread by about 1980, an increase that was correlative with an intensifying culture of pain and the rise of pain medicine in the United States broadly speaking, and more expressly, with the adoption of the MPQ and a new language or vocabulary of pain that would remain unopposed for the next thirty-plus years (see for example Giummarra, et al. 2011).

The Language of Pain

Pain may be a nearly universal aspect of the human condition in that most of us have known transient physical discomfort or distress, as well as the intense suffering associated with excruciating or chronic pain. We know what pain is; it hurts. And, we have over the twentieth and twenty-first centuries developed increasingly "robust" biomedical knowledge about pain, including pain mechanisms, pathways, and centers; the characteristics and qualities of pain; individual and population predispositions and sensitivities; the etiology or cause of pain sensation; the quantification and nosology of pain; and the efficacy of pain interventions, therapeutics, and prophylaxes. We know a lot about pain.

Nevertheless, some scholars have argued that pain resists intersubjective understanding, that we can never really know pain other than our own. Pain is assertedly inaccessible to others because it is fundamentally private (Baszanger 1998a; Hilbert 1984). Being in pain is not obvious or even detectable to others, despite, in some cases, our sincere efforts to clarify, to give voice to, or to express pain. Pain, it is argued, is a primordial state, an antecedent of language. As a result, we lack a vocabulary of pain, a capacity for expression that is intelligible or apprehensible to others, even to those trained to understand it. Most notably, literary critic Elaine Scarry (1985, 4–5) argued,

> Physical pain does not simply resist language but actively destroys it, bringing about an immediate reversion to a state anterior to language, to the sounds and cries a human makes before language is learned. . . . Its resistance to language is not simply one of its incidental or accidental attributes but is essential to what it is . . . for physical pain—unlike any other state of consciousness—has no referential context. It is not of or for anything. It is precisely because it takes no object that it, more than any other phenomenon, resists objectification in language.

Others too have written about the "inarticulacy of pain" (Rivera-Fuentes and Birke 2001, 653), have argued that pain "shatters and resists ordinary language" (Hyden and Peolsson 2002, 326), have proposed that pain is "indescribable" (Mowat 2009), have suggested that pain is "notoriously subjective . . . [because] it is difficult to share" (Siebers 2010, 183), have argued that pain "puts language on trial" (Daniel 1994, 223; Mascia-Lees 2011), or have asserted that pain "resists the objectification of language" (Good 1994, 40; see also Vrancken 1989).

Rather than being private and unsharable, the perception, performance, meaning, and effects of pain are constituted in and through shared discourses; indeed, the intersubjectivity of pain is fundamental to it. Increasingly, the discourses available to people in pain have been those endemic to late-modern pain medicine. With the emergence and entrenchment of pain medicine over the last half of the twentieth century and into the twenty-first, pain has elaborated and, consequently, has been brought more and more into the realm of public discourse.

A number of arguments and observations have been put forward by scholars that could seemingly be harnessed to propose a contraction of the public discourse on pain, rather than an expansion. For example, scholars have argued that modern biomedicine has effectively silenced, discounted, or undermined competing accounts of pain, including pain as meaningful (Morris 1991) or suffering as transcendent (Glucklick 2001). Others have argued that pain has been conceptualized in *narrow* biologic or more specifically neurophysiologic terms (Bendelow 2006) or that patients'/sufferers' opinions, voices, and experiences have been delegitimized (Rey 1993). It is also tempting to argue that pain has been tempered by the discovery and pervasive use of analgesia, anesthesia, and other intervention and prevention technologies. However, this "repressive hypothesis" of pain, the assertion that modern biomedicine has effectively silenced, lessened, or quelled pain, is misleading (Foucault 1978). Pain is in fact everywhere, described by some scholars as epidemic (Morris 1991), and one should not discount the centrality of language for meaning creation, for situating pain within social contexts and social relations (Brodwin 1992; Morris 1998). To suggest that the experience of pain is personal, private, and unsharable is to invoke a conception of pain as it is typically constructed in biomedical practice; this is both uncritical and an illustration of the power and persuasiveness of the expansive biopolitical project on pain.

To be sure, pain sufferers do descriptive work, generating narratives about the origins of pain, the significance of pain, and, importantly, the possibilities for pain expression. And, they certainly try to "wrest control of medical discourse from medical science" (Kroll-Smith and Floyd 1997, 5) and sometimes succeed. I do not want to undervalue the role of sufferers in the work of constructing or more specifically doing pain (Baszanger 1989). Yet, these stories and practices necessarily engage with and invoke cultural resources, resources that in the contemporary context adopt or assimilate a medical vocabulary. We have invented linguistic structures, as Scarry (1985, 6) herself acknowledges, intended to bring "this most radically private of experiences . . . [into] the realm of public discourse." Describing, giving meaning to, and doing pain always involve a specific language and particular practices that delimit the possibilities for the public expression and personal experience of pain. It is precisely this language and these practices that give pain its share-ability. In the case of phantom limb pain, a specific vocabulary of pain quality emerged and became concretized in medical discourse, a vocabulary taken up by researchers, clinicians, and amputees alike, and the widespread adoption of that language effectively accentuated pain.

Dr. Ronald Melzack and the McGill Pain Questionnaire

> The extent to which medical research on the physical problem of pain is simultaneously bound up with the problem of language creation is best illustrated by what may at first appear to be *only a coincidence*: the person who discovered what is now considered the most compelling and potentially accurate theoretical model of the physiology of pain [gate control theory] is also the person who invented a diagnostic tool that enables patients to articulate the individual character of their pain with greater precision than was previously possible. (Scarry 1985, 7; emphasis added)

The impetus for the development of the MPQ was the inadequacy of the dominant medical vocabulary of the time, a vocabulary that captured only one facet of the experience of pain, namely, intensity (Melzack and Torgerson 1971; Scarry 1985). As Dr. Ronald Melzack (2005), famed Canadian psychologist and professor emeritus in the Department of Psychology at McGill University, retrospectively detailed in a 2005 article that revisited the author's now seminal 1975 piece published in *Anesthesiology*, the popular instrument for measuring pain at the time was the dolorimeter. The dolorimeter measured the intensity of a person's pain by focusing radiant heat on the skin in an effort to determine the pain sensation threshold (when the sensation "turned" to pain) and the pain tolerance threshold (how much pain a person would endure before pulling away). This, he recounts, seemed an exceptionally poor mechanism for capturing the multidimensionality of pain in part because the underlying assumption of such an instrument was that there is both "a specific, straight-through pain pathway from skin to a pain center in the brain . . . [and] . . . a one-to-one relation between the magnitude of an injury and the intensity of pain sensation" (Melzack 2005, 199; Melzack and Torgerson 1971).

In his 2005 published recollection of events, Melzack reported that he began collecting the most common pain descriptors used by his patients, such as "burning," "shooting," and "cramping." These terms were eventually organized along sensory, affective, and evaluative (sometimes referred to as cognitive) dimensions. This list of over one hundred words, generated by patients suffering from various conditions such as phantom limb or back pain, he narrated, was returned to again and again over the next few years. Elsewhere, however, Melzack (1975, 278) reported that these descriptors were "obtained from the clinical literature relating to pain," not distilled from his patients' descriptions, and in their original article, Melzack and his colleague Dr. Warren Torgersen reported having started with a list of forty-four words published by Dallenback (1939), to which they added additional descriptors from the clinical literature until the final list contained 102 terms. What I want to highlight is not the seemingly revisionist history that Melzack details some thirty years after his original publication, but rather what this particular story accomplishes. In the mid-1970s, when patients' narratives about pain were constructed as untrustworthy, deriving a set of terms not from the mouths of his own patients but rather from "data" systematically and rigorously accumulated over years of clinical investigation lent legitimacy to the MPQ. The more recent suggestion that the terms were patient-generated, collected over years through direct patient communication, justifies its continued use today. Further, when Melzack proposed that the descriptors tap into something genuine and fundamental about pain (for example, when he reported that the MPQ retains its efficacy when translated into different languages), the MPQ became an ideal tool for all times.

Melzack and Torgerson (1971) refined their list of descriptors, organized them into classes and subclasses, and published on the language of pain in 1971. Their paper attempted to delineate the major properties of the experience of pain and establish the relative degree of pain that was represented by each descriptor. As the authors reported, there was high unanimity on the intensity relationships between the descriptors; they write, "in the spatial subclass, 'shooting' was found to represent

Part 2.   What Does Your Pain Feel Like?

Some of the words below describe your present pain. Circle ONLY those words that best describe it. Leave out any category that is not suitable. Use only a single word in each appropriate category – the one that applies the best.

1	2	3	4
Flickering	Jumping	Pricking	Sharp
Quivering	Flashing	Boring	Cutting
Pulsing	Shooting	Drilling	Lacerating
Throbbing		Stabbing	
Beating		Lancinating	
Pounding			

5	6	7	8
Pinching	Tugging	Hot	Tingling
Pressing	Pulling	Boring	Itchy
Gnawing	Wrenching	Scalding	Smarting
Cramping		Searing	Stinging
Crushing			

9	10	11	12
Dull	Tender	Tiring	Sickening
Sore	Taut	Exhausting	Suffocating
Hurting	Rasping		
Arching	Splitting		
Heavy			

13	14	15	16
Fearful	Punishing	Wretched	Annoying
Frightful	Grueling	Blinding	Troublesome
Terrifying	Cruel		Miserable
	Vicious		Intense
	Killing		Unbearable

17	18	19	20
Spreading	Tight	Cool	Nagging
Radiating	Numb	Cold	Nauseating
Penetrating	Squeezing	Freezing	Agonizing
Piercing	Tearing		Dreadful
			Torturing

Figure 3.1. The MPQ. "What does your pain feel like?" constitutes part 2 of the McGill Pain Questionnaire. (Reproduced from Melzack, Ronald. 1975. "The McGill Pain Questionnaire: Major properties and scoring methods." *Pain* 1:277–99, with permission from the author.)

more pain than 'flashing,' which in turn implied more pain than 'jump-ing'" (Melzack and Torgerson 1971, 278). Not insignificantly, these inten-sity relationships were established by doctors and students as well as by patients. Consequently, how much pain each term denoted relative to the others reflected what "people knew about pain" rather than (exclu-sively) what people in pain reported.

In 1975, Melzack published the now landmark article "The McGill Pain Questionnaire," which reported on five years of clinic applica-tion of the MPQ. The short form was created in 1987 by narrowing the descriptors to include those most commonly selected from the sensory and affective categories, and by adding an intensity dimension to each descriptor (Melzack 1987). Both the MPQ and the short form are prop-erly administered by reading a list of descriptors out loud to patients who then indicate whether or not the words accurately characterize their pain. In his landmark article, Melzack (1975, 283) concluded, "Patients are grateful to be provided with words to describe their pain; these kinds of words are used infrequently, and the word lists save the patients from having to grope for words to communicate with the physician." As Mel-zack acknowledged here, these words were both "gratefully" provided to patients and were words that were infrequently used; they were not what might be generated spontaneously by patients themselves, at least not in the clinical context. Almost contradictorily, he then goes on to argue that these same terms were those that patients use readily in their everyday lives. He wrote, "Furthermore, patients are pleased to see (or hear) words which they use to describe their pain to family and friends but which they would not tell the physician because he may consider them psychologically unsound; the administrator thus often senses the patients' relief at seeing such words in a list, implying that they are acceptable and sound descriptors" (Melzack 1975, 283).

Aside from the unanswered methodological question of how a physi-cian might know the very words that he or she does not have access to, what is of significance here is that these descriptors were constructed as "acceptable" and "sound" on the basis of the administrator's sense of the patients' relief. It is not that one should warily accept that patients were or are genuinely relieved to establish a shared understanding of their pain experience, but rather that the administrator qua instrument is tapping into something authentic, something "out there," something static, when in fact it is more accurate to say that the MPQ functions to construct the qualitative dimension of a language of pain.

The MPQ and the Quality of Phantom Limb Pain

The MPQ established a set of descriptors ostensibly to give people a shared language to express the inexplicable, and to pin down pain for diagnostic purposes, to constitute a "workable object" through the development of a documentation and assessment tool (Whelan 2003, 464). The instrument was certainly intended to give voice to pain (Glucklick 2001; Scarry 1985), but it was also crafted to generate correlations between descriptors and specific disease processes (Glucklick 2001; Melzack 1987), to "discriminate among different pain problems" (Melzack 1987), to suggest treatment modalities tailored to pain types (Scarry 1985), and to legitimate a more multifarious and complex understanding of pain mechanisms (Melzack 2005). The advent of the MPQ was a pivotal moment in the elaboration of phantom pain as well as the maturation of pain medicine. The design and implementation of the instrument was one of the many means through which pain was institutionalized in the United States around 1975 (Baszanger 1992). The development of typologies, tools, techniques, procedures, and practices was core to the legitimation of the nascent field of pain medicine and requisite to its structural organization. As Baszanger (1998a, 34) argued, "Working on pain implies knowing how to recognize it, how to interpret its diversity. It requires classification . . . [which] plays an essential role in creating a community of practice and can become a common basis for physicians to communicate among themselves and with others."

By the late 1980s, the MPQ was one of the most widely used instruments in the United States for measuring pain of all types (Melzack 1987). With the advent of the MPQ, a language of pain materialized, one that could easily be used to capture the qualitative dimensions of phantom limb pain. And, it was. More noteworthy, however, was the rapid and widespread dissemination of that terminology within the medical literature on phantom limb broadly speaking. After 1975, after the publication of Melzack's landmark article, the terminology used in the literature to describe phantom quality was overwhelmingly consonant with the set of descriptors advanced by the MPQ. Even those studies that did not include the MPQ as an element of the study design began to commonly make use of its terminology, whether the description was provided by the researcher, the health care practitioner, or the amputee. The construction of phantom sensation as "knifing," "smarting," "wretched," "lancinating," "lacerating," or "dreadful," for instance, was (and still is) more an artifact of the language advanced by the instrument used to measure phantoms than it was an "accurate accounting" of the quality of those sensations. In effect, phantoms became "vicious," "rasping," "quivering," and "gnawing."

It is important to also historicize the exceptions, the accounts of phantom quality that did *not* employ terminology homologous with the MPQ. The wrinkled, raw, swollen, glowing, dry, and furry qualities of phantoms, for instance, were largely documented prior to 1975, prior to the institutionalization of the MPQ. Using linguistic creativity seldom found in contemporary descriptions, amputees also often gave detailed and frequently macabre descriptions of their phantom pain, including "as though someone were kicking it [the ankle] while he walked" (Morgenstern 1964, 62); "the sensation of his great toenail being twisted off" (Russell 1949, 1025); "[as if] blood [was] swelling between his toes" (Russell 1949, 1026); "as though her right hand were touching hundreds of sharp-pointed pins" (Stone 1950, 746); "as if there were a knife stuck in it and always being turned round" (In Der Beeck 1953, 225); "as if a sharp scalpel were being repeatedly driven into the flesh" (Livingston 1938, 356); "as if there were a wire down the center of his arm . . . [and] some force were pulling on the wire as if to pull the fingers up through the arm" (Livingston 1938, 357); "as if the leg were being squeezed in a pair of pincers, or were lying under a weight" (In Der Beeck 1953, 225); "[as if] ants [were] creeping in his toes" (Beller and Peyser 1951, 433); "as if the flesh

Table 3.2. Phantom Quality: Descriptors Used to Express the Quality of Phantom Sensations Prior to 1975, Those Not Included in the MPQ

Descriptor	Author and Date	Descriptor	Author and Date
Bursting	Cohen et al. 1942	Lightening	Appenzeller et al. 1969
Darting	Parks 1973	Raw	Livingston 1938 Henderson et al. 1948 Stone 1950 Nashold et al. 1969
Empty	Jarvis 1967	Slimy	Henderson et al. 1948
Flashing	Stone 1950	Squirming	Falconer 1953
Floating	Simmel 1956 Melzack et al. 1973	Swollen	Livingston 1938 Cohen et al. 1942 Bors 1951 Bressler et al. 1956 Simmel 1956 Buxton 1957 Weinstein et al. 1970
Furry	In Der Beeck 1953	Tense/Tensing	Harber 1956
Gripping	Harber 1956 Harber 1958	Trembling	Livingston 1938
Hard	Weinstein et al. 1970	Vibrating	Bors 1951 Harber 1956 Pollock et al. 1957 Harber 1958
Kicking	Russell 1949	Wrinkled	Weinstein 1961

References in the medical, psychiatric, and psychological literature to the quality of phantom sensations not found in the McGill Pain Questionnaire (MPQ) by descriptor, year, and author.

were being torn from around the nails" (Livingston 1938, 362); and "as if it had been scratched and skinned from the elbow to the wrist" (Livingston 1938, 358). In fact, for Miles's (1956, 1027) patient, the intensity of the pain was equated to pure hell: "The patient produced . . . a drawing in 'three dimensions' which he had traced from his phantom. He had 'little devils' in his foot who 'hurt him there.' Asked where the devils came from he replied: "From Hell where the rest of the leg probably is."

Most of these richly detailed descriptions are found in the pre-MPQ medical literature.[5] Thus, the role of the MPQ was to standardize and reify a specific language of phantom pain quality, curtailing the kind of linguistic creativity indicative of past descriptions. When asked about the terminology used by amputees, Melzack suggested that the language of phantom pain was very different from that of other pain conditions. He stated, "One of my students did a study on the patterns of words chosen by people with different kinds of pain. Phantom pain was one of those unique pains with a different distribution than other pain conditions" (Melzack 2006). Interestingly, Melzack acknowledged that amputees use a distinctive language to describe their pain, but he attributed this difference to the nature of the pain itself rather than the linguistic structure provided by the MPQ.

In 1989, Dr. Richard Sherman (1989) unabashedly borrowed from the language and organizational structure of the MPQ to advance a tripartite theory of phantom etiology. His argument that there are three categories or classes of phantoms—burning, cramping, and lancinating, each with a unique etiology—did much to naturalize and reify Melzack's terminology. It was not that the terminology advanced by the MPQ was hugely novel. In fact, the MPQ effectively coopted and translated nontechnical vocabulary into that which was subsumed by the discipline. Cooptation is certainly not unique to the case of phantom limb pain; pain medicine has appropriated numerous vernaculars, techniques, practices, and technologies, turning them easily into the stuff of the profession (Kugelmann 1997). Moreover, the complementarity of the MPQ and the new typology of phantoms represented the kind of cross-validation indicative of biomedical knowledge.

Sherman's typology, however, did not go uncontested. For example, Dr. Joel Katz, professor in the Department of Psychology and School of Kinesiology and Health Science at York University, professor of anesthesia at the University of Toronto, and director of the Acute Pain Research Unit, Department of Anesthesia and Pain Management, at the Toronto General Hospital and at Mount Sinai Hospital in Toronto, Canada, was an outspoken opponent of Sherman's typology, suggesting that it "may be

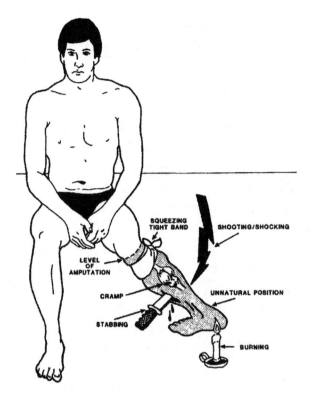

SQUEEZING
TIGHT BAND

SHOOTING/SHOCKING

LEVEL
OF
AMPUTATION

CRAMP

UNNATURAL POSITION

STABBING

BURNING

Figure 3.2. Sherman's Typology. This illustration is a composite of phantom pain sensations highlighting the three symptom classes associated with Dr. Richard Sherman's phantom typology: burning, shooting, and lancinating or stabbing. (Reprinted from Sherman, Richard. 1989. "Stump and phantom limb pain." *Neurologic Clinics* 7:249–64, with permission from Elsevier.)

a misleading step in the search for specific mechanisms underlying post-amputation sensory phenomena" (Hunter, Katz, and Davis 2005, 308).

The classificatory logic engendered by the MPQ was not somehow remiss, inadequate, or erroneous; it did classify phantoms. Still, I want to point out the other ways in which it was "productive." The division of the phantom pain into burning, cramping, and lancinating classes gave way to a set of practices, techniques, and relations that were a logical extension of understanding phantoms in this way. For example, Sherman's typology suggested appropriate treatment approaches for each phantom class, and he argued that the overwhelming inefficacy of the some sixty-eight available treatment modalities employed in 1980 (Sherman, Sherman, and Gall 1980) was the result of not acknowledging separate classes of phantoms (Sherman 1989).

Perhaps more significantly, the utilization of a pain questionnaire to assess phantom limb—justified as an effort to capture what was understood to be an underestimated facet of phantom quality—accentuated pain and consequently, painful phantoms proliferated. One can see how weighty this was for theorizing phantoms when the painless phantom is juxtaposed to its painful counterpart. As painful phantoms proliferated, painless phantoms were entirely reconceptualized. For example, the tingling, prickling sensation—interpreted in the past as pleasant or pleasing—was reinterpreted as a "pre-pain" sensation (Knecht, et al. 1996). As a result, pleasant phantoms became increasingly scarce and a painful-painless continuum emerged along which all phantoms could be plotted. By contrast, early literature characterized phantom limb and phantom pain as distinct phenomena that differed markedly in terms of their features and etiology. For example, Brown (1968, 304) argued that "phantom pain has its own language—a language different from that reported for the non-painful phantom." By about 1980, however, the two were considered expressions of the same phenomenon only with differences in intensity. For instance, Carlen and colleagues (1978, 215) suggested, "It would be wrong to consider the patients during this acute phase as falling into two classes, those with and without pain. Painful complaints were all amplifications of disorders apparent in the noncomplainers." Likewise, Czerniecki described how sensation may intensify, lapsing into pain:

> For some [amputees] the [phantom] sensation may be non-painful. These sensations do not create an avoidance response at low levels, low frequencies, or for shorter durations. But if they persist, the patient interprets them as nociceptive; you end up with a transition from sensation to pain. I think there are also factors—the patient's state of mind, their level of anxiety, their level of distress—that change the way they interpret that sensory phenomenon. It can actually shift between a painful and a non-painful sensory phenomenon. (Czerniecki 2005)

Moreover, contemporary pain medicine has, through instruments like the MPQ and classificatory schemes like Sherman's typology, defined the pained body by means of technologies and techniques intended to visualize, measure, and understand pain, effectively constituting the pained subject. Pain medicine has been pivotal to the embodied self-experiencing as well as the public expression of pain. And, as patient-oriented approaches have become increasingly integral to clinical practice, new forms of pained subjectivity have emerged in tandem with novel approaches to enrolling "patients" in engaging with medicocentric behaviors, practices, beliefs, values, and linguistic structures. Through the instantiation of the pain clinic, the institutionalization of clinical management, the advent and widespread use of a new vocabulary of pain, the pained subject has been brought under the all-seeing biomedical gaze.

Treating Phantom Limb Pain

Until the late 1950s, amputees who lamented their loss and complained of phantom sensations, particularly those who reproached clinicians about their inability to treat intractable pain or amend irregular posture, were regularly regarded as poorly adjusted and psychically compromised, whether the underlying issue was psychosis or neurosis. An organic basis to phantom pain was typically excluded outright in favor of a deficit in mental or emotional well-being. For example, Beller and Peyser (1951, 432) wrote, "PLP is usually not an organic pain, conducted through the spinothalamic tract that bothers the patient; rather, his personality, his emotional tension and his psychic attitude toward his physical incapacity are the bases for the development of a painful phantom."

Still, pain and psychosis were not the only issues warranting aggressive and prompt treatment. Without intervention grave consequences could result. In fact, the "signs of psychopathology," including "personality change, anxiety, emotional instability [and] battle dreams" encouraged alcoholism, which was thought to occur "in a surprising percentage of these men" (Randall, Ewalt, and Blair 1945, 652). Hoffman (1954b, 265) wrote, "In a 'normal' individual a 'phantom grip' on the world can be relinquished to be compensated for by some other defense mechanism. If, however, this cannot be done, severe pain sets in and this, plus bizarre-positioned phantoms, indicates severe psychopathology. This may result in a severe obsessional neurosis, drug addiction, and/or suicide." Immediate treatment was necessary not only because dismemberment disposed an amputee to drug addiction or because an amputee could be driven to suicide by the pain of a disturbed mind but because without intervention, others too could be victimized by the amputee's physical, emotional, and mental deterioration and unfortunately, madness could begin to manifest almost immediately, leaving caregivers and others quite vulnerable to bizarre, exhibitionistic, and unmanageable pathology.

> The patient underwent a below-the-knee amputation under spinal anes-
> thesia. His surgical recovery was uneventful. Within a few hours after
> the surgery, however, his behavior became bizarre and unmanageable;
> he became exhibitionistic, displaying his stump, and exposing himself
> immodestly. He tended to make a great display of his physique, and had
> to be restrained from performing gymnastics in the bed. He spent many
> hours during the night in the latrine in open masturbatory activity or
> posing nude before the mirror. His conversation began to have a great
> deal of sexual content, and he scandalized visitors with obscene stories.
> (Miles 1956, 1027)

If phantom limb was symptomatic of psychosis or neurosis brought on by surgical or traumatic amputation, then a "natural" course of treatment would entail addressing the underlying psychological issue(s). Accordingly, early rehabilitative efforts included psychotherapy, electroshock therapy, and prefrontal lobotomy. Egas Moniz first performed lobotomy in 1935, an intervention that was subsequently adapted for use in the case of phantom limb and phantom pain around 1945 (Beller and Peyser 1951). During the 1940s, after the icepick technique was adopted, some fifty thousand "cost-efficient" operations were performed in the United States and elsewhere (Sargent 2005, 267). Kolb (1950a) identified one case in which a prefrontal lobotomy was requested by the patient after months of unresolved phantom pain. The procedure was performed despite the fact that there was recognition, even at the time, of significant limitations and the inherent risks of the procedure, testifying to the degree of anxiety that phantom limb pain provoked within the medical community. Gutierrez-Mahoney (1944, 447) argued that "unfortunately even this procedure does not truly abolish pain" and may even result in severe personality disorder because of the extensive damage caused to the frontal lobe. One lobotomy patient was described as wetting himself with utter disregard:

> He was apathetic and relatively indifferent to his surroundings. . . . He showed a moderate defect in his fund of general information. He was occasionally disoriented as to time and place and did not remember immediately past events. . . . His wife remarked at length on his emotional lability, his casual indifference to everything but the stimulus at the moment, his new and strange lack of worry about himself and the future of the family. . . . On one occasion while waiting for a bus she noticed that he was unconcernedly urinating. When she remonstrated against his inappropriate behavior he answered with the rhetorical question, "Whose pants are getting wet?" (Pisetsky 1946, 471)

Between 1945 and 1950, psychotherapy, electroshock therapy, and prefrontal lobotomy were the only treatments published in the American medical literature with the exception of neuroma injection, excision, or percussion and nerve block or anesthesia. Lobotomy continued to be advocated until 1953, electroshock until 1968, and psychotherapy (as a sole or joint therapy for phantom sensation and pain) until the mid-1980s. By the mid-1950s, surgical interventions like cordotomy and sympathectomy and pharmacological interventions were introduced as therapeutic options for addressing the onset, persistence, or intensification of phantom limb pain.

Surgical and pharmacological approaches to assuaging phantom pain were inspired by the predominance of specificity theory, which researchers and clinicians embraced until the introduction of gate-control theory advanced by Melzack and Wall (1965) in the mid-1960s (Baszanger 1998a, 1998b). Specificity theory assumed that pain travels along an ascending pathway from the skin to the pain center in the brain; pain is "felt" and then is responded to. Key to specificity theory were two inter-related assumptions: an external stimulus excites specific specialized receptors in the skin; and the extent of pain corresponds to the degree of injury (Melzack, et al. 2001).[6] The introduction of gate-control theory was a move from the periphery to the center in terms of causal explanation (Melzack 1993). Melzack (1976, 138) theorized that

> a gate-like mechanism exists in the somatic transmission system so that pain signals can be modulated before they evoke perception and response. The gate can be opened or closed by variable amounts, depending on factors such as the relative activity in large and small peripheral fibers, and various psychological processes such as attention and prior experiences. By proposing a variable gate, it became possible to attempt to close the gate by various manipulations.

Gate control offered a new heuristic for pain, one that stressed the modulation of pain perception within the nervous system as opposed to pathway disruption, stressed by specificity theory (Baszanger 1998b). Cutting nerves or ablating areas of the cortex, for example, began to be used alongside modulation in the form of transcutaneous electrical stimulation (TENS), hypnosis, relaxation, biofeedback, acupuncture, and numerous pharmaceuticals such as antidepressants. These newly emerging treatment options, however, did not replace earlier approaches. In fact, a review of the literature on phantom pain treatment demonstrates clearly the instantiation of what Baszenger (1992, 182) referred to as the poles of *curing through techniques* and *healing through adaptation*. She argued that the treatment of chronic pain became organized around these two distinct impulses. Practitioners who embraced the approach of curing through techniques sought to cure pain through bio-physical interventions, including drugs and surgery. Conversely, those employing the healing-through-adaptation approach sought to control pain through behavioral interventions that were more global in scope. In the case of phantom pain, treatment options continued to include both approaches even after the turn of the twenty-first century. In fact, some interventions persisted long after there was sufficient evidence to suggest that they were actually exacerbating the problem. For instance, although revision or reamputation of a stump had long been thought to be ineffective (see for example Kolb 1950a), with the potential to effectively multiply the number of phantoms an amputee experienced—what Ramachandran (1998, 33) called "an endless regression problem"—the treatment continued to be either practiced or identified as a potential intervention in cases of pain even into the 1980s (see for example Berger 1980).[7] Jackson (2002, 73) wrote a decade later, "Some doctors have tried to treat phantom pain by . . . doing an additional amputation. Occasionally this helps, but each new amputation can also breed a new phantom, raising the specter of a hall-of-mirrors effect and an infinite number of phantoms-within-phantoms."

Virtually mirroring the trend in increased pain reporting is the pattern of references to treatment options; as the pain prevalence rate increased dramatically, so too did the number of interventions advanced by a burgeoning service industry devoted to and dependent on the commodification of pain. As Kugelmann (1997, 45) noted, "The pain clinic, an institution unique to the second half of the twentieth century, [is] a growth industry, and the place for the professional exploitation of chronic pain." And today, in what Rose (2007) referred to as the new bioeconomy, there is an unending search for biocapital, for that which leads to profitability through health, wellness, cure, hope, treatment, prevention, and others. Pain has become a core biopolitical project of immense consequence for all of us, and its exploitation is part and parcel of a bioeconomic order that continues to reshape the body, life, and living in the name of profit. Rose (2007, 5) wrote of the fundamental intertwining of biopolitics and the new bioeconomy, "Vitality is decomposed into a series of distinct objects—that can be isolated, delimited, stored, accumulated, mobilized, and exchanged, accorded a discrete value, traded across time, space, species, contests, enterprises—in the service of many distinct objectives. In the process, a novel geopolitical field has taken shape, and biopolitics has become inextricably intertwined with bioeconomics."

In the case of phantom pain, by 1980 sixty-eight different treatments were employed by VA hospitals, medical schools, pain clinics, and pain specialists (Sherman, Sherman, and Gall 1980), all of which were reported by clinicians to be at least somewhat successful (Sherman 1994). By 1992, the number had reached eighty-six (Katz 1992b). The majority of these were found to be only temporarily effective in reducing pain in a minority of cases (see for example Sherman 1997) or no more effective than placebo (Sherman, Sherman, and Gall 1980).[8] Sherman, Sherman, and Parker (1984, 93–94; emphasis added) found "the success rate for treatment was dismal. . . . Our survey of physicians treating phantom pain showed that most of them thought their treatments were effective when in fact they were absolutely useless. . . . When the published facts are wrong, ineffective treatments can become *popularized and perpetuated indefinitely.*" The authors reported that only 2 percent of amputees reported any significant benefit from any treatment (Sherman, et al. 1988). Later, Katz (1992b) reported that only 7 percent of phantom pain sufferers received any long-term pain reduction from any of the then available treatment options. And, Mortimer (2002) and his colleagues found that amputees were frequently told that absolutely nothing could be done to help their phantom pain.

Pain Memories and the Decline in Pain

Throughout the 2000s, the phantom pain prevalence rate was typically reported to be between 50 percent and 80 percent (see for example Casale, et al. 2009), a significant decrease from the peak of phantom pain during the 1980s and 1990s. What is particularly notable about this trend is that this substantial decline occurred *despite* the inefficacy of more than eighty-six separate treatment modalities used to treat the often debilitating phantom pain following amputation. How, then, can this trend be accounted for? The abatement of pain was not an effect of successful treatment but rather had its roots in the "discovery" of pain memories. Pain memories had been documented since the late 1800s when Mitchell (1871, 568) wrote,

> The bent posture of the lost arm is frequently that which it had for a few hours or days before its removal. There are some cases of hands which have been crushed or burned, and the fingers remained painfully rigid in life or bound on a splint. Just so for ever [sic] do they continue when the injured limb has been cut off. . . . The latest and most overpowering sensation is thus for all time engraved upon the brain, so that no future shall ever serve to efface it.

References to the persistence of unusual posture, paralysis, or an identifiable pain can be found in the literature throughout the twentieth and twenty-first centuries. A broken arm that necessitated amputation might be sensed in its phantom-ed state as fractured in precisely the same manner, twisted with a bone protruding, for example. The experience of paralysis in a limb frequently persisted so that it was felt as perpetually frozen in the position it occupied prior to amputation. Most commonly, the pain experienced weeks, days, or hours before the amputation, such as the pain of an ulcer, swelling, or gangrene, endured indefinitely. In Der Beeck (1953, 225) relayed the case of pain that continued "exactly as before":

> The amputation of the right lower leg was carried out on 28th September, 1942. Before the amputation there were great pains in the ankle-joint and on the outside of the upper part of the foot. These pains continued after the amputation exactly as before. In my right ankle I have a continual fiercing [sic] feeling, as if there were a knife stuck in it and always being turned round. In this spot I had in 1941 a perforating wound from an infantry gun shell.

And more recently, Giummarrra (2011, 694) and her colleagues wrote of the phenomenon, "One amputee, who lost her leg in a motorcycle accident, described the memory of the pressure of a motorcycle foot-peg under the arch of her foot, and reports that her phantom only feels 'normal' now when she sits on her motorcycle." Phantom pain also emulated the pain of an injury that occurred prior to the amputation, perhaps years before, as well as pain completely unassociated with the amputation itself (Ramachandran 1998; Ramachandran and Hirstein 1998). Long lost reminiscences of a wound, an injury, or pain that transpired many years before the amputation continued to be felt after the limb was removed, such as a sliver under the nail, a bunion, a corn, a blister, an ingrown toenail, carpal tunnel, a gash, or a cut. Henderson and Smyth (1948, 101) elaborated on the qualities indicative of what would later be termed "pain memories":

> The sensation may be divided into three groups, depending on the relationship of the parent sensation to the time of wounding: (1) the revivification of a sensation experienced in the limb before wounding, sometimes even several years previously and apparently forgotten, for example, the discomfort of an in growing toe-nail or a corn, compression of the toes in a tight boot, the impression of a split finger nail, a painful whitlow . . . ; (2) the wound itself; (3) the persistence of a sensation experienced between the times of wounding and amputation, a period often of several weeks['] or months['] duration, for example, the pain of suppurative arthritis, the sensation of a traction pin, pain in relation to pressure points and splints, the sensation of lice crawling under plaster.

Although examples of the revivification of preamputation pain can be found as far back as the late 1800s, it was Katz and Melzack (1990) who coined the term "somatosensory pain memories" in 1990, inspiring a spate of articles on the subject. What distinguishes their article from earlier references to the phenomenon is the authors' explicit proposal that the vast majority of amputees, possibly as many as 79 percent (Katz 1992b; Melzack, et al. 2001), reexperience the quality, location, and/or intensity of pain that occurred in the intact limb prior to amputation. In their seminal paper on pain memories, Katz and Melzack (1990, 332) wrote,

The development and expression of somatosensory memories are intimately tied to the experience of pain. . . .When pain is experienced in
a limb at or near the time of amputation there is a high probability that
it will persist into the phantom limb and continue to cause the patient
distress and suffering. . . .There is [also] a trend for severe pains . . . to be
represented with a greater frequency than mild pains.

More than two decades later, Giummarra (2011, 692) and her colleagues reported the prevalence rate of the "imprinting of past experiences" as up to 79 percent in amputees, especially for those who regain
consciousness during surgery. The "discovery" that pain memories
occurred in the vast majority of amputees corresponded with the peak
of phantom pain, the period from the early 1980s through the 1990s.
As phantom pain became epidemic, pain memories surfaced as a way
of explaining the dramatic rise in pain prevalence. Because preoperative pain was thought to be etched in memory as distortion, paralysis, or pain was endured in the hours, days, or weeks before surgery,
phantom pain would necessarily be pervasive. Still, pain memories also
explained the dramatic decline in the pain prevalence rate around 2000.
Katz and Melzack's (1990, 332) paper pointed to an obvious conclusion:
if clinicians could secure a pain-free interval prior to surgery through
what was termed "preemptive analgesia," phantom pain that mimicked
preoperative pain could be circumvented (see for example Fisher and
Meller 1991). Some researchers and clinicians argued that establishing a
pain-free interval prior to (see for example Katz 1992b), during (see for
example Jahangiri, et al. 1994), and/or after (see for example Weiss and
Lindell 1996) surgery prevented the onset of phantom pain altogether or
at least reduced its severity. The decline in phantom pain prevalence was
partly attributed to the success of preemptive analgesia; researchers and
clinicians expected a lower prevalence rate, and this was precisely what
they began to document at the end of the twentieth century.

However, the efficacy of preemptive analgesia was fiercely debated
during the late 1990s, and by the mid-2000s, the practice was admon-
ished as fruitless and futile (see for example Hayes, Armstrong-Brown,

and Burstal 2004), and pain memories themselves were criticized as far-
fetched. For example, Czerniecki argued that there was no relationship
between preoperative and phantom pain. Indeed, it was pure "dictum":

> For years, people thought there was a relationship between the phan-
> tom pain experience and the pain experienced prior to amputation. It
> was an accepted fact, a dictum that people believed for decades, that a
> memory of pain you had beforehand would sit in your brain somewhere.
> But under objective scrutiny and study, there is actually no relationship
> between the two. (Czerniecki 2005)

Nevertheless, the debate raged on into the second decade of the twenty-
first century despite the fact that McQuay (1998, 595) and colleagues
bluntly argued years earlier that researchers needed to abandon experimentation and admit "when the dodo is extinct."[9]

Researchers and clinicians have always been interested in phantom
limb pain in part because it seemed to communicate something pathological not just about the dismembered body but also about the broken
spirit or the shattered mind. There seemed to be a psychical and moral
as well as a physical dimension to inexplicable pain that haunted some
men and not others, especially fantastical pain—the hand ripped "to
pieces" after a grenade explosion or the bruised and rigid finger crooked
on the trigger of a gun that had cruelly backfired without warning—the
kind of pain that was difficult to imagine, much less trust. Thus, even
when it was considered extraordinarily rare, realized for only a very few
amputees, it was still a predominant theme in the literature. The number
of articles published on phantom pain has always far outnumbered those
attending to phantom sensation or awareness.

Still, interest or even preoccupation within the literature has also
been a consequent of the incredible variability that has characterized
the pain prevalence rate over the twentieth century and into the twenty-
first. Researchers, practitioners, and scholars were pressed to account for
the rise and fall in phantom pain prevalence. Was the erraticism indicative of reports attributable to poor science or unreliable subjects, to the

introduction of a vocabulary intended to capture and examine the qualitative dimensions of phantoms, to a sociocultural milieu within which pain became a serious fascination and problem, to the biomedical commodification of phantom distortion, or to the increased soundness or validity of truly fantastical pain? Indeed, it was. And thus, one might be compelled to ask, "Is it real?" If pain—its severity, frequency, duration, intensity, quality, share-ability, meaning, and the like—materializes with respect to shifts in language, knowledges, practices, techniques, technologies, and institutional arrangements, is it categorically real?

Amputees who reported that their phantoms felt "real good" were not uniformly crazy or lying for fear of reproach by family, friends, and clinicians, and neither were amputees who expressed the agony of the most unrelenting and exquisite torture they could imagine or describe. Instead, the rise and fall in phantom pain prevalence is a classic example of what Hacking (1995, 21) referred to as "the looping effect of human kinds"; he argued, "People classified in a certain way tend to conform to or grow into the ways that they are described; but they also evolve in their own ways, so that the classifications and descriptions have to be constantly revised." In other words, there is a dynamic and co-constitutive relationship between what is known about pain—particularly the ideas that are produced by those in positions of legitimate authority—and how pain is enacted, shared, and embodied. The tendency for the "nature of pain" to evolve both in the public discourse and in the interpersonal narratives of sufferers is a reflection of its sociality. The authenticity, the realness of phantom pain—like other types of pain—is evidenced by "its place in people's lives, by their experiences and convictions, and by the personal and collective investments that have been made in it" (Young 1995, 5).

Historicizing Phantom Pain and the Role of Etiology

Historicizing phantom pain reveals how ethereal appendages have been subject to the institutionalization of pain medicine and the clinical management of pain symptomatology. It exposes the ways in which

phantoms have accordingly been rationalized, categorized, and catalogued. Moreover, it explains the elaboration of pain and the increase
in pain reporting within the medical literature. In fact, given the historical context, the epidemic of pain is easily explicable. What remains
unanswered, then, is not the rise in the pain prevalence rate during the
1980s and 1990s, but rather the decline in reports of phantom pain after
the turn of the twenty-first century. If none of the myriad interventions
employed by clinicians was proven to be a panacea for phantom pain
and if attempts at prevention such as preemptive analgesia were ineffective (equally as fruitful for researchers and others as the illusive dodo),
then how can such a decline be explained?

It is the etiology, the cause, the origin of phantom limb syndrome
that has (1) shaped "knowledge" about the nature of and the relationship between pleasurable, natural phantoms and their painful counterparts; (2) inspired assumptions about the onset, quality, and progression
of phantom pain; and (3) motivated both treatment and intervention
efforts. As pain became a "management" issue of vital import, it was
imperative that those in charge of pain not only effectively measured
(codified and objectified) pain, but that they could say with authority
and conviction where it came from. Only then could phantoms and
amputated bodies be managed well. Only then could the seemingly
bizarre and often otherworldly acts of the "fractioned" body be understood and even appreciated.

4

Phantoms in the Mind

The Psychogenic Origins of Ethereal Appendages

A survey of the major psychogenic theories of phantom limb exposes the palpable uneasiness and even fear that the "fractioned" body and haunted limbs have historically evoked. There is a "profound disquiet stirred in the human soul by bodies that stray from what is typical and predictable" (Thomson 1996, 1). At times, phantoms have made amputees and their families, friends, and communities, as well as clinicians, researchers, and policymakers, uneasy in part because they represented an unsettling alienation from the body while also being profound reminders of the work that embodiment entails. Whether in the form of faithful representations or vehement distortions, phantoms have alienated through emasculation, misbehavior, fraudulence, and lunacy, among others. And still, phantoms have thwarted forgetting. They have been overt reminders that bodies are "accomplished" through attempts to suppress, to make submissive, to harness, and to arouse. At other times, phantoms have incited antipathy and even dread because of the individual and collective guilt that amputation can impart, because of the depths of the anticipated and sometimes realized losses that dismemberment can cause, and perhaps most significantly, because of the utter foreignness that can be exacted from embodied partiality. Without question, there is nothing "natural" about how lived dismemberment is accomplished, about what it does to bodies and how it is done.

Bodies haunted by lost appendages have materialized—have become material and come to matter—through the work of amputees, prosthetists, medical practitioners, researchers, pain clinicians, psychologists, and others, many of whom have had weighty biopolitical agendas. For example, phantoms and amputees have been productively enlisted in the work of re-visioning the field, establishing scientific legitimacy, and determining who can and should be the rightful authors of the phantom origin story. Embodied ghosts have time and again been employed either as proof of prevailing theory or as evidence that theorizing was fundamentally unsound and, consequently, have acted as arbiters in litigious disciplinary turf wars.

Embodied ghosts had long been the province of psychiatry and psychology—they were all in the mind—but they have always been fickle copies, and as such, they have in the contemporary context become the province of (bio)medicine or, more specifically, neuroscience. This shift from the psychologization to the (bio)medicalization of phantom limb syndrome gave rise to a strange politics of susceptibility and contagion, and consequently, phantoms lost much of their "mysteriousness." The emphasis on or attenuation of particular aspects of phantom phenomena engendered by the debates over who was at risk and how amputees might "catch" the syndrome also caused phantoms to proliferate in kind and to spread to vulnerable populations. Likewise, the question of how phantoms should manifest— how "wild" or "domesticated" they should be—and precisely what they could do caused the once exceedingly private and exceptionally uncanny to become intensely public, of-the-social-body, and undeniably "real."

A Ghost Story

In 1551, Ambrose Paré (1509–1590),[1] the exalted French barber and surgeon, made what is regarded as the first reference to phantom limb. He noted a most curious complaint of his patients: continued and often persistent sensation of limbs and digits after surgical removal. He wrote, "Verily it is a thing wondrous strange and prodigious, and which will scarce be credited, unless by such as have seene with their eyes, and heard with their ears the Patient who have many moneths after the cutting away of the legge, grievously complained that they yet felt exceeding great paine of that Leg so cut off" (Paré 1649, 773). Following Paré's reference, the phantom disappeared from the medical literature for the next 320 years until it was resurrected by famed American surgeon Silas

Weir Mitchell (1829–1914) in the late 1800s (Herman 1998).[2] Reports within the medical literature in the interim years were said either to be omitted by practitioners or to be the secrets of amputees because to have made such a claim "would [have been] tantamount to losing one's reason and/or admitting that the devil or some other supernatural forces had gained entrance into the body. This would, because of the status of medicine and society in general prior to the 19th century, leave one's self wide open to all kinds of punishments" (Hoffman 1954b, 261).

Mitchell, the "neurologist extraordinaire," is considered one of the fathers of American neurology (Nathanson 1988, 504). He is credited with coining the phrase "phantom limb" (Postone 1987) and with providing the first modern description (Herman 1998). His first reference appeared in a fiction article published in *The Atlantic Monthly*, where he presented the story of George Dedlow, an assistant surgeon with the Tenth Indiana Volunteers in the American Civil War (Mitchell 1866). Dedlow experienced a horrific series of amputations, losing an arm and both legs to battlefield wounds and his remaining arm to hospital gangrene, after which Dedlow became a fraction of himself, "a useless torso, more like some strange larval creature than anything of human shape" (Mitchell 1866, 4). The following conversation between Dedlow and the hospital orderly revealed his phantoms to readers for the first time:

> "Just rub my left calf," said I, "if you please."
> "Calf?" said he. "You ain't none. It's took off."
> "I know better," said I. "I have pain in both legs."
> "Wall, I never!" said he. "You ain't got nary a leg." (Mitchell 1866, 5)

Dedlow's story ostensibly resolved during a séance when a medium contacted the spirit of his amputated legs using assigned United States Army Medical Museum numbers.[3] He facilitated a brief reunion with 3486 and 3487, after which Dedlow sunk to the floor, left with the sense that he would never be enough of himself, always only a fraction of a man. Dedlow remarked, "I have so little surety of being myself. . . . It is needless to add that I am not a happy fraction of a man, and that I am eager for the day when I shall rejoin the lost members of my corporeal family in another and happier world" (Mitchell 1866, 8).

Unaware of the fictitious nature of George Dedlow, the public sent donations to the "stump hospital"[4] on his behalf and attempted to visit him during his convalescence. This prompted the Surgeon General's Office to search their records in an effort to find this quadruple amputee (Finger and Hustwit 2003) and led Mitchell to publish a clarifying article in *Lippincott's Monthly Magazine*. His scholarly article presented a less "humorous sketch" of phantom limb, including the temporal aspects of "ghostly members," the morphology of "the spirit member," and the kinesthesia of "shadowy fingers and toes" (Mitchell 1871, 564, 566, 567, 568). As Whitaker (1979, 273) concluded, with this article "the literary 'limbs invisible' became the medical 'phantom limbs,' and the term has been with us since, reaching the status of a single category in the *Index Medicus* in 1954."

For Mitchell, phantoms were psychical replacements of lost physical parts, facsimiles that materialized through unconscious attempts at the reparation of broken bodies, minds, and spirits, and were demonstrative of just how gravely the self could be fractioned by dismemberment. Because of their heroic sacrifice, amputees were publicly recognized as deserving of profound gratitude and respect. Still, the Civil War amputee was an "ambiguous citizen" invested with heroisms while also becoming "an object of anguish and horror to himself" (Goler 2004, 174). Exemplified by the torso of George Dedlow, the amputee became fractioned; in his case, one-fifth the weight, one-half the skin, and truncated in all the kinds of movements that mark persons and express selves. The character Dedlow reflected on his condition: "About one half of the sensitive surface of my skin was gone, and thus much of [my] relation to the outer world destroyed. . . . [O]ne half of me was absent or functionally dead. This set me to thinking how much a man might lose and yet live" (Mitchell 1866, 6).

Underlying Dedlow's anxiety is the implicit role that physical wholeness played in the development and maintenance of identity. "Positing an almost arithmetical dependence of subjectivity on the senses, [Mitchell] argues that when the body is incomplete, personality is partial too" (O'Connor 2000, 103). Through an exploration of the lived significance of dismemberment and the origins of the "limbs invisible," Mitchell also exposed Victorian ideas about embodied masculinity. Because the physical body was central to identity, communicating power, vitality, and productivity, dismemberment could effectively undermine manhood. As O'Connor (2000, 104) explained, "Victorian ideals of health, particularly of male health, centered on the concept of physical wholeness: a strong vigorous body was a primary signifier of manliness, at once testifying to the existence of a correspondingly strong spirit and providing that spirit with a vital means of material expression."

Phantom limb was symptomatic of psychic resistance to loss and emblematic of the physical and mental weaknesses that feminize. The amputee lacked physical integrity, productive potential, and masculine vitality, the kinds of deficiencies that could lead to a "falsification of the self"; because he made untenable and insane claims about his body, the Civil War amputee was equated to the female hysteric (O'Connor 2000, 104). Mitchell (1872, 196), in his *Injuries of Nerves and Their Consequences,* published in 1872—a volume that documented an impressive ninety cases of phantom limbs—described how phantom pain reduced even the "strongest man [to being] scarcely less nervous than the most hysterical girl." Like the hysteric whose theatrical displays revealed "a fraudulent body language," the amputee whose stump thrashed about and writhed from excruciating phantom pains, or even simply periodically awakened to preoccupy or misbehave, demonstrated that a man's body could betray him, that it could be deeply inauthentic (O'Connor 2000, 104). When the male body was emasculated, fractioned, and falsified, little could be done to restore its integrity. More disturbingly, his mind was also irreparably damaged by the same bullets that had torn his body asunder. A soldier who confessed of limbs that no longer existed was unequivocally compromised and his phantom was proof of his psychical troubles.

The Lacuna of Phantom Limb Syndrome

Following Mitchell's popular and scholarly publications, few references to phantom limb can be found in the medical literature until around

1935, and none with the descriptive and explanatory depth of that provided by Mitchell. Several researchers commented on and speculated about the dearth of work in this area until well after the turn of the twentieth century. The following account is reminiscent of that offered by Hoffman (1954b) to explain the previous lacuna during the 1700s:

> It is surprising to note the obscuration in medical literature until relatively recent times, because the phantom limb must have occurred in the past as well as in the present. A different attitude of the layman towards mental defects—once regarded as of a mysterious or magic nature—is the only explanation. . . . So the existence of the phantom must often have been the secret knowledge of the amputee only. (Frederiks 1963, 73)

Even when reports of sensation in missing limbs could not be found in the medical literature, even in their relative absence, phantom limbs still exposed how profoundly dismemberment compromised an amputee's mental capacity. He became a mental defect who kept a horrible secret that could never be told lest he become even more uncertain to himself and others.

Phantom limb resurfaced within the psychiatric/psychological and medical literature with the work of Reschke (1934), Molotkoff (1935), and others during the mid-1930s. But, it was Livingston (1938) and Gallinek (1939) who discussed at length what some researchers and practitioners were now referring to as phantom limb syndrome. Consequently, Livingston and Gallinek framed much of the debate about symptomatology (the symptom complex of a disease), nosology (the classification or categorization of a disease), epidemiology (the distribution of a disease within populations), and etiology (the cause of a disease) for the next fifty-plus years. For example, they referenced numerous temporal, kinesthetic, sensorial, and morphologic peculiarities of phantoms, all of which have served as bases for debate. Importantly, Livingston (1938) argued that phantom limbs have their origin in the excitation of the severed nerves of the stump or residual limb, what would later be referred to as nerve irritation theory. Nerve irritation theorists asserted that nerve damage alone could account for the manifestation of phantoms. At the site of amputation, severed nerves were hypothesized to regenerate or heal through the formation of a neuroma because nerves had unusual tenacity. "The skin, the muscle, the fascia and the bone tend toward atrophy rather than toward continued growth, but the individual nerve fibers continue their blind effort to grow down into the absent limb. Meeting with resistance, they snarl up into a twisted mass, which if large enough to be palpated is called a neuroma" (Livingston 1938, 353).

Unlike their parent fibers, these disturbed nerves expressed abnormal activity, in addition to developing an increased sensitivity to a variety of stimuli. In other words, it was the hypersensitivity of a snarled mass or mess of nerves that was considered to be the root cause of phantom sensations and pain. Gallinek (1939), on the other hand, proposed that this relatively parsimonious explanation of phantom etiology was woefully inadequate without the addition of the then increasingly influential body scheme theory. Gallinek (1939, 420) wrote, "Peripheral stimuli are the blood which the sensory ghost must drink in order to be awakened to its phantom existence," but without the activation of "cortical sensory centers" that are the "carriers of the body image," sensory stimuli could not give rise to the phantom limb. Haunted limbs maintained a vampiric relationship with the knotted masses of nerves that formed near the border of the cut; peripheral stimuli may have been the life blood that fed the phantom, but it was vis-à-vis the body image that the embodied ghost materialized with an insatiable thirst.

A Body of Evidence and Body Scheme Theory

The adoption of *body image or body scheme theory* by most researchers and practitioners throughout much of the twentieth century resulted in the emphasis on, minimization of, and even dismissal of various aspect of the body of evidence being compiled on phantom phenomena. First, researchers revealed that body parts other than limbs or digits regularly persisted as phantoms. Although phantoms associated with numerous body parts became increasingly normative, certain body parts such as the

breast were denigrated and assumed to be rarely associated with phantom persistence, a fact that testified to the relative importance and value
of some body parts over others. Second, just as anxiety about the growing
numbers of demobilized WWII veteran amputees escalated, researchers
and practitioners began to fear that phantom pain could be brought on
by exposure to, among other things, another amputee. Even exposure
prior to amputation could cause excruciating, relentless, and debilitating
pain highly resistant to treatment of any kind. Third, the fixed phantom
surfaced as a significant problem in its own right; measures needed to be
taken to prevent the disappearance of dimming ghosts or to reanimate
dead phantoms in order to circumvent or ameliorate the pain brought on
by *learned paralysis*. Fourth, an important aspect of successful rehabilitation became addressing an amputee's tendency to become preoccupied
with the continued care and proper disposal of the amputated part, or
what Scott (1948, 149) termed "the partial corpse." There was growing
concern about handling practices or, perhaps more precisely, with what
amputees should be told about the fate of their severed limbs. Lastly,
dream states surfaced as instrumental to dissecting the body scheme
because amputees' dreams revealed something elemental about its structure and established how phantoms interrelated with the physical body.
Each of these lines of research was engaged at various times in ongoing
arguments concerning the viability of body schema theory and consequently, the problem of phantom susceptibility or the problem of who
was at risk for phantom-ed mimicry and grotesque distortion.

The term "body scheme"[5] has had a "long and illustrious history in
western medicine," particularly within the fields of psychology and neurophysiology (Grosz 1994, 62). At the turn of the twentieth century, Head
and Holmes (1911) advanced a neurophysiological substrate of the body
characterized as a *model* built up from kinesthetic, postural, sensory, and
visual stimuli, the function of which was to register changes in the posture
of the body and localize the body in space. The body scheme was at once
a record of sensorial and kinesthetic histories, the horizon against which
corporeal futures could be considered, and a standard from which both
could be appraised (Grosz 1994, 66). Accordingly, the body scheme was

foremost experientially fashioned with intrinsic plasticity and as such, was intimately ecological. Bodily boundaries, it was argued, do not terminate at the skin's surface or the tips of fingers. Rather, the body is capable of incorporating elements of the external/physical world into the body scheme, a process fundamental to the utility of objects. The body scheme enables

> our recognition of posture, movement, and locality beyond the limits of our own bodies to the end of some instrument in the hand. Without them we could not probe with a stick, nor use a spoon unless our eyes were fixed upon the plate. Anything which participates in the conscious movement of our bodies is added to the model of ourselves and becomes part of these schemata. (Head and Holmes 1911, 118)

Although the body scheme—as a functional *model*—was thought to be constantly modulated through experience, the scheme *template* was conceived as innately acquired. From a Headian perspective, that one has a body scheme is universal, while the exact character of the functional model is idiosyncratic. Thus, the *birthed* physical body was thought to be indelibly "inscribed" on the scheme template constituting the model's foundational structure. For example, researchers argued that congenital amputees (those people born with foreshortened or absent limbs or digits) developed body schemes that necessarily reflected the form and function of their birthed bodies. By way of elaboration, one would not expect phantom limbs to materialize in cases of congenital amputation because the limb or digit was never represented in the maturing or matured body scheme.

Whether or not phantoms *do* or *can* appear in cases of congenital absence is one of the longest running and most acrimonious debates within the phantom literature over the twentieth century and into the twenty-first. Marianne Simmel, who published from the mid-1950s through the late 1960s, was a staunch defender of the position that phantoms do not develop in congenital amputees (although she herself published on a few "rare" cases). She was also one of the strongest proponents of the application of the Headian body scheme to the etiology of phantom limb. Simmel used the *absence* of phantoms in cases of congenital amputation as evidence of the body scheme's explanatory power despite documented reports of their existence as early as 1961 (Weinstein and Sersen 1961). She also proposed that the *presence* of phantoms in those who had lost limbs or digits to leprosy substantiated body scheme theory. She argued that the body scheme was capable of amending itself to the gradual change caused by leprotic absorption, but not to the abrupt change brought on by traumatic or surgical amputation (Simmel 1967). Phantom limb in cases of congenital amputation reemerges throughout the history of phantom etiology as one of the most persuasive ways of either buttressing claims or undermining them, and for that reason, Simmel was one of the literature's most significant interlocutors throughout much of the twentieth century.

Faithful representations of the body scheme as proposed by Head and Holmes (1911) can be found within the literature on phantom limb until the mid-1960s (see for example Gillis 1964). However, the concept was not static or singular. In fact, the body scheme began to fissure and split as early as the 1950s. A psychoanalytically inspired rendering coexisted alongside its Headian double, which was increasingly invoked throughout the 1950s and into the 1960s, and a third version with a purely neurophysiologic structure surfaced around 1980. Let me first turn to what I call the "psychological organ" before elaborating on the *archetypal engram* (or the prototypical memory trace).

The Psychologization of the Body Scheme

Consonant with Grosz's (1994, 67–70) discussion of the psychologization of the concept vis-à-vis the work of Schilder during the 1920s and 1930s and the work of Merleu-Ponty during the mid-1940s, references to the body scheme throughout the 1950s and into the 1960s within the phantom literature became considerably more psychological in nature.

Paul Schilder (1886–1940), Austrian neurologist and psychoanalyst, in his *Image and the Appearance of the Human Body*, advanced a model of the body image as a composite of social, cultural, and interpersonal experiences and investments that were mediated by personality, emotion, and,

in a Freudian sense, one's libidinal attitude toward the body and its performance. Thus, the body image was foundationally relational in that interaction with objects and others influenced evaluative judgments about the
body, its parts, and its capacities, all of which affected and were affected
by sensation, movement, and perception. For Schilder, the phantom represented "a reactivation of a given perceptive pattern by emotional forces. The
great variety in phantoms is only understood when we consider the emotional reactions of individuals towards their own body" (Schilder 1935, 67).

Maurice Merleau-Ponty (1908–1961), the French phenomenological
philosopher, elaborated on the Headain and Schilderian body schema in
his *Phenomenology of Perception*. For Merleau-Ponty, the body schema
was active in a world of objects and relations that were experientially
meaningful not just to the subject but also to the body. However, it is not
that experiences were simply "remembered" by the body, as in acquiring a skill for example, but rather that movement, action, relations, and
experiences were of-the-body as "attitudes" directed toward some purpose or, in Merleau-Ponty's terms, some task. He wrote,

> "Body scheme" was at first understood to mean a *compendium* of our
> bodily experiences. . . .Yet in the use made of it by psychologists, it is
> clear that the body schema does not fit into this associationist defini-
> tion. . . . When we try to elucidate the phenomenon of the phantom limb,
> relating it to the body schema of the subject, we add to the accepted
> explanations . . . if the schema, instead of being the residue of habitual
> cenesthesis, becomes the law of its constitution. . . .We are therefore feel-
> ing our way towards a second definition of the body scheme: it is no
> longer seen as the straightforward result of associations established dur-
> ing experience, but a total awareness of my posture in the intersensory
> world . . . anchoring . . . the body in the face of its tasks. . . . The body
> schema is finally a way of stating that my body is in-the-world. (Merleau-
> Ponty 1962, 113–15)

He considered phantom limb and phantom pain to be an expression
of the refusal of mutilation because the embodied self cannot be lived

through fragmentation or lost integrity. Being-in-the-world, he proposed, refuses partiality, and embodied integrity is consequently maintained through negation, which functions to "keep empty an area which the subject's history fills" (Meleau-Ponty 1962, 99).

The Psychological Organ and Phantom Proliferation

Juxtaposed to Headian versions of the body scheme were references in the medical literature on ethereal limbs to a kind of psychological substrate or organ inspired by Schilderian and Merleau-Pontian theorizing. The psychological organ functioned to inform a person's mental and emotional relationship toward or with the body both in space (a moving, operative body in time and in three dimensional space) and place (an invested body situated within sociocultural contexts). After full development or maturation, the body scheme was thought to operate as a barometer of sorts against which all physical change was "measured" *prior to* entering into consciousness (see for example Weiss 1958). Hence, the body scheme was considered a preconscious formation of the mind that influenced body *consciousness, attentiveness,* and *appraisal* throughout the life cycle. It incorporated all of a person's "exaggerations or diminutions, depending on the subject's particular sensitivities and feelings about his own body" (Easson 1961, 111). Although the theory retained neurophysiological elements, researchers incorporated what might be referred to as a version of the self-concept. In other words, this version of the body scheme was a composite of the neurophysiological body, a person's construal or assessment of his or her body and its parts, and a person's self-feelings about those judgments, all of which were mediated by sociocultural contexts. For example, Frazier (1966, 445) used the psychological organ to hypothesize about the relative scarcity of phantoms in (now commonly acknowledged) body parts other than digits or limbs:

> The meaning of these percepts [phantom sensations] can be modulated by interpersonal and environmental values placed on body parts and body changes. . . . [P]hantoms are frequent in body parts emphasized

by family and culture such as arms and legs, but are rare in body parts deemphasized, such as the genital organs. Certainly the emotional significance of body parts, which is determined early in life, may influence the phantom phenomenon. It may be more difficult to admit a phantom of the breast, penis, or nose because their loss is of greater significance to one's concept of the self.

Although most innervated body parts (those supplied with nerves) were arguably at risk for phantom-ed mimicry, only those parts considered "significant" to the body scheme—or valued by the self, others, or both—were regularly disposed. Because the hand had historically been considered one the most emotive parts of body, a crucial instrument of expression and a "versatile servant" of the organism (Bressler, Cohen, and Magnusson 1956, 184), and because the leg, as Frazier (1966, 445) argued, was emphasized by family and culture, they acquired a level of import that was reflected in their tendency to persist as phantoms. For example, Hoffman (1954b, 265) wrote, "The hand gives more sensations than any other part of the body (in its close relation to the outer world) while the foot gives most intimate touch with the earth. The more distal the part, the more sensitive the end-organ, and the more intimate and more important the contact between the self and his environment."

Breasts, on the other hand, were not regularly disposed.[6] Despite an early reported prevalence rate of 64 percent of mastectomy patients (Bressler, Cohen, and Magnusson 1956), breasts were thought to be infrequently experienced as phantom-ed for one of three reasons. First, employing Frazier's logic, breasts were exceptionally vital aspects of the self concept, so important in fact that a phantom would be difficult to admit. Second, breasts were fundamentally inconsequential in terms of social importance; they simply were not emphasized by society and thus, presumably, the self. Third, breasts were unimportant to the structure of the body scheme. For example, Bressler (1956) and his colleagues argued that in human evolutionary history, the breast appeared late in phylogenic development, and because the breast was consequently un/underdeveloped during the period of body scheme formation and maturation, the breast did not occupy a central or long-standing place in the body scheme and consequently, was rarely experienced as phantom-ed. In fact, women were depicted as naturally inclined to accept loss, leaving them less reactive to amputation generally speaking:

> The female is psychologically and biologically prepared normally to accept that she has no penis, i.e., is castrated, that she must menstruate, and that eventually after impregnation, she must give up a child, i.e., a part of her body. We feel certain that this disposition contributes not only to a lack of perception and reporting of breast phantoms, but helps account for the lesser intensity of phantoms generally in women. (Bressler, Cohen, and Magnusson 1956, 185)

The experience of penis envy and the sense of loss that manifested during the early years of psychosexual development in healthy, young girls was thought to predispose women toward the uncontested forfeiture of "a body part." The fact that a woman would readily give up her endometrial lining, time and time again, as well as any children she might bear, was demonstrative of her consent or acquiescence and primed her both biologically and psychologically to "feel" little to nothing about her breasts in the event of their loss. Anatomy, for Bressler, Cohen, and Magnusson (1956) and others, truly was destiny; her womb was a source of recurring loss and her irrelevant breasts a tangible reminder that she too was inconsequential.

All three arguments utilized the rarity of reports of phantom breast as support for the psychological organ. In this sense, phantom breasts functioned as "evidence" of the explanatory and illustrative power of body scheme theory as much as they were "understood" through body scheme theorizing. Seemingly paradoxically, the rare phantom breast and the universally experienced phantom limb were both offered up as proof of the psychological organ. Despite claims about the rarity of phantom breast, it is important to note that during the 1950s, there was a relative profusion of articles referencing phantom-ed parts other than limbs or digits, including teeth, face, nose, ear, jaw, eye, rectum, breast, nipple, penis, and testes. As researchers anticipated that most body parts were potentially vulnerable to phantom-ed mimicry around 1950, they "found" exemplars and circulated these accounts widely. Phantom limb syndrome, like many other diseases and disorders, spread, proliferated, "diffuse[d] concentrically outward" (Adler and Adler 2011, 2) as the number of authoritative voices advancing innovative and increasingly grand as well as backward-looking and parsimonious origin stories multiplied. The 1950s represents the onset of phantom proliferation, when embodied ghosts began to multiply in kind as a consequence of their relative "normalization," a trend that was effectuated by the active debate had between body scheme theorists and peripheralists on the typicality and susceptibility of phantom limb syndrome.

Proponents of the peripheral genesis of phantoms—most commonly in the form of nerve irritation theory—suggested that one or more of the myriad changes in the residual limb (physical, chemical, and/or structural) after amputation produced what the brain interpreted as noxious input originating from the absent limb. Thus, because phantom limb was a consequent of nerve injury, purportedly any innervated body part was at risk after amputation. Peripheral accounts of phantom etiology were often referenced by scheme theorists as unpersuasive for various reasons. Peripheralists, on the other hand, argued that if parsimony was a guiding principle, one would conclude that the complexity of body scheme theory was simply unnecessary and unconvincing. However, from both body-scheme and nerve-irritation perspectives, phantom limb stemmed from elemental processes of psychoneurologic or neurologic function and thus were basic to human physiology after amputation. It was the debate itself and the increasing import of nerve irritation theory that shaped assumptions about the typicality and susceptibility of phantom limb and caused the proliferation of phantom parts. In other words, once phantom penis or nose became intelligible, reports surfaced and accumulated.

Importantly, from a psychological organ perspective, phantoms were conceived as neurophysiological as well as both psychological and social in origin. The most significant implication of this line of reasoning was that as the personal, interpersonal (especially familial), and social value of physical body parts changed, phantom-ed parts would correspondingly be more or less likely to manifest. Thus, phantoms were considered avoidable despite the fact that phantom limb, in cases of amputation, was thought to be universally experienced at the time (or nearly so). Corporeal ghosts were at once an individual and a societal problem for many reasons, not the least of which was their growing tendency to pathologize, to become painful. However, the painful phantom that connoted poor adjustment to loss could be protected against.

Phantom Exposure and a Contagion of Fear

One means through which protection could be hastened was addressing the issue of contamination, of being "exposed" to the atrocities of war-related amputation. Researchers were particularly keen to investigate how exposure related to the onset, duration, and quality of phantom limb pain in postwar contexts. Approximately 2,610 major amputations were performed on American soldiers during WWI (1914–1918), another 14,912 during WWII (1939–1945), and 1,477 during the Korean War (1950–1953) (Potter and Scoville 2006). Because the survival rate after surgical and traumatic amputation continued to improve over the twentieth century, greater numbers of amputees lived and worked in communities across the United States. "The nurses, physicians, fellow patients, and even the people in the nearby cities have become so accustomed to men lacking one or more extremities that the patients are looked on as other *average citizens*" (Randall, Ewalt, and Blair 1945, 651; emphasis added).

Researchers' anxieties about exposure were predicated on the assumption that seeing or having known another amputee (even past exposure prior to amputation) could profoundly influence an amputee's self-feelings and evaluative judgments about his or her own dismemberment, particularly when either the amputation was perceived to be highly stigmatizing or the amputee was perceived to be excessively well cared for. In other words, phantom pain could result from extreme body consciousness, attentiveness, and/or appraisal, stemming from the perception that amputation was a central concern of others. Kolb (1952, 111) wrote, "Some amputees appear to be predisposed to the development of a painful phantom limb through an earlier association with another amputee. It is probable that such association with an amputee arouses fantasies of personal mutilation which are mastered by repression. These may be relighted [sic] by the threat of the surgical procedure." Two years earlier, Kolb's (1950b, 470) patient reportedly experienced impotence, depression, and suicidal ideation, all of which was brought on by exposure. However, requisite to the psychosomatization of exposure was an overinvestment in the amputated limb, which was typically a consequent of "familial conditioning."

> In the course of growth each person develops through his multiple sensory experiences a concept of his body and its parts which is commonly spoken of as the body image. In addition to the body image, the body and each portion has connected with it some emotional significance derived from early familial conditioning and the later cultural values placed on physical development. The attitude of the mother and father toward the body of the child leaves its indelible impression on that child as far as his later concept of himself as a person is concerned. According to earlier studies of patients with chronic painful phantom limb, the complaint of pain is often intermittent and represents an emotional response, an indication by the patient that he is suffering from the loss of an important part which has significance in terms of his relationship with others. (Kolb 1950a, 110)

Not all exposure was thought to prompt phantom sensations or, more importantly, provoke phantom pain, yet researchers remained worried about the potential, a worry that paralleled the concern that amputees themselves could be unruly and troublesome. In the post-WWII context, for example, professionals of all stripes feared that the demobilized war-wounded would "pathologize" American renormalization efforts. Veterans evoked "a sharply divided consciousness" in the American public, both a sense of honor and a palpable fear of the possibility that they could be consciously and effectively disruptive (Gerber 1994, 545), and experts collectively predicted a postwar "demobilization crisis" (Gerber 1994; Hartmann 1978; Serlin 2002, 2004). "The former soldiers—low in rank, poorly educated, and accustomed to obeying orders—some argued, had *lost the capacity to think for themselves*" and had become "[p]utty in the hands of demagogues seeking to exact revenge on civilians who had profited from the war and calling for violent political mobilization" (Gerber 1994, 547; emphasis added).

Despite the unparalleled efforts of the American government to recruit the well-adjusted and compose an army-of-the-sane through preinduction psychological testing—970,000 men, one of every eighteen men tested, were excluded on the basis of "neuropsychiatry disorders and emotional problems" (Roeder 1996, 62)—millions suffered debilitating psychiatric symptoms, three times the casualty rate (Roeder 1996). The Office of the Surgeon General conducted a "secret" study of active soldiers at the time that concluded, "On average an infantryman could 'last' about two hundred days before breakdown" (Roeder 1996, 62).

American veterans had been wounded physically and psychically in heretofore unimaginable numbers, prompting the Veterans Administration director of Social Work to anticipate an unprecedented national psychiatric problem (Gerber 1994).[7] In the case of dismembered soldiers, the emasculating effects of amputation exaggerated this suspicion (Ott 2002; Peniston-Bird 2003), and amputees who told of sensation in their missing limbs—particularly those who reported painful phantoms—were considered seriously psychically disturbed. The disruptive potential of dismemberment was evidenced by the moniker given to the phantom during this period, "the misbehavior ghost" (Li 1951, 524). As Hermann and Gibbs (1945, 168) concluded, "The clinical syndromes of phantom limb pain and causalgia which may follow the amputation of an extremity should be given serious consideration in this time of war since the victims of these complications are certain to present a major problem for therapy and reconstruction in the years which lie ahead."

The Scheme Gestalt

The body scheme was assimilated into the psychological lexicon with the work of Schilder, among others (Grosz 1994, 67–70) and was key to the etiology of phantoms for most of the twentieth century. However, two other significant conceptual or theoretical influences were also increasingly evident. The first was the concept of the gestalt, which made its way to the United States in the first half of the twentieth century. The gestalt remained a part of the phantom literature even after "extensive theorizing of any kind [from this perspective] had become an unpopular commodity" (Green 2000, 1), in part because the concept functioned as a much-needed theoretical link or ideational bridge between body scheme theory and phantom-ed mimicry.

Second, with the extension and elaboration of her father's work on defense mechanisms, Anna Freud popularized the concept of denial in psychology and beyond. Within the phantom literature, denial functioned to bolster claims being made by proponents of the psychological organ. Because the body scheme was theorized to be a *preconscious* formation, one could be wholly unaware of the ramifications of significant perturbations in its structure. Alterations in the physical body could be compensated for, vigorously resisted, or wholly denied without an individual's conscious acknowledgment. Thus, the concept of denial allowed researchers to explain the relationship between a sudden mismatch of the physical body and the body scheme and the manifestation of unwelcomed phantoms (pathologically painful phantoms, for example). And, it was often the underlying gestalt of the body scheme—the conscious and/or unconscious desire for physical *wholeness*, the experiential "intactness" of the body's psycho-physiological substrate—that was depicted as the impetus for amputee denial. For instance, Hoffman (1954a, 147) argued, "The meaning of the phantom can be understood as the attempt by the ego or the self at reorganization so as to maintain the body image and scheme gestalt. There is a remarkable degree of inability to accept less than totality in his body configuration."

Gestalt psychology emerged in Germany during the early 1900s with the work of Max Wertheimer (1980–1943), Wolfgang Köhler

(1987–1967), and Kurt Koffka (1886–1941) (Green 2000). Koffka is attributed with introducing the concept of the gestalt to the United States with the publication of a paper in 1922 and later with the publication of *Principles of Gestalt Psychology* in 1935. Subsequently, many of the leading proponents of the movement immigrated to the United States to escape the Nazi regime, which further solidified the influence of gestalt psychology in the American context (Arnheim 1986). The gestalt movement peaked in the United States during the mid-1940s, but continued to be influential, particularly in the area of the psychology of perception, until about 1950. Arnheim (1986) argues that the movement's popularity had seriously waned by the mid-twentieth century, after which only traces could be found in experimental psychology and in other, more established theorizing. Despite the widespread abandonment of gestalt psychology by mainstream psychologists, the concept continued to be influential within the phantom literature until the mid-1960s (see for example Ament, et al. 1964).

The concept of the gestalt remained central to phantom etiology at least in part because of the efficacy of the concept. It functioned as a conceptual bridge between the body scheme and phantom mimicry. The body scheme could only be understood as the underlying causal mechanism of phantom limb syndrome if the structure of the body per se was characterized by *intrinsic* wholeness or comprehensiveness. The assumption that living with an amputation (and thus a disjuncture between the corporeality of the present and the schematic body of the past) would only "produce" a phantom (the continuation or copy of the postural, morphologic, kinesthetic, functional, aesthetic, and other qualities of the amputated part) if the scheme was not just experientially "historical" but also resolutely resistant to incompleteness.

A number of phantoms were enlisted during this period in an effort to demonstrate that the body scheme was governed by the gestalt principle or the "scheme gestalt," including paralyzed phantoms and congenital phantoms. First, proponents exploited what has been termed "phantom paralysis" as a means of conceptualizing the significance of part-loss for the scheme gestalt. Hoffman (1954b, 264–65) proposed that the fixed, frozen, or paralyzed phantom was demonstrative of schematic preservation:

> One is accustomed to having a complete body. The phantom of an ampu-
> tated person is, therefore, the reactivation of a given perceptive pattern
> by emotional forces. . . . Since the position of the phantom is often a rigid
> one and that in which the patient lost his limb, it is as if the person were
> trying to preserve the last moment in which the whole body image was
> present.

In the same vein, Zuk (1956, 512) argued that the tendency for paralyzed phantoms to penetrate solids/objects (as opposed to disappearing or shrinking when coming into conflict with, for example, a wall)
was an indication that the body scheme inherently maintained both
material integrity and temporal continuity, what was referred to as the
gestalt "good fit" between the materiality of the body past and present.
Zuk (1956, 512) wrote, "When individuals report that the phantom has
'gone right through' a solid object, it would appear that they do so on
purely logical grounds. How other than by a desire for intelligibility (or
what the Gestaltists called 'good fit') could one explain why an amputee
reports his phantom has penetrated a solid object?"

In contrast, Jalavisto's (1950) work revealed that phantoms had multiple strategies of adaptation when dealing with solids/objects. Her work,
nevertheless, was wholly ignored by Zuk and Hoffman. She wrote,

> The conflict of the actual sensation of a (three dimensional) phantom
> limb, with the experience of objects sometimes occupying the same posi-
> tion in space as the phantom, without, however, eliciting any sensation of
> contact, is felt by most amputees to be very unpleasant. It may therefore
> be regarded as a distressing stimulus requiring adaptation. It can easily
> be seen that there are only three possible modifications of the phantom
> sensation capable of preventing this conceptual conflict between phan-
> tom sensation and physical objects, *the disappearance of the phantom, the*
> *location of the phantom within the stump or the adoption of the behavior*

called obstacle shunning [bending to the side]. Each of these alterations of the phantom sensations forms a perfect solution of the conflict situation and may thus be considered as an equally good adaptation. (Jalavisto 1950, 341; emphasis added)

Jalavisto (1950) showed that penetration was just one way in which phantoms adapted to object conflict. A few years later, however, Jalavisto (1954, 167) had embraced body scheme theory and argued that "the phantom is the most striking illustration of the existence of a 'body image.'" In fact, she began referring to the experimental practice of pitting phantoms against walls as "constancy experiments" and attributing a phantom's low "constancy rating" to insufficient adaptability. Phantoms that had employed one of what she had termed in her earlier article "perfect solutions" to object conflict had been reconceptualized just a few years later through the lens of the scheme gestalt as poorly adapted because they violated schematic constancy and intactness (Jalavisto 1950, 341).

Proponents of the theory also maintained that the absence of phantoms in congenital amputees underscored the persuasiveness of the scheme gestalt. The supposed lack of phantoms in people with congenital amputation was thought congruent with the pre/unconscious egoistic need for wholeness, a need that necessarily accounted for the *precise* form of the birthed body (Bailey and Moersch 1941; Browder and Gallagher 1948; Frazier 1966, 446; Gillis 1964). The congenital amputee who did not report a phantom limb, it was proposed, *had* an *intact* body scheme, one that was *itself amputated*. Many researchers cited an early French article by Pick as the definitive statement on phantoms in congenitally absent limbs, but as Simmel (1966a, 83) argued, "If he had ever examined a group of individuals so affected, he kept it a secret." Weinstein and Sersen (1961) are often credited with the first published description in English of phantoms in children with congenital absences. Five individual cases were included in this "largely ignored" paper (Saadah and Melzack 1994, 479). Simmel (1962) responded with an article suggesting that children who undergo surgical amputation of congenitally malformed extremities experience phantoms only if sensory or motor function was present prior to the surgery and only if the subject was older than four years of age. Two years later, Weinstein, Sersen, and Vetter (1964) presented thirteen new cases of phantoms in congenital amputees who had *not* undergone consequential surgical amputation. Poeck (1964) also reported that same year on an eleven-year-old girl born without forearms and hands who counted with her phantom fingers. Despite these reports, researchers continued to claim that congenital amputees do not experience phantoms, and the matter is far from settled.

Congenital amputees have long represented and embodied the far side of what Thomson (1996) called "freakery." Unlike amputees maimed by war, congenital amputees were demonstrative of the monstrous birth, a form of "enfreakment" (Hevey 1992, 53) that—even in the context of abundant absence, hybridity, excess, and difference—still resided at the very border of dissimilarity and tolerability. Unlike war heroes and even defectors, cheater, liars, and the apathetic who had fought like hell or at least signed up to be in the line of fire, congenital amputees were undeserving of shared gratitude and collective regret. And, even when the manifestation of a phantom was tantamount to a crack (or a comprehensive rupture) in one's psychic armor, those on the far side of freakery did not deserve them. As harmful as they were, phantoms in the form of a badge of courage, a symbol of the toll that conflict could exact, a sad reminder of what was lost and how little was gained from the brutalities of war, were earned and had by those who deserved them.

The purported absence of phantoms in child amputees (typically reported as under the age of five) was invoked by some researchers as a means of intervening in the congenital absence debate (see for example Hoffman 1954a; Weiss 1956).[8] That children did not experience phantoms (an argument that was widespread until about 1960) was assertedly demonstrative of the malleability of the body scheme, both *model* and *template*. If a child amputee did not develop a phantom limb, then the maturing scheme in this instance could be envisioned as *itself* amputated, capable of tremendous revision during development and hardly structurally fixed. Although the research community as a whole was not in agreement on the issue of susceptibility in children, the debate did lead ultimately to a serious revision of body scheme theory. By the mid-1970s, the body scheme had begun to morph into a neurologically based *archetypal engram* or a central representation that operated as a *prototypical memory trace* (or original memory), and it was the congenital absence/child amputee debate that proved to be a prescient indication of the future of body scheme theorizing. Foreshadowing was evident in Weinstein and Sersen's (1961, 910) confession that "at least the framework of the body schema might be 'built-in'" and that phantoms, in cases of congenital amputation, were probably representative of the scheme's overdetermined structure (a supposition that undermined the experiential quality of the body scheme indicative of both the Headian body scheme and the psychological organ).

Egotistic and Secure Denial

The work of Anna Freud (1895–1982) on psychoanalytic defense mechanisms was enormously influential within American psychology, particularly after the 1950s when she began to lecture regularly throughout the United States (Young-Bruehl 1988). "Despite the absence of clear and convincing proof of its validity, psychoanalysis has proven one of the most durable and potent forces in modern culture" (Farrell 1996, 5), and it was Anna's work *The Ego and the Mechanisms of Defense*, first published in German in 1936, that became the principal elaboration of the concept of denial for American psychoanalytic thought (Young-Bruehl 1988). Within the literature on phantom limbs, the concept was invoked (almost exclusively in tandem with the body scheme) from the early 1950s through the early 1980s. However, there were two distinct renderings or applications of the concept that overlapped temporally. For some researchers, denial was depicted as desirable or at least as a favorable sign of adaptation to dismemberment. But for others denial was deleterious, a toxic state that had to be protected against. Denial was either an indication that an amputee was positively attached to or invested in his or her body (a mark of security), or it was a reaction rooted in overinvestment or pathological egotism (a mark of insecurity). The egotistically denied phantom was an artifact of psychoanalytic theorizing that imagined the phenomenon as stemming from a fear of castration, while the securely denied phantom emerged out of theorizing that foregrounded the scheme gestalt. Let me first turn to the securely denied phantom before elaborating more fully on the egotistically denied phantom.

The securely denied phantom first appeared in the work of Kolb (1954), who argued that phantom limb syndrome was a healthy response to the experience of amputation. The phantom relayed a vital appreciation of or regard for the body and was a reflection of the unconscious, primitively motivated persistence of the complete body scheme. Phantom limbs were experienced by the well adjusted and thus denial of the phantom (in contrast to denial of the loss), he argued, occurred in those patients who failed to acknowledge the amputation and the resulting changes in the body image. In other words, those who did *not* report phantom sensations were in denial. Kolb (1954) proposed that the extent of an amputee's denial (manifest in terms of phantom onset, duration, or consistency, for example) was directly proportional to the amount of import or value attributed to the amputated part.

Kolb was one of the few researchers writing against a version of Freudian wish-fulfillment theory (Dorpat 1971), a perspective that dominated body scheme theory until the early 1980s. Some researchers and practitioners of the day theorized that changes in the body's image, form, and function were typically denied by the amputee after significant loss (see for example Weiss 1958) and were more accurately understood as egotistically denied wish-fulfillments (see for example Frazier 1966). Phantoms were pure fantasy and an indication of poor adjustment to dismemberment. As Van Wirdum (1965, 307) proposed, "The phantom is an old 'present' that has failed to become 'past.' But the phantom patient does not accept it; he destroys reality and in magic acts seeks to find a symbolic satisfaction." Egotistically denied phantoms were characterized as narcissistic reactions to part-loss (see for example Gangale 1968), a loss that was often considered tantamount to castration. For example, Weiss (1958, 25) stated, "The amputee experiences feelings of 'castration,' of being 'deprived' or 'half-a-man,'" an account reminiscent of the late-nineteenth-century thought about the emasculating affects of dismemberment and the story of George Dedlow. In this case, however, it was not his productive potential that was compromised; rather, he was deprived of his masculine sexual prowess and the power that his penis commanded.

The painful or "pathological" phantom was considered an apt indicator of a particularly narcissistic personality whose adjustment problems were at times considered indicative of a serious personality disturbance. As Gangale (1968, 426) noted,

> He refuses to accept reality or compromise with it. He is compelled to maintain his former image and, in the case of the painful phantom, serves the function of convincing him that he still has his limb. This denial is on the primitive, unconscious level for the individual would not consciously express the awareness of this form of denial. The painful phantom may also be a form of narcissism, making the amputee unable to accept the permanent loss. . . . There appears to be no question that a patient with a painful phantom is usually a patient with a severe personality disturbance.

In fact, researchers continued to examine the psychological profiles of amputees for the next twenty years, focusing on personality attributes thought to be common among amputees who developed painful phantoms. At various times over the twentieth century, amputees who reported especially horrifying painful phantoms were regarded as poorly adjusted, insecure, delusional, hallucinatory, psychotic, hypochondriacal, obsessional, neurotic, depressive, rigid, compulsive, overly self-reliant, psychopathic, phobic, unstable, passive-aggressive, prone to catastrophizing, drug addicted, and/or suicidal. As phantom pain prevalence rates increased throughout the 1980s, reports of poor adjustment were less frequent, eventuating in their disappearance altogether. Because painful phantoms became typical, work conducted in the 1980s—particularly by Sherman and his colleagues—sought to demonstrate that amputees with phantom pain were no more psychopathological than amputees without pain (Sherman, Sherman, and Gall 1980), no more likely to have emotional problems than other amputees (Sherman and Bruno 1987), no different psychologically than those in the general population (Sherman, Sherman, and Bruno 1987), particularly those experiencing chronic pain (Sherman, et al. 1988), and no more inclined toward personality disorders (Arena, et al. 1990; Sherman, et al. 1989).

What differentiated egotistically denied phantoms from their securely denied counterparts was not just that the former were typically expressive of a serious underlying personality, emotional, or mental issue but also that they were predictably harmful. Egotistically denied phantoms were never functionally adaptive, never neutral, never to be lived with, and must be eliminated once and for all. Hoover (1964, 47) presented an example of a particularly adverse and consequential effect of egotistic-denial, the conviction that the appendage would "grow back," even among the "intelligent."

> This is a psychological reaction to deficiency or incompleteness. . . . This reaction may be so strong as to interfere seriously with personal adjustment to the loss and with the preprosthetic preparation for fitting and the use of a prosthesis. An extreme example is an attractive, intelligent young woman who . . . refused prosthetic fitting because she was convinced that the arm would grow back.

As long as an amputee sensed a phantom, he or she was not cured of egotism, and as long as he or she was not cured of egotism, the phantom would present itself through troubling and injurious effects. Often described as difficult and lengthy, treatment was typically considered successful when the phantom, painful or not, had entirely disappeared. Solomon and Schmidt (1978, 186) offered the following case of a cured patient:

> She stated she would like to have had a funeral for her legs. She indicated that, were her legs buried somewhere, she would go and visit them. She

indicated that, even though her legs are missing, she feels they are still with her and are an important part of her body. . . . [W]ith reinforcement of the idea that the legs were with her in a spiritual sense . . . phantom pain and phantom sensations disappeared completely.

If phantoms were truly egotistic wish-fulfillments, then, as research-ers suspected, one could confirm denial by exploring the nature of amputees' dreams. They assumed that the idealized body would inhabit the dream state and in fact, some reports indicated that amputees' bod-ies always appeared as intact in their dreams (Hrbek 1976). This line of inquiry would, however, never produce definitive results even though psychologists and others pursued the implications of dream morphology into the twenty-first century (see for example Alessandria, et al. 2011). For instance, patient 2 recalled "a dream in which he fought against other people, kicking and punching with both arms. During the fight his right arm was broken and he continued to defend himself with his left [amputated] arm"; the authors concluded that the phenomenological experience of the body while dreaming reflected the true nature of the body scheme (Alessandria, et al. 2011, 1833). The correlation between the body in dreams and the denial of part-loss, however, was complicated by a number of reports that were difficult to resolve, including research demonstrating that only about half of amputees dreamt of their bodies as intact (Chadderton 1978; Shukla, et al. 1982), examples of amputees who dreamt of their dream-phantoms as both similar to and different from waking-phantoms (Frank and Lorenzoni 1989), and cases of amputees who dreamt of amputations that they had never had, such as an upper limb amputee who dreamt of himself as a lower limb amputee (Price 1998). Nevertheless, claims continued to be made about reading suc-cessful adjustment after dismemberment through dream morphology.

There are only a few scientific reports on the dreams of amputees. A look at them shows a range extending from the idyllic fulfillment of wishes to feelings of agonizing fear, like nightmares. Again and again the wish for physical integrity is manifested in dreams. There are parallels to

childhood dreams in which unrealistic wishes represent the latent meaning of the dream. The manifest dream, according to Freud, is the unen-
coded fulfillment of wishes. (Frank, et al. 1989, 182)

From a psychoanalytic perspective —as well as from a Western perspective more generally speaking—sleep is a highly private, "liminal,
unconscious, aspect of bodily being and an 'a-social,' 'in-active' form
of corporeal 'activity'" (Williams and Bendelow 1998, 172). Dreams, on
the other hand, have long had a distinct medical "use-value," even if
those readied for exploitation were not entirely sure how to mine them
for their prize, even if they were inadequate to the task of capitalizing
on their use-value. As an especially insidious form of biomonitoring,
dream "reading"—regardless of its sometimes asserted relationship to
quackery and contested psychic structures like the unconscious—has
long revealed purposes, cross-purposes, raw fantasy, hidden fears, ugly
needs, deep-seated desires—especially as they relate to the form and
function of the body, the nature of corporeal activity, and the will of
the flesh. In fact, the dreams of the dismembered easily revealed that
even the most apparently well-adjusted amputees wished for the kind
of physical integrity that wholeness offered; dream-states operated as a
way into the deepest or the shallowest of egotistic desires. As "unrealistic" as these idyllic dreams—or, for some, agonizing nightmares—were,
they purportedly revealed a universal desire or need to deny the loss of
a limb, a need for physiologic intactness.

One of the other most noteworthy effects of egotistic-denial was the
finding that amputees could become overly invested in or preoccupied
with the care and "proper" disposal of their amputated limbs. The amputee who sought to assure suitable treatment of the amputated limb or
who found solace in knowing its fate had effectively denied the loss; he
or she was in denial. After referencing his mother's refrigerated arm (his
mother intended on preserving the arm until it could be buried with
her), Schwarz's (1964, 52) patient discussed the impending handling of
his own amputated limb: "Although he had initially said with false bra-
vado that the physicians 'could feed it (amputated hand) to the chickens,'

the patient's words dissolved into a pool of tears when he expressed the wish for his arm to be buried with him at death."

Phantoms are quite distinctive in that they maintain a rare ambiguous status residing contentedly in the realms of both the living and the dead, a state that precludes them from being fed to the chickens or other fowl. Dead or detached parts of the physical body are often assigned a lesser meaning and value than vital parts, pieces, and bits (Lock 2001) despite the fact that dead parts are more central to our experience and understanding of the cadaver, dissection, anatomy, blood and guts, disease and dying, and the incarnate (Walby 2000). Living parts, on the other hand, have "a pulse" even when they are detached from bodies because they are vitalized by personhood and an immediate corporeal history; living parts are treasured and treated with care, but dead parts are more easily discarded. It is not that phantoms are alone in occupying this status—residing between worlds, perhaps with something interesting to "say" about both—but we are less troubled by embodied ghosts and their ambiguity than we are about living cadavers, scavenged or salvaged parts, or other forms of crossover. We are less troubled even when amputees seem to have a sustained relationship with dead parts and a preoccupation with their continued care.

Scheper-Hughes (2011, 175) referred to bodily preoccupations of this kind as stemming from what she termed "body love"; she wrote, "Body love [is] understood as an intuitive, existentially given, sense and appreciation of the body's design and of the inalienability of its parts, both the visual and obvious head, trunks, limbs, and skin, and its silent and 'absent' organs and tissues." During the 1950s and 1960s, amputees were regularly concerned with the handling practices of severed body parts. In fact, not knowing whether the limb—even if diseased or deformed— found its way to an incinerator, the trash heap out back, or the resident laboratory in the name of medical inspection and experimentation was for some amputees utterly unbearable. But, preoccupation of this sort unquestionably did not communicate "body love"—at least not to others. Rather, those who pleaded passionately, inquired subtly, or appealed rationally to their handler about the whereabouts of dead parts communicated to practitioners, as well as family and friends, a disturbed curiosity and morbid attachment to something that was better off left alone and forgotten.

Moreover, if interest in disposal practices is an expression of body love, then those in the contemporary context do not share the kind of sentimentality, appreciation, and intuitive "inalienability" that was expressed so readily in the past. Indeed, by the late twentieth century, stories of unrelenting interest and continued connection had been reduced to pure myth (Mortimer, et al. 2002) or to "well published folk-lore" (Davis 1993, 80).

Prior to this, becoming unduly anxious, expressing pity, and needing to engage in ceremonialism was a mark of true neuroticism. Kolb (1952, 17) argued,

> The patient, almost with panic, fantasies [sic] about whether the ampu-
> tated hand will be handled with respect and tenderness by the surgical
> team. . . . This one question they fear to fade in their own minds and they
> may secretly weep or become unduly anxious. They express it to us as
> almost a feeling of pity and protectiveness toward an old familiar some-
> thing that is being cast out. Of course, it is the highly neurotic persons
> who have a need for any complicated ritualistic burial ceremonial.

Whether in the form of burial, cremation, freezing, stuffing, or pickling, preoccupation often had its origins in the unrealistic hope of a reunion with the severed limb. Parks (1973, 346) wrote of one man's naive and troubled fantasy, "'Outside the ward there's a great chimney stack. . . . I thought it was all the limbs burning but I thought they might have kept mine for medical research.' . . . His fantasy [was] that someone would find a cure for his illness and then put the leg back on again." A particu-larly pathological consequent of egotistic-denial, however, was the ten-dency for an amputee to mistakenly associate the quality of his phantom pain with the handling or fate of the amputated limb during and after surgery or with respect to the circumstances surrounding its traumatic loss. For example, Kolb (1952, 111) relayed the story of a limb burial after which his patient began attributing his stinging phantom pain to the conditions of his limb's grave:

> Previously his school teacher had told the class of a story of a man who had an amputation and then developed a severe stinging pain in his phantom limb. Nothing was found to relieve the pain in his phantom until the man was told that if his amputated leg were disinterred, the cause for his pain would be found. When this was done, it was discovered that ants were stinging the amputated part. The man's pain ceased when the ants were removed and the leg was carefully reburied.

Preoccupation could be particularly disruptive if an amputee believed in a spiritual or otherworldly connection that could manifest in phantom pain, especially pain that emulated the experience of the severed but not disembodied limb. Preoccupation was evidence that egoistic-denial was fundamentally maladaptive and phantom pain was unfortunately a likely sequela of exceptionally poor adjustment to limb loss.

The Medicalization of Phantom Limb Syndrome

The establishment of medicine as a primary apparatus of social control (Zola 1972) through the rationalization of scientific medicine and the institutionalization of the medical model of illness, injury, disease, wellness, healing, death, dying, and disability has engendered the medicalized body—the body, its processes, and its structures reduced to a biophysical machine (Weitz 1996)—and the medicalization[9] of most aspects of life, living, and social organization—including those facets of social life that were previously relegated to other institutions or social spheres such as childbirth, inattention, drug use, sexuality, aging, disability, sleep, death, and many others—such that it has become virtually impossible to escape the biomedical gaze.

Embodied ghosts have long been all in the mind, but in the contemporary context they have undeniably become the province of (bio)medicine. Phantom limb syndrome is certainly not unique in terms of its history being defined by a profound nosological shift; behaviors, acts, thoughts, feelings, and the like that were once considered criminal or psychogenic have time and again become irrefutably medical matters. In fact, history is replete with examples of the categorical transition of behavior from badness to madness (from the sinful or the criminal to the psychologically pathological), from badness to illness (from the sinful or the criminal to the physically pathological), and from madness to illness (from the psychologically to the physically pathological) (see for example Conrad 1975, 2007; Conrad and Schneider 1980; Foucault 1965; Shorter 1992; Szasz 1974; Young 1995).

In the case of ghost stories told by wounded and "damaged" soldiers in the postbellum context—many of whom were accused of the unconscionable practice of malingering—the only appropriate diagnosis was madness, the kind that was intimately entwined with the dire problems of dependency and emasculation. As psychoanalytic thought gained traction in the United States, pre/unconscious denial, narcissistic wish-fulfillment, and symbolic "castration" surfaced as the principle underlying causes of limbs that haunted good and bad soldiers alike. Men's minds, like their bodies, were compromised by mortar shells and the cutting tools of battlefield surgeons, and any evidence to the contrary was systematically ignored, roundly attacked, or relegated to the category of "contributory."

As soldiers began to survive battlefield amputation with increasing frequency and greater numbers of dismembered boys and men were demobilized, the logic of war-induced madness gave way to increasingly persuasive accounts of shadowy limbs being roused by chemical, physical, and structural changes in the residual limb, changes in the sympathetic or/and autonomic nervous system, the limbic system, the vestibular system, and/or the central nervous system,[10] and consequently, by about 1960, critiques of the psychogenesis of phantom limbs began to appear in the literature with growing regularity. Increasingly, phantom limb syndrome was considered physiologic or more specifically neurologic in origin.

The tension between neuroscience and psychology/psychiatry, which had heightened over the first half of the twentieth century as the disciplines jockeyed for position as the legitimate arbiters of the diagnosis and treatment of war-related injuries, began to give way as psychology itself became progressively more influenced by the growing authority of the neurosciences. Noteworthy critiques of the psychological origins of phantom sensations have, since the mid-1950s, coexisted alongside dominant theorizing. However, by the mid-1960s, these critiques became both more overt and more derisive. Early critiques surfaced during post-WWII renormalization; renormalization efforts included the orchestrated rehabilitation of the demobilized war wounded, significant state investment in the then nascent field of prosthetic science, and the strategic conflation of dismemberment with military-inspired technological liberation (Serlin 2002, 2004). This was a national program that was incommensurate with the association of dismemberment with mental instability, with wish-fulfilling hallucinations, with narcissism, or with egotistic-denial. In the literature, this incongruence played out in the tension between the "facts" that phantoms were demonstrably psychogenic in origin, phantom limb syndrome was universally experienced by amputees (or nearly so), and phantom sensation, especially pain, could persist indefinitely. If amputees invariably developed phantom limbs and if phantom limbs were rooted in minds deeply troubled by profound physical loss, then amputation and by extension war and the state were the cause of potentially permanent and debilitating mental instability. We were "knowingly" subjecting the best and bravest of our young sons, our dear brothers, our darling husbands and partners, and our beloved fathers not only to the possibility of death and serious physical disability but also to a lifetime of mental torment. Not surprisingly, scathing critiques of psychogenesis began to emerge by the late 1960s.

In an appraisal of the psychoanalytic theory of denial, Simmel (1959) argued that what was known about phantoms was simply not congruous with the theory. She suggested that phantoms often persisted in amputees who had successfully adjusted to amputation and were thus not in need of a psychical defense. Further, phantoms often telescoped, a morphologic phenomenon incommensurate with a theory of denial.

Simmel (1959, 605) wrote, "If denial leads to such distortions, then, I would think, this turns out to be a very inefficient defense which does not even protect the individual at the level at which it is supposed to." Finally, she surmised that because phantoms did not develop in cases of congenital amputation and "the individual with congenital absence of a limb, be he child or adult, has as much need to defend himself as the amputee," denial was simply unpersuasive (Simmel 1959, 605).

One of the most influential assaults came from Kallio's (1952, 112) examination of amputees who had undergone kineplasic surgery to produce a forearm stump cleft, what is referred to as Krukenburg's operation. The purpose of the operation is "to transform a forearm stump, by cleaving it, into a forcepslike gripping organ with sensation." During the surgery, the ulna and radius are essentially divided, along with the accompanying musculature and tissue, to produce a cleft between the two bones, a tong-like structure (Gangale 1968, 426) that resembles a "lobster claw" (Weiss 1956, 670) and is capable of manipulation with training. Interested in the nature of phantom limbs in cases of cleaved arms, Kallio (1952) questioned dozens of amputees, revealing an extraordinary trend. He noted,

> In the majority of cases the [phantom] hand was reported to have been cleft. In three cases there had been loss of fingers: in one the middle finger had disappeared, in another both the middle and the ring finger, and in the third case all that remained was the thumb and the little finger. Four patients reported that it felt to them that the ulnar fingers of the phantom hand were tied together. (Kallio 1952, 117)

In other words, the majority of amputees who had undergone Krukenburg's operation consequently felt their phantom hands as cleaved, with fingers absent or fused and palms split. Given his findings, Kallio (1952, 117) described the denial-based intact body scheme as "downright impossible" and provided the following reasoning: "The present writer emphasizes the fact that the Krukenberg (cleft) hand is in point of fact a new organ with no preexistent engrams or central representation. How could one imagine the presence of any sort of body scheme for straight, hinge-like movement between the radius and the ulna, which no human being has by nature?"

Others too increasingly argued that the available data were simply not consistent with the supposition that phantoms were a product of denial, wish-fulfillment, or the like, pointing to reports that experimental phantoms could be induced in "normal" subjects (Melzack 1973) or that some amputees "not only accept but are relieved by amputation" (Postone 1987, 63). Kellye M. Campbell, nurse practitioner in the Department of Rehabilitation Medicine at the University of Washington in Seattle, argued, "We have some folks who come in after living with a bad leg for some period of time. It is usually between one and twenty years and those people are eager to get rid of that leg. Generally they are well adjusted after that" (Campbell 2005). During the 1980s through the 2000s, references to psychological mechanisms appeared chiefly in terms of psychic contributions to the intensification or interpretation of phantom pain or the psychic consequences of living with chronic pain. By 1990, even amputees with chronic phantom limb pain were thought to have measurably "normal" psychological profiles.[11]

This shift from the psychologization to the medicalization of phantom limb syndrome is a significant event in the modernization of amputation; phantoms were no longer found in the dark recesses of the disturbed or repressed mind but rather in the pink, convoluted folds of the cerebral cortex. Medicalization has had myriad effects, not the least of which has been the relative normalization of phantoms. As they became an ordinary consequent of amputation or deafferentation, their historic mysteriousness eroded; their long-recognized strangeness was a product of ignorance, not abnormality, aberration, or defect. Most notable, perhaps, their normalization caused phantoms to spread to vulnerable populations. Because phantoms became understood as a consequent of the brain's response to deafferentation or the loss of nerve supply, a number of populations were identified as at risk for phantom-ed mimicry. In the 1950s, reports of phantoms in cases of paraplegia, spinal cord injury, paralysis, tabes dorsalis, cerebral lesioning, brachial plexus avulsion or lesions, and "feeblemindedness" surfaced, and throughout the 1960s, phantoms began to manifest in congenital amputees and patients under anesthesia. During the 1970s, there were reports of phantoms in cases of multiple sclerosis, leprosy, and gangrene. Phantoms were becoming more and more difficult to protect against.

This propensity for risk to spread to vulnerable populations is one of the central functions of risk discourses. Because risk identifies and defines what is imperative—what we should and should not attend to—it distinguishes between the benign and the potentially dangerous, maintaining a durable and often enduring tension between the two. Risk operates on the principle of fear. It differentiates, separates, stigmatizes, and hierarchizes, creating a border between the contaminated, the polluted, the infected, the infested, the morally repugnant, and "the rest." And, because risk identifies the *potentially* dangerous while instilling fear and often disdain, it spreads, seeps, widens, deepens, elaborates, and amplifies. Risk enlists more and more of the population into joining or consenting to the feverish search for those who are vulnerable, susceptible, or exposed so that fear itself becomes the most potent contagion (Giddens 1991; Lupton 1999).

Dr. Ronald Melzack and the Archetypal Engram

By the mid-1970s, Melzack himself began to argue against the persuasiveness of the psychological organ. He and his colleagues resurrected a more Headian version of the body scheme. Like its Headian predecessor, the *archetypal engram*[12] functioned as a postural guide based on cutaneous, kinesthetic, and visual input. However, they proposed that the engram was not experientially derived; rather, they concluded that "the nature of the schema is fixed, archetypal and possibly inherited; rather than plastic and acquired" (Bromage and Melzack 1974, 268). In other words, as opposed to the experientially based, developmentally secured, malleable structure envisioned by earlier proponents of body scheme theory, Melzack proposed a much more static structure with a genetic basis that was relatively invariant from person to person. And because the engram was a built-in structure, Melzack (1973) envisioned that "our perceived limbs are, at least in part, images based on central neural activities and are not solely the result of feedback from our real limbs."

Table 4.1. At Risk Populations: Populations Recognized as Vulnerable or NOT to the Manifestation of Phantoms

Earliest Date	Author	Population	Reported or NOT FOUND
1939	Gallineck	Congenital amputation*	NOT FOUND
1941	Riddoch	Spinal cord injury	NOT FOUND
1948	Browder & Gallagher	Children	NOT FOUND
1948	Henderson & Smyth	Gangrene	NOT FOUND
1950a	Kolb	Spinal cord injury	Reported
1951	Li	Paralysis	Reported
1951	Harrison	Tabes dorsalis	Reported
1954a	Hoffman	Leprosy	NOT FOUND
1956	Harber	Anesthesia	NOT FOUND
1956	Simmel	Feebleminded**	NOT FOUND
1956	Simmel	Cerebral lesions	Reported
1956	Simmel	Brachial plexus lesions and avulsions	Reported
1957	Buxton	Children	Reported
1959	Simmel	Feebleminded**	Reported
1961	Weinstein & Sersen	Congenital amputation*	Reported
1963	Frederiks	Mutilation, Memory disappearance	NOT FOUND
1966a	Simmel	Anesthesia	Reported
1976	Price	Leprosy	Reported
1976	Hrbek	Gangrene	Reported
1978	Wilson et al.	Paralysis	NOT FOUND
1979	Mayeux & Benson	Multiple Sclerosis	Reported
1993	Halligan et al.	Stroke	Reported
1995	Spitzer et al.	Dementia	NOT FOUND
1998	Ramachandran & Hirstein	Spinal Block	Reported
1999	Fisher	Blind	Reported
2001	Andre et al.	Replantation	Reported

*Congenital aplasia includes both phocomelia (a congenital deformity in which the limbs are extremely shortened) and peromelia (congenital malformation).
** Included under this category are references to mental defectives and low intelligence.

Thus, unlike earlier versions of the body scheme, the engram was able to conceptually account for phantoms in cases of congenital amputation, at that point well documented. Melzack and colleagues (1997, 1618) wrote,

> It may be, then, that previous reports of phantom experience [in congenital amputees] were rejected in part because there was no conceptual framework to make sense of the data. Simmel (1961) had espoused the concept that the phantom is produced by the body schema described by Head and Holmes . . . as the product of continuous proprioceptive and other somatic input. The idea of an innate structure for the neural basis of the phantom was, therefore, not considered. Yet, this is precisely where the data point.

Melzack's reinvention of the body scheme was largely a corollary of the discovery of *experimental phantoms,* or phantoms that were induced in "normal" subjects as well as paraplegics, typically by anesthetic block.[13] In an early experiment, seventy-seven patients being prepared for surgery were given an anesthetic block of the motor and sensory nerves of the arm and were then asked to identify the position of the affected limb. Patients reported

> a sequence of experiences [that] was essentially the same for all subjects. . . . [T]he anesthetized arm felt normal in terms of its position in space; using his tracking arm, he generally showed it to be at the side of the body and bent at the elbow, or above the abdomen or lower chest. The real arm at this time lay flat beside the body. Sometimes the experimenter moved the anesthetized arm slowly until the lower arm and hand were beside the head. When the subject opened his eyes, he was astonished to find the discrepancy between the real anesthetized arm and the perceived arm. The reality of the phantom arm to the subjects was unequivocal. Most of them searched actively for their arm in the area where they felt it to be. . . . [S]ome of them failed to recognize their real arm when it was raised above their head, and stared in disbelief at it and at the place where they perceived it to be. (Melzack and Bromage 1973, 263)

The authors argued both that patients' reports of arm positioning bore no relationship to the actual location and posture of the affected arm and that they demonstrated remarkable constancy across subjects. Experimental phantoms assertedly revealed the stereotyped quality of the body scheme, one associated with the male and undeniably masculine body readied or poised for action. Bromage and Melzack (1974, 273) wrote,

> The body schema is subservient to and waits upon objective reality. The nominal internal standard proposed by Head and Homes is set at its most efficient point, and is poised for phenomenal instruction. . . . [T]he final possibility for our phantom origins is one of inherited neural memory from postural patterns laid down and selected throughout the history of man. We have pointed out that the position-of-rest is also the position of alert for instant action. Indeed, the posture of repose adopted by the phantom homunculus is strikingly similar to the stance of a wrestler or knife fighter balanced and crouched to spring. Such an internal standard would have great functional value as an instrument for swift response in a dangerous environment, and it is tempting to see it as a kinesthetic legacy in our inherited repertoire for violent survival.

The engram was a product of the evolutionary history of "man" and, as such, its very structure and form reflected man poised for action. The pose of the knife fighter coiled to strike or, more accurately, crouched to spring emulated primitive man's "kinesthetic legacy" in his quest for "violent survival." This pose of man readied for violent action, Melzack proposed, was preserved in the universally acquired, archetypal engram and became man's "natural" position-of-rest. The masculine quality of the innate engram (relatively invariant from person to person) was unremarkable and thus, the phantoms that materialized vis-à-vis these genetically acquired memory traces conveyed masculinity (rather than emasculation). Phantoms actually testified to an amputee's fundamental manliness, and they were a reminder of the inherent power of primitive man.

By the 1990s, Melzack had abandoned body scheme theory altogether, arguing that it was too vague and that there was no cortical equivalent, no identified underlying neurological mechanism (Melzack 1989).[14] As an alternative, Melzack proposed what he termed the "neuromatrix," a "network of neurons that extends throughout widespread areas of the brain, composing the anatomical substrate of the physical self" (Melzack 1990, 91), which produces both "overt action patterns" and "awareness of output" (Melzack 1995, 78). He hypothesized the integration and parallel processing of three major neural circuits: (1) the sensory pathway through which information from the periphery travels via the thalamus to the somatosensory cortex; (2) the emotion pathway in which signals travel through the reticular formation to the limbic system; and (3) the "sential neural hub" through the parietal lobe producing conscious awareness (Melzack 1995, 76).[15] In many respects, the neuromatrix was equally as elusive as the body scheme. In fact, Davis (1993) interpreted the neuromatrix as a contemporized version of the body scheme, and others used the two terms interchangeably (Czerniecki 2005). Like the engram, the neuromatrix was genetically acquired and phylogenic. But, unlike the engram, the neuromatrix was capable of generating all the sensations felt by the body without sensory input.

> [The neuromatrix] . . . can generate every quality of experience which is normally triggered by sensory input. . . . Phantom limbs are a mystery only if we assume the body sends sensory messages to a passively receiving brain. Phantoms become comprehensible once we recognize that the brain generates the experience of the body. Sensory inputs merely modulate that experience; they do not directly cause it. (Melzack 1993, 620, 629)

Into the twenty-first century, the neuromatrix has remained one of the most frequently referenced theories of phantom limb etiology (see for example Giuffrida, Simpson, and Halligan 2010). That is not to say that the neuromatrix has been without critics. In fact, it has been criticized as unable to account for phantom limb pain, distorted phantoms, supernumerary phantoms, the absence of phantoms, delayed onset, the spontaneous cessation of pain, or the elimination of pain through cortical lesioning. Others proposed that there was simply no substantial direct evidence to support the theory (Sherman and Sherman 1983). For instance, Dr. Edward Taub, behavioral neuroscientist in the Department of Psychology at the University of Alabama–Birmingham, argued that the neuromatrix was highly speculative:

> There's not a great deal of evidence for it. I think that Ron Melzack, who's a good friend, is absolutely convinced that he has found the answer. In fact, I wrote a laboratory analysis of it and the evidence for it is very weak. There was never any doubt in my mind that he was smart, but smart people can get diverted by their pet hypotheses. (Taub 2005)

Regardless of its speculative nature, the neuromatrix was representative of a new line of argumentation that surfaced around 1990 and claimed that phantoms found in the brains of amputees demonstrated quite compellingly that corporeality was epiphenomenal. The mind was capable of generating, of creating, of "manufacturing" sensation, so that the body was "not essential for any of the qualities of experience . . . from excruciating pain to orgasm" (Melzack 1989, 1, 9); the undeniable cruelty of stabbing, burning, or lancinating pain, the utter bliss of the perfect orgasm, the sweetness of a soft and tearful kiss, the true remorse of that left undone or behind—all of the qualities of human experience, it seems—begin and end in the brain.

As the concept of the epiphenomenal body spread, phantoms and amputees were catapulted into a position of unprecedented neuroscientific importance. Although the syndrome, as Melzack argued, had apparently lost its mysteriousness when the phantom puzzle had effectively been solved, haunted parts nevertheless reemerged as exceedingly valuable "experimental objects" and consequently, after the turn of the twenty-first century, phantom phenomena would once again become quite mystifying indeed. Moreover, amputees themselves became remarkable in their own right, operating as conduits who—with the help of neuroscientists and visualization technologies—could expose some of the most extraordinary promises and possibilities that the human brain and humanity had to offer.

5

Phantoms in the Brain

The Holy Grail of Neuroscience

Since the late nineteenth century, ethereal traces of once physical parts have become substantive. They have come to, in Young's (1995, 6) terms, "penetrate people's life worlds, acquire facticity, and shape the self-knowledge of patients, clinicians, and researchers." Phantoms have become substantive not because of their physical properties per se but because of their power-as-effect (Harré 2002). Phantoms bridge corporeal biographies of the past with those of the present. Phantoms inhabit brains in order to be seen, and they skillfully animate prostheses in order to be felt. In fact, they can be seen quite clearly using neuroimaging technologies—often in vibrant and stunning color—and they can be felt quite keenly as vital body parts rather than defunct remains when they occupy or inhabit prostheses, bringing "dead wood" and "cold steel" to life. Moreover, phantoms remake the morphology of human bodies—sometimes in bizarre and very distorted ways—and they remap the geography of human cortices, effectively disturbing what was once considered immutable. Phantoms are imbued with social substance and material integrity because they are at once work objects (Casper 1998a, 1998b) and actants (Callon 1986, 1999; Latour 1987, 1991; Law 1992, 1997).

Casper (1998a, 19) defined a work object as "any material entity around which people make meaning and organize their work practices . . . [the] constructions of [which] vary depending upon who cares about it, who is attributing meaning, what the work goals are, and material contingencies." The peculiarities of phantoms have been of interest to researchers, clinicians, and scholars of the brain sciences because these cortices allow those who are curious, authoritative, and skilled to answer some of the most elemental questions about human ontology, questions that can only be explored through highly technologically mediated forays into the body-in-the-brain, the kind that are never innocent, dispassionate, or benign. It seems that there is little that we cannot derive from the neuronal activity of some of society's most valued and valuable brains; all of that which is consequential and mysterious—the last of the unknown frontiers—is apparently assessable from inside of the right human skulls.

As work objects, phantoms have been entrenched in the practices and knowledges endemic to the discipline. Phantoms have been sensitive to, for example, changes in corporeal ideology, the biomedical institutionalization of pain, and attempts at re-visioning the research on phantom etiology, epidemiology, nosology, and symptomatology. And, because they have become a clever and productive way into (and a way around) the body-in-the-brain, phantoms have also become a biopolitical tool for dissecting, understanding, appraising, and intervening in the "natural" or biologic/biomedical body, the dismembered or "disfigured" and "functionally impaired" body, the prosthetized or hybridized body, the epiphenomenal or "superfluous" body, and the collective or social body.

While historicizing and contextualizing phantom limb syndrome—situating ethereal appendages within the social worlds of psychology, medicine, and biomedicine—I also highlight the fact that phantoms have clearly been the source of and a resource for embodied recalcitrance. Corporeal transgressions are, of course, not new. Many scholars have detailed accounts of and theorized about the leaky (Shildrick 1997), unruly resistant (Mitchell 2002), recalcitrant (Williams and Bendelow 2000), seepy (Lawton 1998), and transgressive (Monaghan 2001) aspects of bodies. Bodies as well as body parts (haunted limbs that "belong" to amputees and are embodied or lived) transgress because they always "themselves hold an unspoken knowledge" (Kosut and Moore 2010, 2) and because they meaningfully act as relational partners when associating with objects and others—even in the context of biomedical attempts to construct these same limbs as productive technologies of the body. To be sure, corporeal transgression or recalcitrance is always relationally accomplished; the leaky nature of bodies materializes in response to attempts at containment, control, regimentation, management, or, in the case of phantoms, (bio)medical rationalization.

I do not mean to suggest that phantoms have been indifferent or impervious to orchestrated and vehement attempts at rationalization. Rather, I want to underscore the fact that phantoms are not simply objects that can be made "explicit" once and for all as science "progresses," as measurements become more sensitive and researchers more discerning, as the naivety of the past transitions into the deep insight of the present or potential future. Indeed, the qualities and peculiarities of phantoms are not merely uncovered or discovered with wonder because phantoms are actants as well. An actant is "any agent, collective or individual, that can associate or disassociate with other agents. Actants enter into networked associations, which in turn define them, name them and provide them with substance, action, intention and subjectivity" (Crawford 2005, 1). Bodies—like artifacts, things, substance, and matter, as well as the ostensibly discursive or ideational—are mediating objects in social relations and are understood as one dynamic element in a heterogeneous network that is historically situated and nested in broader dynamic networks.

Many scholars invested in actor-networks advance a form of relational materialism that is concerned with the material aspects of social life, how these are brought together, and the implications of such associations. Networked elements are made meaningful only in relation to other elements in the network (and as a consequence of the network's nature or features). Importantly, because they embrace agnosticism, any a priori assumptions about "objects" and "matter" are avoided, and in fact, assumptions like these are thought to be in need of critical examination. Accordingly, bodies or even body parts (cells, genes, organs, tissues, phantom limbs, etc.) are objects of importance that are "dissected" in an effort to expose the processes underlying their emergence as interactional effects. In other words, the qualities and characteristics of the network, the processes and practices that make up networking, and the networked objects themselves are all of interest and foci of analysis.

As actants, as adept transgressors, phantoms have been the force behind many transmutations within the field of neuroscience, within the bodies, minds, and brains of amputees and others, and between bodies and prosthetic technologies. In fact, as we shall see, often what is rendered collective originates with (and inside of) bodies through corporeal transgression or the myriad means through which the body and its parts resist biopower. In short, I embrace what Barad (1999, 3) referred to as "agential realism," an approach that acknowledges the "material-discursive" nature of a "world [that] kicks back." Phantoms have unequivocally kicked back.

Chasing the Phantom

The history of phantom theorizing has time and again been described as rife with controversy. In the latter half of the nineteenth and the first half of the twentieth centuries, the "organicists"—proponents of the physiological origins of phantoms, whether attributable to peripheral or more central mechanisms—were depicted as engaged in a "long and bitter" controversy with the "psychopathologists"—advocates of the psychogenic origins of phantoms (Hoffman 1954b, 263; Riscalla 1977). Over the second half of the twentieth century, the peripheralists—champions of nerve irritation theory—were engaged in impassioned debate with the centralists—exponents of the primary role of the central nervous system (including the spinal cord and/or cortex). Since the turn of the twenty-first century, although remnants of the other debates remain, phantoms have been definitively situated in the brain and dispute has primarily focused on exactly which structure or structures are implicated (the localizationists versus the diffusionists) (Star 1989), as well as precisely how change in cortical geography occurs (neural sprouting versus unmasking).

Although accounts of the peripheral contributions to the etiology of phantoms have existed alongside psychogenic explanations since the first half of the twentieth century (see for example Livingston 1938), the role of what was termed "nerve irritation theory" was at times characterized as insignificant or as simply playing a part in the exacerbation of phantom pain. Nonetheless, nerve irritation theory continued as a widely acknowledged explanation for phantom phenomena and as a guide to treatment for practitioners into the twenty-first century despite the fact that scathing and pointed critiques were increasingly common throughout the 1960s, 1970s, and 1980s and despite the fact that by the 1990s, some of the most prolific and prominent researchers in the field asserted that there was "virtually universal agreement that phantom limb phenomena cannot be explained in terms of peripheral mechanisms such as neuromas or other pathological activity of the stump" (Melzack 1989, 7). Researchers argued that nerve irritation theory was an untenable explanation because (1) phantom pain did not follow a known peripheral nerve supply; (2) surgical revision of the residual limb or the proximal nerves did not alleviate pain or produce change in the painless phantom; (3) neuromas developed gradually, while phantom limbs often appeared immediately after surgery; (4) phantom pain persisted long after adequate healing had occurred; (5) local anesthetic did not produce pain relief; and (6) complex perceptual, kinesthetic, and kinetic qualities could not be modified at the periphery.

Despite the evidence, however, nerve irritation theory persisted. For example, nurse practitioner Kelly Campbell argued that "phantom limb and phantom pain arise from a common source; I think it is just disrupted nerves" (Campbell 2005). Melzack complained about the "absurd" persistence of the "neuroma issue" among the many practitioners he had worked with. He said,

> I have actually found practitioners who still predominantly think that phantoms are a neuroma issue. Most of them—most physicians—do believe in it even though that should have gone out the window with the article that John Moser and I published in 1978. Even in cases where the spinal cord is completely broken, they still tell you it's a neuroma. [In one case a practitioner said], "God, we took out an inch of spinal cord." It can't possibly get beyond that break which is at about navel or nipple level, let's say. And he said, "They still feel their feet and they're burning."

People will still tell you that it's a neuroma issue which is an absurd idea. (Melzack 2006)

Nerve irritation theory retained widespread support among the "ill-informed" because it had face-validity and because it was parsimonious so that both research and therapeutic interventions could be relatively straightforward. In fact, it was—in Fujimura's (1986, 1987) terms—the inherent "doability" of the phantom pain problem from a peripheralist perspective that enabled the theory to endure with such tenacity. When patients presented with unrelenting and debilitating pain, practitioners could present both a feasible origin story and much-needed hope for relief.

Consequently, during the second half of the twentieth century, researcher and practitioners were keen to identify and catalogue events, states, substances, and the like that exacerbated phantom sensations (or more often phantom pain), as well as provoked phantom reoccurrence (after having "disappeared") or induced phantom onset (in amputees who had not experienced sensation or pain previously). Documented irritants included seemingly benign events such as falling asleep, writing, or smoking, in addition to pain or injury. However, much of the research centered on neurological, biochemical, and physiological changes at the periphery, such as fluctuations in skin temperature or the growth of neuromas. The condition of the residual limb was a core concern so that the onset of phantom sensation as well as changes in phantom morphology or the quality of awareness was often attributed to the treatment of the stump.

Despite the fact that nerve and/or tissue damage as the sole explanation of phantom etiology had arguably been debunked, the legacy of phantom peripheralism remains evident in the contemporary treatment of phantom pain. Treatments aimed at mediating the effect of nerve and other tissue damage, such as peripheral stimulation or other local interventions, are still commonly employed (see for example Casale, et al. 2009). This trend can at least partly be attributable to the work of Sherman (1994), who was the strongest proponent of conceptualizing phantom pain as a *class of symptoms*; he advanced a model or typology of phantom pain that has also persisted into the twenty-first century (see for example Giummarra, et al. 2007). Sherman proposed that at least two of the three classes of phantoms he identified were physiologic in origin. Burning phantom pain resulted from reduced near-surface blood flow, and cramping phantom pain resulted from muscle tension in the residual limb. His typology was consistent with the peripheralist argument that ethereal appendages must have their origin in the ill health of the stump or residual limb and hence, his work established what Rodgers (2008) termed a "legitimating loop." A legitimating loop connotes "a sense of mutual influence as well as impl[ies] the potential benefits this connection would provide" (Rodgers 2008, 23). The association or connection between peripheralism and the typology of phantom classes suggested a clear strategy for the amelioration, cure, and prevention of phantom pain, while also justifying the practice of surgical and rehabilitative techniques intended to, first and foremost, protect and advance the health of the residual limb rather than the phantom or artificial limb (which presupposed that the three were distinctively embodied). Other scholars and practitioners, however, have prioritized friendly phantom-prosthetic relations or a lived intimacy among the stump, the phantom, and the prosthesis.

By the early 1990s—what Congress had declared the decade of the brain—phantom limb syndrome, like many disorders, diseases, illnesses, syndromes, and conditions, had been definitively located in the cortices of amputees. No longer originating in psychosomatization or denial, no longer the product of the hyperexcitability of damaged nerves and tissue, the phantom had been "chas[ed] . . . up into the brain itself" (Shreeve 1993, 3). As Wade (2003, 17) recounted, "Phantoms once lurked at the extremities of the human body—now they are invading the brain."

The brain became a viable site in part because of the emergence and proliferation of medical imaging technologies during the 1970s and 1980s (Dumit 2004; Joyce 2006; Kevles 1997; Pasveer 1989), technologies that procured very provocative and persuasive pictures.[1] In fact, neurophysiologic research on phantom limb tripled during the 1980s, 1990s, and

2000s, with dozens of articles written every year on some aspect of the visualized neurology of brain-based phantoms. Visualization technologies of various kinds are commonly employed in biomedicine and technoscience in an effort to produce justifiable work and legitimate findings; they bring a sense of definitiveness and an impression of accuracy to that which is often categorized as problematic. As Moore and Clarke (2001, 58) argued, "Scientific accuracy has been constructed historically as the ability to create the one singular representation of a given phenomenon which fully 'captures' it. This is accomplished by normalization, standardization, deletion of range of variation or difference, and deletion of the mediation of the observer," as well as though the use of trustworthy technologies that seem to never lie. They are "technological tellers of profound somatic truths [whose] compelling images come to mediate wider interactions between doctors, patients and society and gain further salience in the process" (Pickersgill and Van Keulen 2011, xv).

In the contemporary context, neuroimaging has ensured that the brain is everywhere, and needless to say, as a collective, we are completely captivated. These representations are so ubiquitous that without them, the brain sciences are ill equipped to provide persuasive and robust claims. For example, using wet brains from brain banks—floppy grey slices of tissue saturated in toxic chemicals of preservation—seems comparatively limiting and barbaric when contrasted to the manipulative potential and commanding expressiveness of crisp images colored by brilliant blues, sunny yellows, and fiery reds. Moreover, as Dumit (2004, 15) warned, these technologies have without question transformed the way we think about—among many other things—our minds. We can observe and intervene into anything assertedly brain based, and it is by way of imaging technologies that, as Casper (1995, 84) proposed, "The representation becomes the phenomenon." Accordingly, the mind in Western medicine has become conflated with the brain, with cortical tissues, structures, and processes. It has become what Beaulieu (2002, 76) called "the mind-in-the-brain," and the phantom has surfaced as confirmation that, like the mind, the body too is all in the brain.

The New Holy Grail

As it began to be argued around 2000, study devoted to this illusive and obscure phenomenon has provided heretofore unimaginable and invaluable insights into the functionality and organization of the human brain. Phantoms are exceedingly fruitful experimental objects, and the researchers dedicated to their investigation are serendipitously in a position of unprecedented exploitation. Dr. Vilayanur Ramachandran, professor of psychology, biology, and neuroscience at the University of California–San Diego, published the popular science text *Phantoms in the Brain* with Sandra Blakeslee in 1998, a text that has been translated into eight languages.[2] Ramachandran, arguably one of the most widely known contemporary figures in the field, proposed that the study of phantoms has allowed us to

> address lofty "philosophical" questions about the nature of the self. . . .What brings about the seamless unity of subjective experience? . . . Philosophers love to debate questions like these, but it's only now becoming clear that such issues can be tackled experimentally. By moving these patients [amputees] out of the clinic and into the laboratory, we can conduct experiments that help reveal the deep architecture of our brains. Indeed we can pick up where Freud left off, ushering in what might be called an era of experimental epistemology . . . and start experimenting on belief systems, consciousness, mind-body interactions. (Ramachandran and Blakeslee 1998, 3)

Brain-based body parts, researchers implored, should be brought into experimental contexts in an effort to answer some of the most elemental and lofty questions about human sensation, perception, experience, and much more—a truly neuropolitical plea and project. In fact, we would be remiss if we do not give phantoms the chance to show us that cartographers of the brain can expose what even the most formidable architects of the mind could not. In an interview appearing in *Discover* a few years before the above claim was made, Ramachandran was quoted by Shreeve (1993, 2), who wrote,

> While chasing the phantom, neurobiologists have thus been led to a solid revelation: the sense of touch, and the physical world it ushers into existence, has much more to do with what is going on in our heads than at our fingertips. The illusory sensations may even be on the verge of revealing one of the brain's most powerfully guarded secrets. If neuroscientists like Ramachandran . . . are correct, the exotic phenomenon of phantom limb offers one keenly magnified perspective on what routinely happens in the brain as we engage the world around us. . . . We're looking at a new route to the *Holy Grail of neurobiology*, says Ramachandran.

Because they are conduits of valued "research material," amputees have occupied the often unanticipated role of pioneer. By exposing the shifting geography of their brains to neuroimaging and neuroscientists, by "consenting" to the experimental exploitation of their (fractioned) brain-based bodies, amputees are necessarily positioned at the center of efforts to intervene in the biopolitical order vis-à-vis the exploration, territorialization, classification, and representation of cortices of interest. In the name of science—and because embodied apparitions, like windows, can apparently be as transparent as the clearest paned glass—amputees must be brought into experimental contexts for their own good, as well as ours.

Dr. Joel Katz, professor in the Department of Psychology and School of Kinesiology and Health Science at York University in Toronto, said, "I think that whoever solves the puzzle or problem of the phantom limb will also solve the problem of perception. . . . That is what I like so much about the phantom: I think of it as *a window* into the central nervous system" (Katz 2005; emphasis added). The eerie appendages of the past—those that Michell (1871) argued betrayed so many good men—were being touted as the Holy Grail of neurobiology, providing a window into the very secrets that the brain had always so fervently guarded, a window into "the last great-unsolved problems in science" (Ramachandran 2009, 777). Phantoms became invaluable, enabling revolutionary insight into—among many other curiosities—the true nature of the mind-body connection.

For instance, Melzack (1993, 620) boldly proposed, "You don't need a body to feel a body," and he argued that the phantom functions as quite compelling evidence of the body's epiphenomenal quality. He wrote, "The brain itself can generate every quality of experience which is normally triggered by sensory input" (Melzack 1993, 620), and told me, "The brain is a structure which generates and *creates everything we feel*" (Melzack 2006; emphasis added). Thus, the body is "not essential for any of the qualities of experience . . . from excruciating pain to orgasm" (Melzack 1989, 1, 9). Ramachandran and Blakeslee (1998, 58; original emphasis) took this supposition to its logical extreme when they argued, "*Your own body* is a phantom, one that your brain has temporarily constructed purely for convenience." By extension, the self too is all in the brain. Dr. Burgess was quoted in the *New York Times* as saying, "The research shows that the self can be detached from the body and can live a phantom existence on it own" (Blakeslee 2006, D6).

Contemporary phantoms may not be as mysterious as their predecessors but, by the turn of the twenty-first century, they were exotic and truly precious, enabling revolutionary insight into the most pressing questions of human ontology. Far from being psychic baggage—the manifestations of wish-fulfilling denial buried deep within the disturbed mind the purpose of which was seemingly only to torture and horrify— far from being "dead weight"—defunct or silent cortical tissue taking up valuable neural space in those rare brains "fractioned" by dismemberment—today phantoms are the Holy Grail of neurobiology, sacred objects with wondrous and enigmatic qualities that assertedly deserve our collective curiosity and concern. They are unique neurologic windows that allow us to peer intently and with awe into the cortical processes that are considered constitutive of human experience and the very essence of our humanity. Indeed, they assertedly make known one of the most profound revelations of our time: "we are our brains."

Many scholars have critically engaged with this notion that we are reducible to our most revered organ (see for example Dumit 2004; Fein

2011; Rose 2003, 2007), that "the brain is the only part of the body we need in order to be ourselves" (Vidal 2009, 6). The way neuroscientists envision and visualize the structure or architecture, the function or processes, the maturation or development, the dysfunction or maladaptation, the plasticity or malleability, and the many other fundamental aspects and features of the brain has enormous implications for interventions both cortical and biopolitical. For example, the long-celebrated hard-wired brain, one that is fixed at birth, presupposes a decontextualize organ (and self) because it is necessarily "impervious to social and cultural life" (Fein 2011, 47). This vision or version of cortical structure and function allows researchers and scholars to absolve themselves of moral culpability when "knowledge" about the brain is harnessed for the purposes of surveillance, control, valuation, intervention, and more. Moreover, those born with a "disturbed" or "disordered" brain or those with acquired disease or dysfunction are in need of biomedical and neuroscientific management. And, to whom else would we turn?

As a distinctively productive way of tapping into the most vital and compelling mysteries of the human cortex, as persuasive evidence of the brain's ability to generate the most complex of sensory experiences, as clear proof that the body has always only been a phantom constructed by the brain for our convenience, embodied ghosts have secured a prominent place in the history of neuroscience and have become entirely indispensable. Moreover and paradoxically, phantoms have become more real than real, more substantive than the intact limbs they have at times mimicked with such meticulousness and ease. In fact, intact limbs have become superfluous to corporeality, as well as comparatively fruitless in experimental contexts, while phantom limbs have become, at least in some respects, better than the best fleshy limbs because they are brain based.

The Sensory and Motor Homunculi

A neurologist might conclude that God is a cartographer. He must have an inordinate fondness for maps, for everywhere you look in the brain maps abound. (Ramachandran and Blakeslee 1998, 39)

Canadian neurosurgeon and director of the Montréal Neurological Institute, Dr. Wilder Penfield (1891–1976) was "widely recognized as one of the great neurosurgeons and neurologists of all times" (Feindel 1977, 1365).[3] Among many other accomplishments, Penfield initiated groundbreaking research during the 1930s and 1940s into intractable epileptic seizures (Finger 1994; Restak 1984). Using cortical stimulation during neurosurgical operations, Penfield was able to induce what is termed the "aura stage" in his patients, a state that is typically felt by epileptics just prior to the onset of a seizure.

With the surface of the subjects' brain exposed, he used electrodes to pinpoint and excise the section of brain matter that caused replication of the aura stage, effectively curing some patients of their seizures.

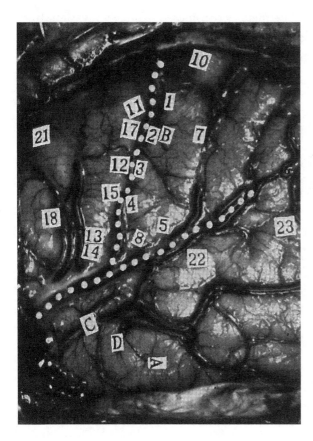

Figure 5.1. Penfield's Map. Tiny numbered tickets indicate the area of the cortex that produced a specific response (a sensation, memory, etc.) in his patients. (Reprinted from Penfield, Wilder, and Edwin Boldrey. 1937. "Somatic motor and sensory representation in the cerebral cortex of man as studied by electrical stimulation." *Brain* 60: 389–443, with permission from Oxford University Press.)

Serendipitously, he also made a discovery that would profoundly impact the then nascent field of neuroscience. With fully conscious patients, a stenographer, photographer, electrodes, and tiny numbered tickets dropped onto the brain, Penfield constructed maps of human sensory and motor function, maps that have remained virtually unchallenged since.

Equipped for exploration with his tiny territorializing flags, Penfield localized what are commonly referred to as the sensory and motor homunculi (Penfield and Boldrey 1937; Penfield and Rasmussen 1951). In the depiction of the homunculi in figure 5.2, a little man's distorted and reorganized body lies stretched across sections of each of the cerebral hemispheres, representing topographical maps of sensory and motor function.[4]

The gross layout of the maps is considered relatively invariant from person to person (Ramachandran and Blakeslee 1998), suggesting that "man's" primordial body-in-the-brain is foundationally male. Consistent with Grosz's (1994, 71) observation that "'the' body that is generally

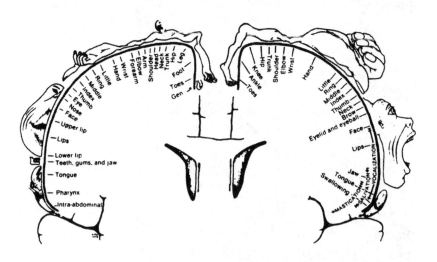

Figure 5.2. The Somatosensory and Motor Cortices. These schematic representations of the sensory and motor homunculi indicate the proportion of cortical area devoted to each body part within the brain's primary sensory and motor maps.

addressed by neuro- and psychophysiology is implicitly the male body," as well as with the anatomical essentialism of genital depictions found, for example, in anatomy texts (Moore and Clarke 1995, 2001), representations of the homuncular body within the medical literature are unmistakably anatomically male. The unacknowledged imbrication of maleness with the primordial brain-based body is demonstrative of the fact that the modernization of amputation has always been a project in the instantiation, institutionalization, and defense of a particular form of hegemonic masculinity, one that prioritizes potent and industrious manhood.

These maps have also been depicted as bilaterally reversed (the left side of the homunculus corresponds to the right side of the body), upside down (the homuncular feet are at the "top" of the brain), and not fully continuous (from homuncular head to neck to shoulder, etc.). For example, the area corresponding to the genitalia in the sensory homunculus can be found located next to the feet, the face next to the hand, and the breast next to the ear. The sensory homunculus is considered to be a relay center that receives and processes sensorial information from the periphery, while the motor homunculus precipitates movement by sending signals directly to the muscles, and the two are hypothesized to integrate in the parietal lobe (Metman, et al. 2005; Penfield and Boldrey 1937; Penfield and Rasmussen 1951).

Penfield's research demonstrated that when the physical hand is introduced to heat, pressure, or pain, for example, the sensation "registers" in the cortical area of the somatosensory cortex known as the "homuncular hand." Likewise, stimulation of the homuncular hand in the brain (using an electrode) is felt by subjects as sensation originating in the physical hand (Bolderly and Penfield 1937).[5] Because some body parts are more densely innervated (they have more nerve fibers) than others, they are accordingly associated with larger cortical areas; they take up more "space" in the brain. These are body parts that are more sensitive to touch, temperature, pressure, and pain and are capable of finer degrees of discrimination. For example, the tongue and hands of the sensory homunculus and the hands and lips of the motor homunculus correspond to or occupy disproportionately larger cortical areas because of their relative sensitivity and because of their physical import. Miller (1978, 21) offered the following metaphor:

> It is like an electoral map as opposed to a geographical one. Because of their functional importance, the hand and the mouth have more sense organs per square inch than the leg or the trunk, and since all of the parts of the body are clamoring for attention, they have many more Members representing them in their Parliament, that is to say, in the brain.

This image of the sensory homunculus illustrates the asserted proportional association between brain area and body surface. In other words, if the body were shaped in accordance with the brain's representation, we would look something like this relatively well-endowed guy.

Illustrations like these do more, however, than reconstruct a topographical map of the homunculi in three-dimensional terms for instructive or even voyeuristic purposes; they suggest that women's "internal" genitalia are not sensorial in the same way or to the same extent as men's "external" genitalia and are therefore less integral or less central to human experience. By implication, the brain-based body-maps of women are constructed as simply derivative, and perhaps most significantly, one of the essential attributes of the female homunculus is its inherent deficiency.

Penfield first published on the homunculi in 1937 (Penfield and Boldrey 1937), but it was his *Cerebral Cortex of Man* (Penfield and Rasmussen 1951) and *The Excitable Cortex in Conscious Man* (Penfield 1958) that were among his most significant contributions to modern neuroscience (McNaughton 1977). And, although there were correspondingly early references to the sensory (and sometimes motor) cortex during the 1940s, 1950s, and 1960s within the medical literature on phantom limb, it was not until the mid-1980s that the role of Penfield's homuncular maps in the etiology of phantom limb was widely acknowledged. In these early references, the homunculus typically acted as a heuristic accounting for one aspect of phantom morphology, the dropping out of parts (gapping) or phantom telescoping, and they tended to merely state

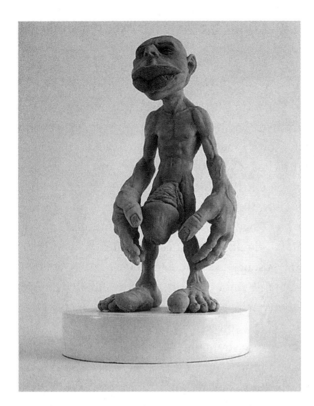

Figure 5.3. The Sensory Homunculus. This illustration of the sensory homunculus is a representation of the male body if proportionality were consistent with the relative "size" or the amount of cortical area devoted to each body part in the somatosensory cortex.

that the most vivid phantom sensations originated in body parts associated with the largest cortical representations. The homunculi were not engaged as theory proper, as a means of explaining phantom phenomenon in toto, but rather as the structural correlate of the body scheme and a way of substantiating that body parts (homuncular, scheme-d, physical, or phantom-ed) have differing degrees of import and vibrancy relative to one another.[6] These references also typically invoked the work of Head and Holmes (1911) and/or Schilder (1935) on body scheme theory rather than Penfield's somatosensory and/or motor homunculi, and they read as affirmations of what researchers had already "known" about the structure and function of the body scheme.

For instance, Simmel (1956) argued that telescoping was the perceptual correlate of the differing degrees of import of parts within the body scheme, as well as the larger cortical areas devoted to the body's periphery. She argued that phantom-ed parts that had greater schematic significance and homuncular representation, the fingers and toes for example (distal parts), were actually felt more vividly (a tendency that was commonly acknowledged in the literature). The more proximal areas or parts, on the other hand, forearms and shins, or upper arms and thighs "dropped out" over time because they were less vivid experientially, because they had less schematic significance, and because they had less homuncular representation. Indeed, proximal parts often faded and even disappeared altogether. Fingers and toes were consequently sensed as disconnected or floating, a state that was both perceptually disturbing (because digits should be attached to bodies) and antithetical to the lived scheme gestalt (an embodied sense of being whole). The "answer" to this type of embodied dissonance—floating fingers or detached toes—was either the body stretching toward the hovering part or the part moving closer to reestablish a vital connection. Simmel (1956) argued that because stretching would entail a fundamental change in body shape and proportionality, floating parts would naturally telescope toward the body. Not insignificantly, the homunculi in these early references explained what denial could not. Body parts suspended in space returned to the body even if this meant that feet would be directly attached to thighs and wrists secured straight to shoulders. From the perspective of wish-fulfilling denial, this kind of embodied experience would be denied by the amputee; it would be too disquieting to be lived with, too antithetical to corporeality, too disturbing for conscious awareness.

Because early references to Penfield's somatosensory and motor maps were imbricated with body scheme theorizing, the homunculi were conceived of as among the many places where the body schema could be found or, more accurately, among the many spaces of influence. The body scheme, even when conceptually well defined, was an elusive formation and was often intimately intertwined with a number of other psychic structures, including the body ego, the body concept, and the body ideal, other structures that were equally as ill defined. At the time, accepted wisdom was consonant with what Star (1989, 176) termed "dif-fusionist localizationism," an approach first advanced within the nascent field of neurophysiology by Charles Scott Sherrington at the turn of the twentieth century. Sherrington asserted that the brain was not com-posed of discrete functional areas but rather was a matrix of integrated functions and formations, processes, and structures. Consonant with this logic, researchers envisioned the body scheme to be a multifari-ous process/product with psychological, physiological, neurological, and experiential features, and the homunculi to be ancillary structures that were accordingly vulnerable to revision by way of psychosocial practices and events.

The work of Pons and others, however, transformed the sensory homunculus into a purely neurophysiologic substrate and phantoms into evidence of the geographic quality of the brain, a shift reflective of the rising predominance of "explicit localizationism;" this was an approach that "reached its apex" with the work of Penfield and others around 1950 (Star 1989, 179). Star (1989) argued that explicit localization-ism became entrenched in the institutions, practices, and knowledges of modern neuroscience by the mid-twentieth century. Although dif-fusionist localizationism predominated in the late-twentieth-century literature on phantom limb syndrome, explicit localizationism also remained clearly evident.

Because neuroscientific knowledge has implications for the way health, wellness, disease, disability, and death are defined, for how dis-ease and dysfunction are diagnosed and treated, and for how wellness, disease, and disability are experienced, expressed, and made intersub-jectively meaningful, disciplinary re-visioning of this kind necessarily has profound consequences for the field, research, patients, and the public. Disciplinary re-visioning in this case ultimately led to a decisive paradigmatic battle, and the controversy left phantoms both everywhere in the human cortex (or nearly so) and nowhere in particular. Some researchers argued that the body-in-the-brain could be found in dis-tinct cortical areas, while others suggested that it was a nebulous circuit woven through many structures and spaces of influence. Accordingly, phantoms became fundamentally protean in nature and as such, more and more difficult to protect against. In fact, phantoms, once again, began to proliferate with abandon.

Dr. Timothy Pons and the Silver Spring Macaque Monkeys

By the 1990s, monkey cortices and Dr. Timothy Pons would offer unequivocal proof that Penfield was one of history's most masterful cartographers of the human brain. In 1991, Dr. Timothy Pons (1956–2005),[7] a neuroscientist at the Laboratory of Neuropsychology at the National Institute of Mental Health, conducted a series of experiments with the now infamous fifteen Silver Spring macaque monkeys (Holden 1989; Ramachandran and Blakeslee 1998; Schwartz and Begley 2002; Sideris, McCarthy, and Smith 1999).[8] In the summer of 1982, in an unrelated rehabilitation experiment of Dr. Edward Taub's (Barinaga 1992; Elbert and Rockstroh 2004), the monkeys underwent rhizotomy, a procedure in which the nerves from the arm are completely severed from the spinal cord. Years later, with the help of animal rights activists and a court order, the research was discontinued and Taub was charged with six counts of animal cruelty (Holden 1989; Sideris, McCarthy, and Smith 1999).[9] The monkeys were seized by police but languished in the custody of the National Institutes of Health until the court demanded that three be humanely euthanized (Shreeve 1993).[10] In an ironic twist of fate, Pons was given permission to examine their brains before their euthanasia, and the monkeys spent their last days back in the laboratory (Pons, et al. 1991; Shreeve 1993).

During his examination, Pons found that in each of the monkeys, the cortical area previously corresponding to the arm (the homuncular arm/hand) was not dormant or inactive as one might assume after all those years of paralysis but instead responded to stimulation of the *face* (Pons, et al. 1991; Ramachandran, Stewart, and Rogers-Ramachandran 1992). Pons argued that because the homuncular face and the homuncular hand were adjacent to one another in the somatosensory cortex (the sensory homunculus) and because the neuronal region belonging to the homuncular hand "sat unused," the homuncular face began to encroach upon or make use of the idle region. In fact, the deafferentated area of the brain had purportedly been reorganized "at least an order of magnitude greater than that reported previously," suggesting the growth of new connections between neurons, a phenomenon referred to as neuronal sprouting or arborization. As Shreeve (1993, 3; emphasis added) concluded, "In effect, fully a third of the entire touch map—over half an inch of cortex—had switched its allegiance. With no orders coming in from the numbed limb, it had married its fortunes to those of the face instead. This is neural reorganization on a *massive scale, unimaginable in a hardwired brain*."

Pons's speculation that the cortex was amenable to reorganization through the growth of new connections contrasted with the notion of "hard-wired" cortical organization and development that then prevailed in the neurosciences.[11] For instance, Gillis (1964, 89) wrote about the inherent rigidity that exemplified the adult human brain, "As we know, adult cortical processes are notoriously rigid in their processing of new information; where an established interpretation of sensory data exists, further information tends to be similarly interpreted, and therefore a phantom limb in an adult becomes a likely consequence of amputation." Researchers assumed that new neural connections are never (or rarely) formed in the mature mammalian brain, that connections established in fetal life or in early infancy are the only ones to manifest over the life course (Ramachandran 1994).

Phantoms visualized through the reorganized somatosensory cortices of macaque monkeys had further legitimated Penfield's maps and solidified his reputation as one of the brain's most notable cartographers, but more importantly, phantoms had effectively shaken the foundation of modern neuroscience, eventuating in the hard-wired brain being all but abandoned (at least in some circles). Ramachandran and Blakeslee (1998, 31) enthusiastically explained, "The implications are staggering. First and foremost, they suggest that brain maps can change, sometimes with astonishing rapidity. This finding flatly contradicts one of the most widely accepted dogmas in neurology—the fixed nature of connections in the adult human brain."

Pons proposed that the brain was amenable to dramatic remapping through the growth of new connections, and accordingly, researchers in the field began to argue that if the sensory and motor maps of the brain were reorganized in response to limb loss there would likely be a sensorial equivalent. In other words, cortical reorganization or remapping must somehow be *felt* by amputees.

Mislocation Phenomenon

Researchers have long documented what has been termed "mislocation phenomenon" or "referred sensation" in cases of major amputation, describing the "projection" or mislocalization of sensation from a *trigger zone*[12] located on the residual limb onto or into the phantom (see for example Cronholm 1951). For instance, a light touch, a breeze, a thump, or a painful pinch on the stump could be referred to or projected onto a phantom foot, producing "separate sensations in the [phantom] foot and stump which appear to come from the same point" (Katz 1992b, 286). This depiction of the volar (palm-side) and dorsal (back-side) view of a residual limb (on the left) and phantom arm (on the right) shows how precisely trigger points could be mapped onto phantoms. Amputees sometimes reported in remarkable detail a direct one-to-one correspondence between distinct points or regions on the stump and very precise referral points on the phantom. At times, referred sensation was spontaneously reported and at other times, it was elicited by researchers or clinicians. For example, Doetsch (1997, 10) described how, when prompted, one patient reported that sensation "retreated up the limb": "When asked whether he could elicit sensations referred to his PH [phantom] by self-stimulation, he replied that he had always been able to do so—and proceeded to demonstrate the location and size of each of his TZs [trigger zones] by touching or lightly scratching his left forearm [stump] with his right index finger."

These "dual percepts," as they were sometimes called (see for example Hunter, Katz, and Davis 2005), remained a relatively unexplored phenomenon until around 1990 because they were thought to be the

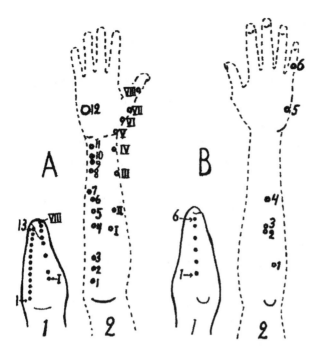

Figure 5.4. Referred Sensation. This illustration shows the pattern of referred sensation in the phantom hand felt when the stump was stimulated at each of the points indicated on the volar (A) and dorsal (B) regions of the stump.

byproduct of the (over)activity of residual nerves (a supposition rooted in nerve irritation theory).[13] In the case of an above-elbow or AE amputee, the nerves that previously supplied the lower arm and hand terminate in the upper arm, and when stimulated, these residual nerves were thought to give rise to sensation felt as originating in both the stump and the amputated hand (after all, these were nerves that once terminated in the hand). Mislocation from this perspective was simply a byproduct of the continued activity of severed nerves attempting to do their job. The logic was straightforward and thus remained relatively unchallenged until the discovery of what were referred to as "remote trigger zones."

By 1990, researchers began to document cases of far-removed or remote trigger zones, and they used cortical reorganization to explain this curious form of mislocation phenomenon. Without warning, faces, mouths, and lips were being referred to phantom hands (see for example

Barinaga 1992), ears were referred to phantom breasts (see for example Aglioti, Cortese, and Franchini 1994), and genitalia were referred to phantom feet or feet to phantom genitalia (Aglioti, Bonazzi, and Cortese 1994).[14] Within the somatosensory cortex, the homuncular hand is adjacent to the homuncular upper arm, and thus, a stimulus applied to the upper arm (the residual limb or stump) would expectedly be referred to the phantom hand. However, because most homuncular parts are flanked on either side,[15] two separate referral zones theoretically exist, both of which should produce referral to the phantom. In fact, in the case of amputation of the hand (and lower arm), researchers found that stimulation of the upper arm/shoulder/trunk, as well as the *face*, produced sensation referred to or felt in the phantom hand (see for example Knecht et al. 1996). Ramachandran (1998, 1853) explained what one would expected if the inactive homuncular hand territory in the brain were "invaded" by two adjacent homuncular parts: "Because the hand area in the Penfield map is flanked on one side by the upper arm and the other side by the face, this is precisely the arrangement of points that one would expect if the afferents from the upper arm skin and face skin were to invade the hand territory from each side."

This same process of invasion or takeover also occurred in cases of phantom breast and homuncular ear, as well as phantom feet and homuncular genitalia because these body parts reside next to each other or occupy neighboring zones in the somatosensory cortex or the sensory homunculus. For example, Aglioti, Bonazzi, and Cortese (1994, 273) reported three cases of "bizarre" far-removed mislocation. They found that both sexual intercourse and defecation induced phantom sensations in the feet of two men and a woman because "both anus and genitals are mapped medially to the areas formerly subserving the amputated lower limb." The woman described the sensation she experienced during intercourse as "a tiny, painless 'electric current' sliding from the stump to the phantom" (Aglioti, Bonazzi, and Cortese 1994, 275). Like all dual percepts, sensation was often felt as strangely exaggerated, remarkably intense, or exceptionally vibrant. For example, Ramachandran (1996, 123; 1998) wrote of the erotic effect of cortical remapping or invasion for one of his patients whose orgasm was actually "bigger" than before because the sensation was felt *in his foot,* offering more terrain for pleasure; no longer confined to his genitals, both the tactile sensation and the erotic sensation of sexual pleasure were transferred to his phantom foot: "In the Penfield homunculus, the genitals are adjacent to the foot and, as one might expect, we found that two patients reported experiencing sensations in their phantom foot during sexual intercourse. One of these patients, a 60-year-old engineer, reported actually feeling erotic sensations in the foot so that his 'orgasm is much bigger than it used to be.'"[16] Likewise, Aglioti, Cortese, and Franchini (1994) found that almost half of the women in their study of mastectomy patients who reported persistent phantom sensations experienced stimuli to the ear as referred to the phantom breast. The tingling that was elicited from

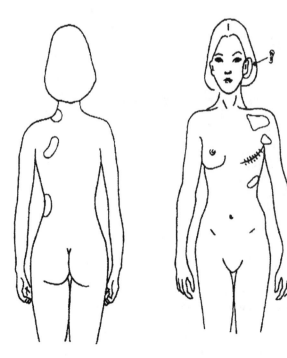

Figure 5.5. Mislocation in Phantom Breast. This rendering shows the areas that invoked phantom sensation in the breast when stimulated. (Reprinted from Aglioti, Salvatore, Feliciana Cortese, and Cristina Franchini. 1994. "Rapid sensory remapping in the adult human brain as inferred from phantom breast perception." *NeuroReport* 5(4):473–76, with permission from Wolters Kluwer Health.)

stimulation of the earlobe produced an erotic sensation referred directly to the nipple (Ramachandran 1998).

Just like early reported trigger zones, remote trigger zones were characterized by an incredible degree of topographical precision. For example, Ramachandran and Blakeslee (1998, 29) found two distinct trigger zones on Tom. When Ramachandran brushed a common household Q-tip across various parts of Tom's body while he was blindfolded, he found one "beautifully laid out 'map' of [Tom's] missing hand" on his upper arm (his stump) and another complete map of Tom's phantom hand superimposed on his face. In a similar study, Halligan (1994) and his colleagues provided

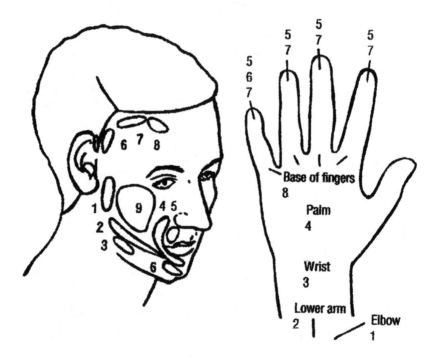

Figure 5.6. Mislocation in Phantom Hand. This rendering shows the regions on the right side of the face of D.M. that elicited precisely localized, modality-specific, topographically organized sensation in her phantom hand. (Reproduced from Halligan, Peter W., John C. Marshall, and Derick T. Wade. 1994. "Sensory disorganization and perceptual plasticity after limb amputation: A follow-up study." *Neuroreport* 5:1341–45, with permission from Lippincott Williams & Wilkins.)

the illustration in figure 5.6 of an intricate map of D.M.'s phantom hand, which they had discovered splayed across the side of her face.

These topographically precise maps, characterized by a one-to-one systematic correspondence between very precise points on a trigger zone and defined points on the phantom, Ramachandran and others insisted, were the perceptual correlate of neuronal invasion and proof that phantom limb phenomena had their origins in cortical remapping. For example, as the homuncular face invaded the dormant homuncular hand, the phantom hand became perceptually superimposed on the physical face. Researchers also reported that these referral maps were modality specific, that temperature, pressure, vibration, as well as the sensation of metal, tickle, itch, massage, or a breeze could be transferred to or mislocalized to the phantom. For example, Ramachandran (1998, 1613) wrote,

> On one occasion when the water accidentally trickled down his face, he exclaimed, with surprise, that he could actually feel the warm water trickling down the length of his phantom arm! . . . We tried applying a drop of warm (or cold) water on different parts of the face and found that the heat or cold was usually referred to individual fingers so that there was a sort of crude map of referred temperature that was roughly superimposed on the touch map.

One of Ramachandran's subjects was able to trace the illusory trickle with astonishing specificity as it meandered down the side of his face, and others could accurately discern temperature. When, for example, warm water was applied to the thumb reference field (on the face) and tepid water to the fifth finger reference field (on the face), the subject reported warmth only on the phantom fifth finger. Moreover, when hot water was applied to the thumb reference field (on the face) and ice-cold water was applied to the thumb reference field (on the shoulder), the subject experienced "a flash of heat followed by a flash of cold" (Ramachandran 1994, 300). Others have used iced test tubes, pinpricks, and deep pressure to elicit "mysterious and amazing . . . cool spread-out areas" and deep or fleeting pain (Aglioti, Bonazzi, and Feliciana 1994, 275).

What is so remarkable about these far-removed, topographically pre-cise, modality-specific trigger zones is their complete absence from the literature until around 1990. Incredibly, just as visualizing technologies began to be used regularly to peer into the brains of amputees and just as cortical remapping surfaced with the work of Pons and others, embod-ied ghosts morphed once again and trigger zones spread to the very places that they were "supposed to." They should have been captured within the visualized images of sensory and motor function in ways that abided by Penfield's homuncular geography. And, in fact, they were. Phantom breasts lay across the ears of mastectomy patients, phantom feet spread their toes along genitalia, and phantom hands reached their fingers nimbly over jaws and across cheeks. In other words, just as Pons's remapped somatosensory and motor cortices were being imported into experimental and clinical contexts, researchers found and amputees described far-removed, topographically precise, modality-specific, trig-ger zones. Amputation no longer entailed the perceptual loss of a limb but rather its reduplication, making phantoms easy to feel and hence, easy to find. As Shreeve (1993, 4) argued, "The hand was not missing at all—indeed, it was now a pair of left hands one meticulously laid out across [the] face, the other wiggling its digits just below the shoulder."

Despite attempts by researchers and practitioners to rationalize phan-toms, to delimit the parameters of phantom morphology, embodied ghosts morphed or shape-shifted once again. First, they proliferated and spread to occupy new and "erroneous" body parts just as they were being "captured by the camera" and just as they were being "pinned down" by neuroscientists in an effort to buttress claims about cortical structure and function. Consequently, as phantom parts became understood as brain rather than body based—and hence, severed or detached from the laws that had always governed human morphology—phantom distor-tion spread, becoming more and more intelligible. Embodied apparitions were no longer simply mimetic of fleshy limbs. They were restructured or more accurately, destructured, becoming progressively more bizarre.

Second, even when in the "limelight" of visualization technologies, phantoms continued their transgressive ways. The remainders, the mongrels that did not find their way across bodies to sprawl across the square of jaws, the lobes of ears, or the soles of feet, became the rule rather than the exception. By the turn of the twenty-first century, intricate maps of haunted fingers strategically or arbitrarily splayed across faces sensing the icy cold rigidity of metal or the sharp prick of a pin were considered to be relatively rare. As quickly as they had come into view, they started to vanish.

Though referral has remained a common phenomenon, far-removed, topographically precise, modality-specific referral became exceptional, found in roughly 7 percent of amputees by 2000 (Flor, et al. 2000) and in only 3 percent of amputees by 2005 (Taub 2005). Once again researchers had to explain a glaring contradiction. If homuncular invasion was the cause of phantom limb syndrome and if mislocation was the quintessential perceptual correlate of remapping or cortical geography taking place in the brains of amputees, why did topographically precise, modality-specific referral become so rare? What happened to those phantoms that wandered across corporeal terrains to cozy into faces, ears, and genitals?

Some researchers argued that it is the very process of procuring viable research material that is to blame. For instance, Taub suggested that Ramachandran was mistaken about referred maps precisely for this reason:

> The actual point-to-point facial remapping that Ramachandran found is very rare. In our research, we had one patient for whom there was facial remapping. But, we had four other patients with cortical reorganization and no facial remapping. It was a good hypothesis and actually, it was Ramachandran's hypothesis that inspired me to work on cortical reorganization. We had a public interchange at a meeting in 1993, where he said that his facial remapping phenomenon was the perceptual equivalent to Pons's physiological data. I pointed out that it was an excellent hypothesis, but it was still a hypothesis that required demonstration, to which he got very excited and he said, "It isn't a hypothesis. It's true. What else could it be?" To which I said, "I don't know what else it could be but there

is no evidence that your assertion is correct." What actually happened with Ramachandran was interesting. There's no question in my mind that he was reporting accurately what he had observed; he wasn't falsifying anything. But he chose to emphasize the subjects who experienced facial remapping. He's a very personable individual and his friends in the San Diego area sent him the very patients he was interested in. At first he got a large number of patients with facial remapping and then as time went on, he began to recruit people from the general amputee population. In the last ten patients, there was not a single case of facial remapping and that's about what we got, maybe 3 percent of the population. Now, what is evident is that you cannot have a theory on the nature of phantom limb based on 3 percent of amputees. So I mean you put it all together and it's sort of an historical accident. (Taub 2005)

In her analysis of the developing field of reproductive science, Clarke (1995b, 183, 187) argued, "in order to observe or produce the phenomena they study, all working scientists must obtain and manage research materials." She described the "catch-as-catch-can ethos" that predominated materials acquisition at the turn of the twentieth century. In the neuroscientific study of phantoms, this catch-as-catch-can ethos gave way mid-twentieth century to a *quality-catch ethos.* Researchers were increasingly interested in acquiring or enlisting remarkable phantoms: phantoms that shrunk (telescoping); phantoms that remained fixed (paralysis); phantoms that penetrated objects; phantoms that retained the contorted posture and sensorial quality of the intact limb prior to amputation (pain memories); and, as Taub intimated, phantoms amenable to topographically precise, modality-specific referral.

Taub argued that personable researchers can at times unwittingly produce erroneous historical "accidents" that at first blush seem to be accurate, factual, and valid. However, I would suggest that this type of disparaging "narrative of blame" is a cousin to the "great mind" account of biomedical and techno-scientific innovation; scientific discovery, in fact, is not a product of the indomitable, independent, and naturally generative (and mostly male) mind, and it is not the byproduct of personable researchers who attract precisely what they want and need. Indeed, Ramachandran and others were not mistaken about topographically precise, modality-specific mislocation. To be sure, the phenomenon was as "real" a chapter in this ghost story as furry, raw, and petrified specters of limbs, as denial-based misbehaving ghosts, as limb facsimiles that waved good-bye in earnest, or as grotesque and painfully contorted "memories" that haunted "for life."

As the implications of cortical reorganization became the subject of debate, what researchers expected to find or not find changed dramatically. Cortical reorganization became conceptualized as dynamic, as a product of activity (of adjacent homuncular parts) rather than of inactivity (a lack of sensory input from the periphery), and consequently, referred maps only made sense as short-lived, indistinct, and perceptually vague phenomena. If remapping occurred as a process over time (whether gradual or rapid), one would expect a referral map (superimposed on a face, for instance) to move, to morph, to change size and shape as the cortex gradually or rapidly reorganized, and referred sensation would expectedly be sensed in the same way, as dynamic and thus indefinite and elusive.

In fact, researchers since the mid-1990s have found dynamic maps, maps that disappeared, expanded, or shifted over time. For example, Halligan (1994, 1342; emphasis added) and his colleagues wrote about D.M.'s precise topographic mapping a year after their initial evaluation: "Unlike the original assessment [of D.M.], the referred sensations were now less reliable and did not constitute a stable topographic mapping between specific regions of the face and localized parts of the phantoms limb. . . . Reports of the little finger, found reliably a year before at one specific location, were now found at *seven different locations.*" It appears that surveying the geography of fractioned bodies-in-brains was more difficult than researchers and others suspected. The crossing over of brain-based body parts was a dynamic process that prevented researchers from definitively locating phantoms once and for all. Indeed, D.M. lived not with one phantom situated appropriately within her brain-based body-map sharing space with neighboring body parts. Instead, she lived with seven of her littlest fingers scattered arbitrarily across the surface of her face.

Cortical Plasticity

References to the causal role of cortical plasticity in phantom manifestation after major amputation began to emerge with increased frequency around 1990. Sometimes termed "neural remodeling," "neuronal/neural rearrangement," "neural plasticity," "neuronal colonization," "synaptic remodeling," "cortical reorganization," "cortical remapping," or "cortical invasion," reorganization of the cerebral cortex in neurophysiologic terms referred to changes in the cortical geography of the brain, principally within the primary somatosensory (see for example Karl, et al. 2001) and motor cortices (see for example Dettmers, et al. 2001)[17] on a scale often described as massive or dramatic. Over the next few decades, researchers found both immediate and long-term changes in cortical structure and function after deafferentation and debated the degree to which these changes were permanent and stable; idiosyncratic or universal; preventable; and/or reversible.

The widespread acceptance of the malleability of the sensory and motor homunculi by the turn of the twenty-first century was contributory to and consonant with a larger trend in neuroscientific research at the time of challenging the relative stability of neuronal connections in the adult human brain, a trend that necessitated the development of a new model of cerebral function. For instance, Ramachandran (1998, 1859) argued that advances made in the area of cortical reorganization after deafferentation mandated the abandonment of antiquated theory: "The modular, hierarchical, 'bucket brigade' model of the brain popularized by computer engineers [needs] to be replaced by a more dynamic view of the brain in which there is a tremendous amount of back-and-forth interaction between different levels of hierarchy and across different modules." The illusive, shape-shifting phantom forced researchers to envision the brain as dynamic rather than relatively static. And, if the embodied ghost could not be imagined as an artifact of too-full buckets spilling over into one another, there must be other processes as work.

Assumptions about the structure, functionality, and organization of the human brain had to be entirely rethought, and as some researchers zealously argued, the remapped brains of traumatic, surgical, congenital, and elective amputees provided some of the most fruitful insights. Perhaps most notably, some asserted that reorganization itself had to be reconceptualized as basic to human cortical development and function. Among those at the forefront of this research was Taub, whose work was based on both amputees and stroke patients. He asserted that the brain should be appreciated by neuroscientists as amenable to experientially based reorganization. In fact, it should be understood as "built for" restructuring (Taub 2005). Such ideation led him to ask, if the brain is capable of remapping itself in response to the absence of sensory input, how might the brain respond to "excessive" sensory input and, by implication, "novel" sensory input? In line with this query, Taub and others demonstrated that cortical remapping occurred under conditions of both reduced and enhanced peripheral input or stimulation, what have been termed "injury-related" and "use-dependent" reorganization (see for example Elbert and Rockstroh 2004).[18] Taub explained,

> There are two kinds of reorganization, afferent increase and afferent decrease, one might say injury-related and use-dependent cortical reorganization. For a few years, no one recognized that these were behaviorally different causations. But, in 1994, I starting thinking, "Wait a second; there are two separate things going on." The mechanisms may be similar. You have injury-related cortical reorganization where the lip invades the former hand area and now presumably the other extremity has to do the work of both, so you get an increase in the size of the cortical representation of the intact hand. You have two kinds of cortical reorganization in a single brain. (Taub 2005)

Indeed, it was the experimental investigation into and conceptual elaboration of the relationship between use- and injury-related reorganization that prompted researchers to conceive of phantom limb as a product of neuronal *activity* rather than of *inactivity*, a proposition that had significant implications both for the treatment of phantom pain and for facile prosthesis use. Let me elaborate on the relationship between

cortical reorganization and phantom pain before discussing the implications for prosthetization in more detail.

In the early 1990s, researchers characterized cortical reorganization as
a dysfunctional process, one that was beneficial to the organism during
early development but in cases of deafferentation was quite maladaptive.
It was a capacity never "intended" for the adult human brain. In an interview for *Discover*, Kaas elaborated on this position: "I doubt that it does
anybody any good to have their missing arm mapped out across their
face, or to suffer from extreme pain. . . . But these things demonstrate
that the adult brain has far greater flexibility than we thought. They are a
result of brain plasticity that works against the person" (Shreeve 1993, 6).

By the mid-2000s, cortical reorganization was decidedly functional,
in fact beneficial (Mercier, et al. 2006) and fundamentally adaptive
(Elbert and Rockstroh 2004). Even by the mid-1990s, the language that
researchers used to describe the process began to change. What had previously been described as dramatic reorganization or reorganization on
a massive scale became cortical modification or remodeling. And alongside characterizations such as "invasion," "occupation," and "takeover"
were descriptors like "recruitment," "expansion," "cohabitation," "overlap,"
and "shift." For example, Reilly and Sirigu (2008, 197) wrote, "The well-
documented postamputation reorganization—in which remaining body
parts expand their representations to include the cortical area that previously controlled the amputated limb—appears to be less of an aggressive
takeover of the amputated limb's cortical territory than a peaceful cohabitation of remaining body parts' muscle representation with the amputated body part's movement representation." Moreover, Taub elaborated
on the significance of such a dramatic change in perspective:

> The idea was that there was a functional correlate of cortical reorganiza-
> tion. Up until that time people had worked primarily with animals, who
> can't talk. And that is one of the reasons that there was no strong evidence
> of the functional significance of cortical reorganization. Phantom pain
> had previously been considered adverse, but if we thought of it as func-
> tional we could imagine advantageous consequence. (Taub 2005)

Remapping became "advantageous" because the process was found to be correlated with the amount and intensity of phantom limb pain, with telescoping, and with pain memories (Flor 2003, 2002a, 2002b), but not with phantom sensations (Flor, et al. 2000).[19] That reorganization resulted in (or was the consequent of) phantom pain and pain memories would seem to signify dysfunction, so why was this finding the impetus for such a profound shift in perspective, for remapping becoming advantageous?

The productive link between phantom pain and cortical reorganization seems at first glance to be quite tenuously made until the legacy of explicit localizationism (Star 1989) is taken into consideration. Even if regions of the cortex could/did switch their functional and structural allegiance from one body part to another, researchers did not abandon the presupposition that space was equated with purpose, that function could be localized, that certain areas or parts of the brain carried out specific functions. In the early 1990s, research surfaced on what was described as "electrically 'silent' zones, or islands . . . found within the reorganized region of cortex" (Katz 1992a, 286). At the time, these islands of inactivity were thought to be simply too far from the neighboring areas of vibrant neuronal activity to be recruited by other homuncular areas, by other cortical regions; they were for all purposes dead zones. By the late 1990s, these dead zones were recharacterized as pockets of allegiance, atrophied homuncular areas that retained at least some of their original sensory and motor function. For example, Doetsch (1997, 13, 15; emphasis added) wrote,

> Although physiological reorganization takes place—in the sense that previously ineffective sensory inputs gain excitatory access to a set of cortical neurons—this physiological remapping apparently is not accompanied by significant functional remapping. Activation of a set of cortical neurons appears to retain its *original meaning*! . . . The trick is to identify the positive and negative features of brain plasticity, and to develop ways (physiological, pharmacological, behavioral, etc.) to enhance the former and diminish the later.

Taub elaborated on how these pockets of allegiance worked advantageously in the case of both stroke patients and amputees:

> In our research, we were able to show that after stroke the cortical representation of the affected hand shrinks by a half, and then through constraint-induced movement therapy [when the "good" side is prevented from movement, forcing use of the "bad" side], it will expand back to normal size. What everyone typically points to, which is a fascinating phenomenon, is Mike Merzenich's invasion. But, I will be willing to lay ten-to-one odds that the cortical area shrinks but remains. Not all of the synaptic space has been taken up by the axonal sprouting and there is still representation of the limb there; it just hasn't been demonstrated. What happens in amputees is you get this referral to the phantom but the referral is not stable, which suggests a rapid alteration of the balance of excitatory/inhibitory factors in different parts of the body projecting to the area. And, the area will keep shifting. (Taub 2005)

Because these islands retained the capacity to receive input from the periphery, because they remained at least somewhat allied to the amputated limb, researchers speculated that phantom movement and/or sensation could return input to these silent cortical islands of allegiance—"normalizing" homuncular geography and consequently, preventing phantom pain (see for example Mackert, et al. 2003)—and in fact, less cortical reorganization was found to be correlated with less phantom pain.

This was an incredibly old idea in a very new package. Purposeful movement of one's phantom had always been advised because it was considered restorative and crucial to prosthetic animation, and because it was indispensable to the treatment of phantom pain and/or key to its prevention. Phantoms animated, vitalized, gave life to prostheses and therefore, keeping one's phantom fit was historically thought of as essential to facile prosthesis use, as well as to adequate prosthetic investment, incorporation, or coupling. And, such coupling, clinicians argued, helped to stave off pathological pain. At the turn of the twenty-first century, keeping the phantom fit allowed neural connectivity between the periphery and the somatosensory and motor cortices to remain active and healthy, readied for "reexpansion" or "reactivation."

Interested in the role of phantom-use in stimulating or "reawakening" deafferentated areas of the cortex, researchers explored these cortical islands of allegiance (see for example Ulger, et al. 2009). Brain imaging studies demonstrated that movement of the residual limb or stump produced a pattern of cortical activity that was dissimilar to what was termed "virtual" or "willed" movement of the phantom and demonstrated that phantom movement more closely approximated the pattern of activity produced by the intact limb than by the residual limb. In other words, moving the phantom "looked" in the brain more like moving the intact hand (on the other side) than it did like moving the stump. Sumitani (2010, 338) and his colleagues wrote, "In terms of the perception of limb movements in the brain, there may be no discrimination between phantom and healthy limbs." The supposition that the deafferentated brain responds differently to stump activity than it does to phantom activity had significant implications for the treatment and prevention of phantom pain. In fact, phantom "exercise" became requisite to reawakening cortical islands of silence and staving off pain.

Brain imaging may have aided researchers in the reincarnation of lifeless "partial corpses," but targeting allied islands of silence through phantom exercise also reinvoked the time-worn concept of explicit localizationism—the notion that the brain is composed of discrete functional areas—an idea that supported the biopolitical "mission of reading the internal through the external, thus bringing the invisible into sight" (Gross 2011, 108). Pictures of the brain's deep interior or even convoluted surface, just like all images of the body's viscera, make the exceedingly private and once unseen open to public consumption and vulnerable to scrutiny; in fact, the interiors of some bodies have become of-the-social-body in this way, and consequently, they belong to all of us. And as Casper (1998a) argued, when the viscus is rendered visible, something uncertain is often given substance, legitimacy, and purpose while something else is often concomitantly subject to conceptual and material erasure.

Vis-à-vis the neuroimaging of haunted and prosthetized cortices, the brain has become an ever more productive and powerful signifier of who we are and what we can become. However, these images also expose the fact that we can no longer "discriminate" between healthy, natural limbs and other brain-based limbs. Limbs are just that, limbs. Fleshy, haunted, reattached, residual, as well as homuncular, willed, artificial, virtual, and other appendages have become integral to understanding the nature, features, and potential of the body-in-the-brain.

We Are Smarter Than Our Brains

> We know that the source of phantom limb is in the brain itself, he says
> [Ramachandran]. Far from being deadweight in the brain, the cortex
> associated with the lost limb is alive and well, passing messages further
> on up into the system. The messages may not be originating in the limb
> anymore, but the rest of the *brain doesn't know that.* (Shreeve 1993, 5;
> emphasis added)

Researchers disagreed about the process by which neighboring or adjacent areas of the homunculi (and other cortical areas) began to utilize the "fallow" regions left silent by deafferentation. In contrast to the theory of neural sprouting or aborization proposed by Pons and others, Ramachandran advanced what has been termed the "unmasking hypothesis," emphasizing the role of hidden circuitry.[20] Because cortical remapping occurs within weeks of deafferentation, he speculated that the reactivation of dormant circuits, rather than the laying down of new circuits, was taking place in the brains of amputees (Ramachandran and Rogers-Ramachandran 1996). The adult human brain, he proposed, is predominantly characterized by redundancy, by latent neuronal connectivity that is typically inhibited and hence, nonfunctional (Ramachandran 2005). As a consequence of neuronal competition, stronger synapses dominate weaker adjacent synapses, effectively "masking" their activity. However, in the brains of amputees, weaker neurons are unmasked, becoming active and functionally significant. Ramachandran argued that far from

being stagnant, "each neuron in the map is in a state of dynamic equilib-
rium with other adjacent neurons; its significance depends strongly on
what other neurons in the vicinity are doing (or not doing)" (Ramachandran and Blakeslee 1998, 35). Neuronal *activity*, he asserted, was the
primary source of phantom sensations, not neuronal *inactivity*. Ramachandran (1998, 33) wrote in the case of his patient Tom,

> To put it crudely, the phantom emerges not from the stump but from the
> face and jaw, because every time Tom smiles or moves his face and lips,
> the impulses activate the "hand" area of his cortex, creating the illusion
> that his hand is still there. Stimulated by all these spurious signals, Tom's
> brain literally hallucinates his arm.

Because the brain can be stimulated by "spurious" signals, it can literally be outwitted, a tendency that Ramachandran exploited in his effort
to treat phantom limb pain. For example, in cases of phantom paralysis
or painful flexion (a tightly clenched phantom hand with fingers digging
into the palm, for example), Ramachandran placed amputees' hands (the
intact hand and the phantom hand) into a mirror box. The mirror box
was a simple cardboard square with a mirror inserted down the middle,
allowing the intact hand to be projected onto the phantom. "The reflection of his [intact] hand is optically superimposed on the . . . phantom
limb so that he has the distinct visual illusion that the phantom limb had
been resurrected. If he now made . . . movements while looking in the
mirror, he received visual feedback that the phantom limb was obeying
his command" (Ramachandran and Rogers-Ramachandran 2000, 319).

According to Ramachandran and others, this crude device was
extraordinarily effective in producing change in phantom morphology
and movement. It caused telescoping and reversed telescoping, led to
impossible posturing or the normalization of posture, prompted feelings
of movement and enhanced awareness, produced other morphologic
distortions, and caused phantoms to disappear. In terms of the latter,
Ramachandran exclaimed, "What we had achieved, therefore, may be the
first known case of an 'amputation' of a phantom limb!" (Ramachandran

and Rogers-Ramachandran 1996, 382). Because "the brain doesn't 'know' that the hand is missing" (Ramachandran and Rogers-Ramachandran 1996, 379), it could easily be tricked with carnivalesque mirror illusions. Remarkably, by the end of the 1990s, we had truly become smarter than our brains, and it was the phantom that showed us how.

On the basis of the idea that the brain can be deceived, amputees were also trained to use "augmented" or "immersive" reality to treat their phantom pain. For example, training that required an amputee to move his or her phantom to match prerecorded movements of a hand both resulted in pain reduction and, importantly, showed reversed cortical reorganization (Bergmans, et al. 2002). Employing the concept of the mirror box, others have created virtual reality environments that allowed amputees to both view and control the motion of their phantoms in order to reawaken paralyzed phantoms (Murray, et al. 2007), alleviate phantom pain, and reverse cortical reorganization (Brodie, Whyte, and Waller 2003; Giraux and Sirigu 2003; O'Neill, dePaor, and Mac Lachlan 1997). Because the deafferentated area of the brain was thought to remain functional (or functionally allied) for years or decades after amputation, phantoms could be utilized for pain prevention or amelioration even long after amputation. This line of argumentation is another aspect of the discourse on *phantom utility*. Because they assertedly produce a unique neurophysiologic signature (different from use, movement, and sensation of the residual limb or intact limb), phantom limbs became eminently productive phenomena with astonishing potential readied for harnessing. In fact, it was argued that phantoms should be protected from "learned non-use" and should be resurrected whenever possible. For example, Ramachandran and Hirstein (1998, 1625) wrote, "We are now exploring the possibility that a long-lost phantom that has faded many years ago in an arm amputee or even one that never existed (e.g. in some patients with a congenitally missing arm) may be lying dormant somewhere in the brain. If so, can it be revived?"

Still, it was by way of prosthetic animation that phantom utility could be fully realized, and it was this relationship with and to prostheses that solidified the phantom's indispensability to amputees, as well as to neuroscientists.

Phantom Utility

Phantom limb pain was a correlate of cortical reorganization, and the most effective means of treating the widespread and often unendurable pain brought on by the embodied ghost was the prevention of reorganization (see for example Huse, et al. 2001). If sensory and motor cortices remained amenable to the reestablishment of a connection with the periphery, then the truncated nerves of the residual limb retained access to the deafferentated cortex, to islands of allegiance (Mackert, et al. 2003). Like phantom exercise, sufficient stimulation of the stump provided input that thwarted reorganization and averted the onset of phantom pain by reawakening or reactivating silent cortical islands and normalizing homuncular geography (Fraser, et al. 2001). In other words, both phantom movement and stump stimulation, researchers argued, had the capacity to prevent and even *reverse* cortical remapping (Mercier, et al. 2006). In fact, researchers demonstrated that prosthesis use (prosthesis-induced increased use of an amputation stump) decreased cortical reorganization (Weiss, et al. 1999) and that decreased or reversed reorganization was correlative with pain reduction and elimination. Indeed, the extent of cortical reorganization after amputation was reportedly directly related to daily prosthesis use (Karl, et al. 2004) and to the frequency of phantom pain (Fraser, et al. 2001).

Dhillon (2005) and his colleagues surmised that functional connections between the periphery and the cortex could be strengthened with training and suggested that prostheses could potentially interface directly with residual nerves to allow an amputee to have closed-looped control of a prosthesis with significant implications for prosthetic facility but also for pain prevention. And, the "gullible" brain could with little difficulty be fooled into adopting an alternative limb as its very own. The authors wrote, "Our study implies that if a neuroprosthetic arm were to be interfaced to the residual nerve stumps, amputees might be able to improve control over its movements and incorporate it into their body image through the effects of training, learning and central plasticity" (Dhillon, et al. 2005, 2631). The use of upper-limb functional or myoelectric prostheses, rather than purely cosmetic alternatives, was found to permit more extensive use of the residual limb, reduce phantom pain, and correlate with less cortical reorganization. For example, Flor (2003, 69) reported,

> The provision of correlated input into the amputation zone might be an effective method for influencing phantom pain. FMRI was used to investigate the effects of prosthesis use on phantom limb pain and cortical reorganization. Patients who systematically use a myoelectric prosthesis that provides sensory and visual as well as motor feedback to the brain showed much less phantom limb pain and cortical reorganization than patients who used either a cosmetic prosthesis or none at all.

Even long after amputation of a limb, the use of functional prostheses—not the cumbersome deadweight of realistic but passive alternatives—assertedly led to decreased pain in amputees who may have been tormented for years by unrelenting and unbearable agony. In other words, functional prostheses provide peripheral stimulus, producing use-dependent reorganization that researchers argued countervailed injury-related reorganization (Elbert and Rockstroh 2004; Weiss, et al. 1999).

Spatiality and Phantom-Prosthetic Relations

At the turn of the twenty-first century, prosthetization was thought to effectively ameliorate phantom pain through the prevention or even reversal of cortical remapping after amputation. And, because phantoms were considered vital to prosthetic animation, they became a necessary or at least a desirable precondition for harnessing the curative properties of artificial limbs. Embodied ghosts had undeniably secured a prominent place in the history of neuroscience and had become utterly indispensable to amputees (who should keep them healthy in order to promote facile prosthesis use), prosthetists and other practitioners (who should use virtual and artificial reality, among other means, to coax phantoms into friendly phantom-prosthetic relations), and neuroscientists (who should use the phantom "window" to peer into the fractioned and prosthetized body-in-the-brain).

Cortical mapping and neuroimaging allowed researchers to see the utility of phantoms—to appreciate their curative, animating, affiliative, and generative properties—as well as to further territorialize the body-in-the-brain. Like the physical body, the brain-based body has been dissected, territorialized, and employed as resource. It has been surveyed, marked, plotted, charted, and appraised by those who are committed to "seeing" and understanding its features and functions. The body-in-the-brain has, in Foucault's (1973, 3) terms, become "a space, whose lines, volumes, surfaces, and routes are laid down, in accordance with a now familiar geometry, by the anatomical atlas" (Foucault 1973, 8). As a centerpiece of bio-monitoring, the anatomical atlas imposes spatiality onto the human body, whether in its fleshy or brain-based form, in order to strategically represent its interior, surface, processes, and structures in classificatory terms. Because "Classificatory thought gives itself an essential space" (Foucault 1973, 9), the body exists only in relation to that space, and its existence reaffirms the historicity, the rational order, and the taxonomic logic that governs the anatomical atlas, neuro-politics, and techno-corporeality, among many other aspects of the biopolitical order.

Visualized maps of cortices are persuasive and rarely challenged because they have both defensible credibility and dramatic appeal, because they are easy-to-read records of where we have been and optimistic charts of where we might go, and because images like these are presumably characterized by clarity, accuracy, and truth. Seeing, after all, is tantamount to knowing (Lynch and Woolgar 1990; Dumit 2004; Joyce 2006). Consequently, embodiment and corporeality—like behavior, drive, emotion, temperament, and much more—are increasingly understood in distinctly neurophysiologic terms. In the same way that the "mind seems visible within the brain, [as] the space between person and organ flattens out—mind is what brain does" (Rose 2007, 198), the body too seems reducible to the brain "as increasingly more human attributes become folded into neurocognitive spaces" (Williams, Katz, and Martin 2011, 238).

Neuroimaging undoubtedly produces provocative and persuasive pictures, but the practice also creates "remainders," residues, remnants that are resistant to biomedical rationalization because the body and its parts are quintessentially recalcitrant. As Van Loon (2002, 111,112) explained, "Modern technoscience is centrally concerned with 'presenting,' that is the making visible of phenomena. . . . [B]y the same token . . . it can only do so by creating another *remainder*: of that which defies visualization" (Van Loon 2002, 111,112; emphasis added). Phantom distortion, phantom proliferation, phantom mislocation, phantom shape-shifting, phantom disappearance, phantom reawakening, phantom utility, and phantom animation are all exemplars of visualization defied.

The recalcitrance of embodied ghosts has materialized out of friendly and contentious networked relations with neuroscientists, psychoanalytic theory, macaque monkeys, postwar renormalization policies, epileptics, cortical cartographers, malingerers, brain imaging technologies, mirror boxes, and artificial limbs, to name a few. Misbehaving ghosts are meaningful interactional or relational partners for individuals, collectives, objects, and the like. Phantom limbs have always been historically situated, relational, or networked *effects* with affiliative qualities and transgressive tendencies that have been the impetus behind many transformations within and between technologies and bodies. Indeed, phantom-prosthetic relations have been pivotal to dramatic shifts in neuroscientific thought and have, in the contemporary context, undeniably taken center stage. Because prostheses assuage phantom pain while intervening in cortical reorganization, and because phantoms are so amenable to technologic conjoin-ment, these ghosts have become coupled to machines "in theory" with the same intimacy to which they had long been coupled "in practice." This, however, may prove in the coming decades to be a lethal joining.

6

Phantom-Prosthetic Relations

The Modernization of Amputation

Prostheses and phantoms are "objects" that have what Lucy Suchman (2005, 379) called "affiliative powers"; neither the prosthesis nor the phantom are in her terms "innocent"; rather, they are "fraught with significance for the relations that they materialize." They facilitate and enter into affiliations of various kinds, and accordingly, they are much more than mere instruments or tools adopted for the purposes of restoring or enhancing the functionality of limbs and, by extension, bodies. They are much more than commodities exchanged or valued with the intent of satisfying human want or need. They are much more than pathology or sensation belonging only to the partial body. They are much more than hypotheses or knowledge residing contentedly in the realm of pure ideas.

Even as they at times "present themselves to us as self evident" (Suchman 2005, 381), as "black-boxed" (Latour 1987, 2) such that their controversial histories, their biopolitical origins, and their inner workings are reduced to mere "output," prostheses and phantoms alike have refused to be fixed or determined. And, even when they are made by biomedicine and technoscience to appear concretely synthetic, decidedly inert, entirely ideational, or fundamentally natural, objects with affiliative powers refuse to be overly determined material or abstract "things" designed with intent or discovered with wonder. In fact, the "malleability" of these objects enables people to establish and renew social relations and identities, and in some cases, it is through such affiliations or associations that "objects displace human beings as relationship partners . . . or . . . mediate human relationships" (Knorr-Cetina 1997, 2).

Accordingly, amputees, prosthetists, surgeons, neuroscientists, as well as other individuals and collectives, have developed prosthetic-centered and phantom-centered affiliations or, in Knorr-Cetina's (1997, 1) terms, "object-centered socialities."

However, it is not just the affiliations that prostheses and phantoms have developed with amputees and others, not just the practices or relational trajectories that these affiliations promote for people, but rather the capacity for objects to affiliate with one another and the concomitant effects that those affiliations have for objects themselves that is the frame of this chapter. Phantom limbs are "dissected" and prostheses "dismantled" in order to reveal the ways in which phantom-prosthetic relations have shifted over the twentieth and into the twenty-first century from (1) the prosthetization of phantoms to (2) the phantomization of prostheses to (3) phantom-prosthetic reciprocity. Thus, I take seriously Moore and Casper's (2009, 9) call to commune with ghosts in order to see which aspects of their history have begun to fade. But, I also commune with machines in order to see how the successfully transcendent might have been otherwise.

Often considered in isolation from the very bodies they mimic—as disembodied—often theorized as distinct from the very machines they inhabit—as dissevered—often removed from the very history that established their legacy—as decontextualized—phantoms have also time and again been cut off from the social milieus in which they materialized. Here, phantoms are reattached to dismembered bodies, reunited with artificial limbs, and are reminded of where they have been. The modernization of amputation is a complex history: amputation surgery transitioned from barbaric to constructive; a collaborative relationship between prosthetic science and amputation surgery was forged; the field of prosthetic science matured and "militarized"; the "meaning" of dismemberment for individuals, families, communities, and the nation shifted time and again; amputees surfaced as icons of progress, hybridization, and technologic liberation; and phantoms developed a fundamental utility that was antithetical to what seems to be their impending displacement.

The Modernization of Amputation

Historically, amputation had been a last resort for the management of severely damaged limbs. Because the patient would be likely to die from blood loss or sepsis, early interventions were always desperate measures. For example, Porter (1997) characterized the incidence of hospital gangrene, one of the most troublesome of the septic diseases during the nineteenth century, as endemic to the procedure. In fact, the introduction of antiseptics in the mid-1800s significantly improved survival rates (Meier 2004), but prior to their use, surgeons did little to curtail the onset of infection. For instance, Vitali (1978, 3) noted, "It is difficult to realize that surgeons seemed almost to glory in avoiding even normal social cleanliness in their professional work." Despite many medical and surgical advances, however, including the advent of anesthesia (Meier 2004), the practice of amputation throughout the nineteenth century remained commonly fatal.[1] "It was said that it was less dangerous for a patient to have his thigh amputated by gunfire than by a surgeon" (Vitali 1978, 3), and "the public at large [were] apt to call amputation the opprobrium of surgery" (Figg and Farrell-Beck 1993, 456). If one survived amputation, there were available few and often crude prosthetic options, which began to change somewhat after the Civil War (1861–1865) with the government provision of prostheses to Union Army Civil War veterans, a policy that spawned the entrepreneurial design of manufactured limbs (McDaid 2002).[2]

In the postbellum context, the medical literature emphasized the role that prostheses played in returning an amputee to productivity and to physical normalcy. However, despite claims that amputees were readily accepted by the public as well as their families and that they had no need to hide their "deformities," despite claims that the visible wound was a badge of courage on and off the battlefield (Figg and Farrell-Beck 1993), despite claims that amputees were icons of the "the triumph of a nation" (Goler 2004, 179), physicians still advocated the use of prostheses to stave off the harmful effects of pity and "unwanted stares and questions" (Ott 2002, 11).

Artificial limbs restored mobility, but this was a *prima facie* goal; the restoration of mobility fooled others into looking past the loss in a context in which the integrity of the physical body was a reflection of the quality of one's character (Mihm 2002). As Ott (2002, 28) argued, "Not only was it natural to conceal physical defects, but also a conspicuous 'deficiency of the body' attracted attention and invited sympathy, and such reactions from others were inimical to maintaining self-respect." Prosthetization dissuaded others from attending too ardently to an amputee's losses; physical degradation, when given too much attention, could easily lapse into a more serious degradation of the self. Still, prosthetization was motivated by more than replacement or restoration. In fact, artificial limbs enabled technological salvation because prosthetization was tantamount to a "conversion experience" (Herschbach 1997, 31). The unsightly, the pitiful, the debilitating were utterly transformed by the miracle of prosthetization. Dismemberment by way of technologic salvation could open up a world of possibilities. "Amputation . . . could lay out new paths, voyages of discovery, and . . . science and technology would show the way" (Herschbach 1997, 25).

Importantly, the rhetoric of technologically mediated salvation vis-à-vis prosthetic conversion enabled guiltless condemnation. As Stiker (1997, 4) rhetorically inquired, "People have never felt comfortable with what appears deformed, spoiled, broken. Is it because they never knew whose fault it was?" Dismemberment was the price paid for reckless behavior, careless soldiering, sinful deeds, or some other act deserving of public disapproval, but prosthetization had the effect of absolution. The sinful, the unlucky, the unfit, the stupid, and the foolish were forgiven, and the public too was absolved, released from the guilt that judgment exacted. The disfigured may have been to blame, but through technologically mediated salvation everyone could put the idea of "fault" behind them. Moreover, prosthetization brought these bodies into "a regime of tolerable deviance. If disability falls too far from an acceptable norm, prosthetic intervention seeks to accomplish an erasure of difference altogether; yet failing that, as is always the case with prosthesis, the minimal goal is to return one to an acceptable degree of difference."

Because prostheses were thought to "competently" replace a missing limb, they fooled those who might stare and question, they transformed disability through erasure, and they "saved" the amputee—body, mind, and spirit. Prostheses had the capacity to deceive others and the self, but they also had the power to trick the body. Artificial limbs coaxed the body into productivity, cajoled it into successful ambulation by provoking and fooling the phantom. In the following case of reverse telescoping, for example, the phantom was "continually antagonized" until it eventually submitted to coordinated locomotion with the artificial limb. Mitchell (1871, 567) wrote,

> When we replace the lost leg by an artificial member—which for purposes of motion competently supplies the place of the missing limb—such feelings as result in the notion of shortening [telescoping] are continually antagonized . . . [and the phantom] acts in locomotion with the acquired member. It is then found that by degrees the leg seems to lengthen again, until once more the foot assumes its proper place.

Artificial limbs coaxed phantoms into their proper place, restored normalcy by hiding disfigurement, and returned efficient, autonomous productivity to males who had lost limbs in conflict with bitter enemies, while also redefining national losses and revitalizing a pained nation. "Potentially helpless and unproductive cripples [were] transformed [when prosthetized] into independent citizens, restored to their masculine role as worker . . . [becoming] safeguards of national (even cosmic) pride and progress" (Herschbach 1997, 23).

In spite of the rhetoric of pride and progress that debatably epitomized public sentiment, Civil War amputees, as Goler (2004, 161) argued, were unequivocally "ambiguous figures," visible reminders of the price paid for battle who "provoked a profound mixture of love and horror, fascination and anxiety . . . ambiguous figure[s], simultaneously epitomizing survival and death, victory and bereavement."[3] They, like all soldiers, embodied bravery and cowardice (Wiley 2002), fearless dedication and unchecked recklessness (Donald 2002). They were honored and pitied, respected and feared. They may have been icons of progress, but they were also overt reminders of the brutalities of war.

Innovations in prosthetic technologies after the Civil War were welcomed but were also thought to have detrimentally affected surgical advancements. For instance, the use of muscle-flaps over bone to increase weight-bearing potential and the practice of disarticulation (amputation through the joint) were abandoned because they resulted in bulbous stumps that were not compatible with the conical shape that limb manufacturers preferred (Vitali 1978). Thus, amputation surgery at the turn of the twentieth century was largely a continuation of practices adopted during the Civil War, when over sixty thousand amputations were performed (Figg and Farrell-Beck 1993). The principle aims of battlefield surgery were to control bleeding and prevent infection (Helling and Kendall 2000), an approach that neglected postoperative concerns, including the shape of the stump, and as a result, many veterans were unable to wear prostheses (Figg and Farrell-Beck 1993, 464).

Despite the lack of coordination between amputation surgeons and limb manufacturers, prostheses were regularly hyped as miraculous, extraordinary, and just like the real thing. They were touted as truly transformative, making over the cripple so that he was equally unimpeded in all walks of life. In fact, he was afforded the opportunity to embody "perfection." For example, Smith (1871, 54) wrote, "In our time, limb-making has been carried to such a state of perfection that both in form and function they so completely resemble the natural extremity that those who wear them pass unobserved and unrecognized in walks of business and pleasure."

In the decades after the turn of the twentieth century, the survival rate after amputation improved dramatically.[4] This was partly a consequence of advances in amputation surgery (Ott 2002), but it was also a result of the modernization of combat. Soldiers in modern warfare were targets of intentional injury and disfigurement by means of the technologies-of-mutilation indicative of conflict from WWI (1914–1918) onward (Bourke 1996; Koven 1994); modern weapons were designed to maim and mutilate but not to kill so that precious resources would be expended on the wounded. Once again, however, during WWI, when more than forty-four hundred amputations were performed (Hermes 2002), the primary concerns of battlefield surgeons were bleeding and shock, "a damage control" philosophy (Helling and Kendall 2000, 935), which resulted in residual limbs that were frequently incompatible with the requirements of prosthetists. As Thomas and Haddan (1945, 11) complained, "There was little or no cooperation between the limbmakers and the surgeons; in fact the surgeon often looked upon the limbmaker as some sort of shyster preying on the amputee, and avoided contact with him whenever possible."

In the wake of the postwar "crippled soldier problem," the then fledgling field of prosthetic science continued to be concerned with restoring an amputee's productive potential (Brown 2002, 263) because of the association of the working male body with masculinity and of the idle, disabled male body with problematic manhood (Brown 2002). In this context, many practitioners and policymakers alike were worried that demobilized disabled veterans could become overly dependent on the state and that if dependency became widespread, disabled veterans could tax an already impoverished nation. Moreover, there was concern that they could also become overly dependent on their families and communities, effectively undermining their own manliness, which, as Brown (2002, 263) argued, had "been consolidated, in large part around the role of the male bread-winner." Prostheses were consequently envisioned as "supplementary limbs" meant to return amputees to the workplace in order to minimize dependency and circumvent the crippled soldier problem (Brown 2002, 270).

In the same way that the rights of women, their very citizenship, has often been "doled out on the basis of how well she conforms to societal norms about 'womanly' or feminine behavior" (Flavin 2009, 182), men's citizenship has often been predicated on their deep and demonstrable devotion to their country and to the ideals of freedom, democracy, justice, and the like. A man's commitment to the nationalistic, war-inspired rhetoric that "framed" his service was always a reflection of the kind and the extent of masculinity he embodied. Indeed, the widespread dissemination, adoption, and institutionalization of a particularly loathsome form of hegemonic masculinity was more central to war-based policy than "winning" ever was.

Although WWI did stimulate the establishment of the artificial limb lab at Walter Reed Hospital and amputation centers across the country managed by the Veterans Administration (VA), only about two hundred independent limb manufacturers existed in the first decades of the twentieth century, and they were characterized as "an unorganized group of rugged individualists, each going his own way" (Thomas and Haddan 1945, 11). In 1917, the surgeon general invited limb manufacturers to Washington, DC, a meeting that "no doubt, contributed more to the development of the science of prosthetics than any other occurrence in history" (Thomas and Haddan 1945, 11). As a result, the American Orthopedic Limb Manufacturers Association was established, and manufacturers began to work collaboratively in an effort to supply veterans with artificial limbs.

Provocation and Cure

From about 1940 to 1950, while coordination between prosthetists and amputation surgeons improved and prostheses grew increasingly sophisticated, practitioners and researchers debated the nature of phantom-prosthetic relations, a debate that was engendered by two apparently contradictory findings: prostheses both provoked phantom limbs and cured phantom limb syndrome. Some studies demonstrated that when donned, prostheses provoked or incited phantoms, causing the intensification or exaggerated vividness of phantom awareness, sensation, and/ or pain; the reawakening or reappearance of previously disappeared or faded phantoms; and reverse telescoping, or the restoration of shrunken or foreshortened phantoms. For example, in terms of the latter, Weiss (1956, 673; original emphasis) wrote,

> The patient stated that when he was without a prosthesis, or when he was
> wearing his cosmetic hand, he felt the phantom as a miniature, tightly

clenched fist which was attached to the end of his stump. When a hook or the *miracle hand* [functional prosthesis] was used, the phantom lengthened and resumed a more normal, open-handed position. . . . [I]t is interesting to note that without the prosthesis, or with the cosmetically acceptable but *functionless* hand, the phantom was felt as a shriveled-up, miniature appendage dangling from the end of the stump. The hook, which did not resemble a hand at all but which restored function, brought the phantom hand back to its normal position. The same was true of the miracle hand.

At the same time, modern prostheses were considered extraordinary for their capacity to cure phantom limb syndrome. Some studies demonstrated that early, regular, and continued prosthesis use caused the phantom to fade, becoming a faint apparition of itself or, in some cases, caused its disappearance altogether (see for example Herrmann and Gibbs 1945; Hoffman 1954b). Both of these findings—cure and provocation—were explained by appealing to the exceptional quality of modern, miraculous, prosthetic technologies. Prostheses that restored function caused phantoms to "naturalize" by re-growing, reappearing, or returning to a vibrant state, effectively curing distortion. And, prostheses that caused phantoms (painful or otherwise) to weaken or vanish effectively cured the syndrome itself. From both perspectives, prostheses were quite transformative to be sure.

Still, it was not until WWII (1941–1945), when fifteen thousand amputations were performed (Thomas and Haddan 1945) that some of the most significant gains in prosthetic science (Northwestern 2002), as well as rehabilitative medicine (Ott 2002) and amputation surgery (Meier 2004), were made. After WWII America celebrated the most wealth and prosperity the country and the world had ever known. Americans considered the modern world to be one "in which people would be free to create themselves anew . . . the world of new opportunities, new possibilities, and limitless hopes" (Farber 1994, 17). Within this milieu of abundance, hope, and renewal, the then entrenched war culture[5] became material in numerous ways, including through the maturation of prosthetic science. The late 1940s to the mid-1950s was considered the peak of prosthetic innovation in the United States until the turn of the twenty-first century, during which quantum leaps were made in technique and technology (Northwestern 2002). The "key findings from this era still provide the conceptual basis for virtually all contemporary techniques" (Michael and Bowker 1994, 100). The U.S. government was the central player in the transformation of the prosthetic industry from a loose assemblage of uncoordinated craftsmen[6]—typically considered ambulance chasers—to an organized and legitimated profession.[7] In April of 1945, U.S. Surgeon General Norman T. Kirk requested that the National Research Council establish the Committee on Prosthetic Devices (CPD), a prosthetics research and development program funded jointly by the Veterans Administration (VA)[8] (Northwestern 1995) and the war department (Kurzman 2003). In July of 1947 the CPD founded the Advisory Council on Artificial Limbs (ACAL), which initiated the Artificial Limb Program (ALP) (CPD 1946; Rang and Thompson 1981). The surgeon general had also gathered prosthetists, surgeons, and engineers together in 1946 to discuss the state of the science (Northwestern 2002),[9] a meeting that marked the establishment of the American Orthotic and Prosthetic Association (AOPA) (Pike and Nattress 1991). The founding of the AOPA acted as a stimulus for the instantiation of ethical standards, educational programs, and university-based research in the field of prosthetic science (Northwestern 2002). Sixteen universities and industrial laboratories were enlisted or organized and funded under the ALP, including Northrop Aviation, Catranis, the U.S. Navy Hospital, the University of California–Berkeley, and the University of California–Los Angeles (Rang and Thompson 1981).[10]

State intervention in prosthetic science was consistent with a larger trend in the United States at the time of blurring the boundaries between science/medicine and the state. "Medical men and scientists were absorbed into the wider machinery of the state in ever-increasing numbers. In this process, medical science became a constitutive force in the creation of a 'knowledge society' built around the functionality of the body" (Goodman, McElligott, and Marks 2003, 5; Pickering

1995). The productive, efficacious, and decisive functionality of the body, especially the male body, became central to American citizenship and a crucial facet of one's social responsibility. Not inconsequently, medicine and science were largely responsible for defining what functionality, and therefore citizenship, entailed.

Governmental response to what was termed the "demobilization crisis" (Gerber 1994, 547) took the form of establishing the CPD and facilitating coordination among limb manufacturers, but it also took the form of censorship. The Office of War Information (OWI), established by executive order in June of 1942, was mandated to coordinate the dissemination of war information intended to assist the public in understanding war-related progress and policy (Blum 1976; Roeder 1996).[11] The OWI emphasized both the production of particular themes within wartime media (Blum 1976)—including movies, comics, and magazines—and the suppression of what Roeder (1996, 51–62) categorized as confusing, disrupting, and disordering imagery. Censored material was housed in the then new Pentagon in a room referred to in internal documentation as the "chamber of horrors" (Roeder 1996, 49). Efforts to eliminate disordering imagery included the deletion of photographs depicting dismemberment because images "could document meaningful sacrifices that Americans made for the larger cause, eventually including even death, but could not demonstrate how thoroughly war could disorder—rip asunder—their individual lives and bodies" (Roeder 1996, 59).

Moreover, in the war's aftermath, in an ever more visual culture—as television began to be marketed starting around 1950—images of amputees were widely circulated in propagandist efforts to promote patriotism; "persuade able-bodied Americans that the convalescence of veteran amputees was not a problem"; and demonstrate a commitment to rehabilitation, while foregrounding American technologic ascendancy (Serlin 2002, 28). What made these images so potent was their relative absence from public consumption during most of the war. "Such photographs are powerful because they appear to telegraph all their meaning to the viewer; they are immediately identifiable signifiers and substitutes for the war itself" (Koven 1994, 1193). Representations of resilient war-wounded veterans were increasingly disseminated as Cold War tensions rose, "transform[ing] amputees into powerful visual and rhetorical symbols" (Serlin 2006, 53). As Serlin (2004, 33–35) deftly argued in his *Replaceable You*, the circulation of these provocative images and captivating stories had myriad effects, not the least of which was the resultant hierarchization of disability. Bodies disabled by modern warfare were considered remarkable, demonstrative of an individual's service and commitment to the state, while bodies disabled from birth, by accident, or by self-mutilation either were associated with the antiquated notion of the "monstrous birth," were considered inept and culpable, or were labeled cowardly and were thought of as undeserving of pity. "In the aftermath of the war . . . veteran male amputees constituted a superior category on an unspoken continuum of disabled bodies" (Serlin 2004, 35).[12]

Amputation Surgery and Techno-Induced Liberation

Massive amputation casualties and related governmental intervention prompted collaboration between the fields of amputation surgery and prosthetic science, fostering common restoration goals, namely, mobility and the reestablishment of "normal" appearance (Vitali 1978). Prior to this point, the two disciplines had fundamentally conflicting objectives. Surgeons prioritized speed and the maintenance of viable tissue at all costs, while prosthetists wanted to ensure postoperative mobility, which necessitated the loss of viable tissue when the shape of the residual limb would be incompatible with subsequent prosthetic replacement (Hughes 1996). Further, surgical amputation produced a residual limb that was simply a passive attachment site for prostheses, a site that did not "actively" participate in ambulation (Ertl 2000). From the prosthetist's perspective, despite the widespread circulation of knowledge concerning the import of stump shape and health for postsurgical prosthetic fitting, during the first half of the twentieth century, amputation surgery was commonly performed without such considerations. In fact, prescriptions provided by surgeons often simply read "fit with artificial leg" (Pike and Nattress 1991, 2). By the mid-twentieth century, amputation surgery was no longer fundamentally barbaric. As Slocum (1949), who published *An Atlas of Amputations,* based on his WWII experience, indicated, amputation was "no longer ghoulish cutting off of a part, but rather it [was] a phase of reconstruction" (Meier 2004, 2).

Clinicians working with amputees to address issues related to rehabilitation or postoperative care in the post-WWII (1941–1945), post–Korean War (1950–1953), and post–Vietnam War (1955–1975) contexts advocated the use of prostheses to prevent or minimize social stigma. If an amputee could hide his deformity, he would give others little reason to be judgmental or disapproving. For instance, Hoover (1964, 48) wrote, "In general, there is very little prejudice toward an amputee who learns to function well with his prosthesis." Amputees were envisioned as "normalized" through prosthetization because artificial limbs had the power to convert the useless and unsightly into the functional and sensible:

> With the development of modern prostheses, most amputees, who only recently were rejected as cripples, are now *accepted by society and by industry as normal persons.* Thus when both the stump and the prosthesis are designed for function, the amputee soon ceases to regard himself as abnormal in any way. . . . Where amputations were once considered only as a life-saving measure they are now performed yearly by the hundreds in a deliberate attempt to substitute a useful prosthesis for a useless, unsightly, or hopelessly deformed extremity. (Thomas and Haddan 1945, 12; emphasis added)

Since the turn of the twentieth century, prostheses had been glorified as normalizing (restoring productivity and combating emasculation and/or stigma) and as transformative (saving the body, mind, and spirit). Yet, by around 1950, prostheses were considered irrefutable marvels of the modern era. As Serlin (2004, 36) argued, "What made new prostheses different from earlier models is that they represented the marriage of prosthetic design to military-industrial production." In the "hyperpatriotic" (Serlin 2002, 35), "hypernationalistic" (Serlin 2004, 2) "Victory Culture" (Engelhardt 1995) of post-WWII America, the correlation of military prowess with prostheses converted amputees into "tools for consensus building . . . [an] apotheosis of domestic engineering" (Serlin 2004, 3).

As a result of the state-sponsored cross-pollination of biomechanics, cybernetics, materials science, and industrial robotics, the then fledgling field of prosthetic science was catalyzed into a biomedical discipline (Serlin 2004). In this context, intense and extensive efforts were undertaken by the state to rehabilitate the war wounded, and the miracles of modern, militarized medicine and science promised to be the tools of renewal. Further, "the association between amputees and state-of-the-art prosthetics research may have been an intentional strategy to link disabled veterans with the positive, futuristic aura surrounding military-industrial science" (Serlin 2002, 55), a strategy that effectively transfigured amputees into icons of military-inspired, technologically induced liberation. They were envisioned as liberated from the physical constraints of disfigurement, from the dire hazards of maladjustment and self-pity, and from the emasculating effects of immobility and lost productivity. For example, Serlin (2004, 29–30) relayed the story of Jimmy Wilson, who became a "poster boy" for the liberating effects of American, militarized prosthetization. He was the sole survivor of a ten-person flight that crashed over the Pacific Ocean who was found after an incredible forty-four hours. In a story reminiscent of George Dedlow's, all four of Jimmy's limbs had to be amputated, but through prosthetization he was not only rehabilitated; he was catapulted into fame. A *Philadelphia Inquirer* campaign raised $105,000 for Jimmy, testifying to his celebrity status, which peaked when he posed with Miss America, Bess Myerson, to advertise the then-new Valiant, a General Motors special designed specifically for lower-limb amputees[13] and, of course, named to glorify them.

The image of the prosthetized soldier, the cyborg[14] warrior, was circulated in the post-WWII context in a propagandist effort to communicate a national commitment to the rehabilitation of demobilized veterans injured in combat, to secure the public's confidence in the state, and to flaunt the technologic prowess of the military—its ability to destroy and to rebuild. This image of the hybridized "killing machine" devoted to the protection of nation and neighbor was vital to establishing and maintaining the conceptual and practical link between masculinity and militarism and consequently, it was a crucial weapon in the state's arsenal.

> If the reciprocal relationship between masculinity and militarism is weakened, so too is the power of the state to manipulate public support for its right to use violence to pursue its policies at home and abroad, as well as to encourage young men to join the armed forces. Thus, the state has a vested interest in maintaining strong ideological links between militarism and masculinity. (Hopton 2003)

The hybridized soldier, the cyborg warrior, embodied technologic transcendence, patriotism, and national consensus building, but he did so only through the exploitation of a particular expression of hegemonic masculinity. The cyborg warrior was stoic, imposing, authoritative, unassailable, and conspicuously powerful. He exemplified what Mellström (2002) termed "homosociality," a techno-masculine sociality that was expressive of *man's* proclivity for techno-corporeal con-joinment. He expressed calculable bodily precision, self-imposed discipline, as well as an adventurous and courageous spirit. And, as "one of the central images of masculinity in the Western cultural tradition . . . the murderous hero, the supreme specialist in violence" was efficiently brutal and effectively terrifying (Connell 1995, 126). He was resolutely masculine and decisively male, evincing the kind of manhood that was far removed from "lily-livered effeminates" (Connell 1995, 127) and emasculated cripples (Siebers 2008).

It is only by engendering, distinguishing, and valuating different styles or forms of masculinity, by constructing and hierarchizing *masculinities*, that hegemonic forms of maleness can come to dominate while other forms are subordinated and marginalized. As both an extension of the remasculinization of amputees in the postbellum and post-WWI contexts, and the centerpiece of renormalization in the hyperpatriotic context of celebrated, military-industrial technologic innovation, the cyborg warrior had a commanding presence, and we cannot underestimate the impact that widely circulated images, stories, ideas, and logics indicative of the battle-ready, hypermasculine male had on dismemberment, phantom limb syndrome, and prosthetization.

Prosthetization became a pivotal and productive project in the surveillance and regulation of male bodies—an unapologetic form of biomonitoring qua the politics of national defense—through the instantiation and spread of this particularly loathsome but decidedly influential version or expression of masculinity, the legacy of which is evident today in the form of the "wondrous," out-jutting, homuncular penis; the primordially male brain-based body scheme, homunculi, and neuromatrix; the rhetoric on the natural and easy affiliation had between "men" and machines; the fetishization of the cyborg warrior readied for violence; and many others.

Coinciding, Embodiment, and the Vital Phantom

As prostheses grew increasingly remarkable, amputees were more fervently encouraged to become invested in their artificial limbs. Ready adaptation and successful embodiment facilitated integration of the new limb into the body scheme and self-concept. Importantly, it was the extraordinary military-inspired prostheses that had the most promise of full integration because they epitomized the complexity of the lost limb.

> Can a simple prosthesis, a piece of wood or plastic, really ever satisfy the amputee as a replacement for a limb? Do we not hear amputees joking about such things as the "splinters" in their legs? It seems to me that a complex prosthesis, such as a hydraulic leg, the mechanism of which in some ways resembles the complexity of a real leg, may be more readily integrated into the body concept of the amputee. Give him a wooden or plastic leg, and he feels that it is artificial. Give him a well-functioning complicated mechanism and, to some extent, you may approximate the complexity of the natural limb he has lost. (Weiss 1958, 28–29)

Adequate investment in one's prosthesis could be determined by the degree to which the phantom and prosthesis *coincided* or were felt as superimposed. Although consistently lauded since before the turn of the twentieth century, the importance of coinciding intensified during the 1950s and 1960s because it was vital for both amputees and the state to invest in the rehabilitative process after WWII and Korea and during Vietnam.[15] Investment was symbolic of the state's capacity to restore productivity to the war-wounded and to rebuild in postwar contexts. It was also demonstrative of the amputee's commitment to embracing renormalization efforts, and thus, phantoms became key to "reading" an amputee's dedication to the rehabilitative process. Coinciding testified to the authentic embodiment of an artificial limb and for some amputees, this was facilitated by purposive training and "exercise." In fact, over the latter half of the twentieth century, clinicians increasingly advocated regular phantom exercise as a means of keeping the phantom fit and thus, capable of coinciding. For example, Stattel (1954, 156; emphasis added) wrote, "When the phantom limb is trained the individual retains the totality of their physical experience. . . . [I]f a healthy phantom feeling exists or is regained by training then it is *brought into line* with the artificial arm." The healthy phantom kept mobile and experientially vibrant by use, training, or exercise could and was harnessed in the service of facile prosthesis use. Ethereal appendages aided amputees in the rehabilitative process because they had an undeniable utility. "Phantom sensations can be kept more 'natural' and more vivid if soon after amputation the patient takes daily exercises in 'willing' phantom movements; such exercises are said to make a patient better able to use a mobile (cineplastic) prosthesis" (Harber 1956, 625).

Phantoms enabled successful prosthetization because coinciding entailed *animation*. Although phantoms had long been thought to occupy or inhabit prostheses, during the 1950s through the mid-1960s, phantoms were characterized as having innate animating properties; they had the intrinsic ability to vivify, to literally bring prostheses "to life," and it was at this time that phantom sensations were most commonly found to be more vivid when a prosthesis was donned than when it was doffed. Although this finding was consistent with some earlier studies, the implications had changed quite radically. It was not the prosthesis that incited the phantom, but rather the phantom felt "at home" when it was allowed to animate, when it was given the opportunity to express its essential attribute. Prostheses did not call out phantoms. Phantoms motivated prostheses. And, because phantoms had the capacity to animate woods, rubbers, metals, and plastics, researchers viewed them as integral to proper prosthetization. Accordingly, they became absolutely indispensable. This period marks a dramatic change in phantom-prosthetic relations, a shift from the *prosthetization of phantoms* to the *phantomization of prostheses*. The literature at the time frequently highlighted the astonishing aspects of phantoms. Rather than being coaxed, cajoled, or fooled, phantoms were depicted as active, as doing "all the work," while the prosthesis became passive, lucky to be animated when donned by an amputee committed to rehabilitation.

As the utility of phantoms began to be widely recognized, clinicians advocated exploiting the ability "to move the phantom voluntarily . . . in training them [amputees] in the use of the prosthesis" (Weiss 1956, 673). It is through coinciding or coalescing—as it was sometimes called—that amputees were thought to appropriately and effectively embody their prostheses so that they became taken-for-granted aspects of corporeality, the body scheme, and the self-concept. This is why practitioners began advocating immediate postoperative fitting—so that "the patient is aided in assuming the standing position as early as possible" (Weiss 1956, 673)—and fitting for children within the first years of life. Kyllonen (1964, 20) wrote, "From the standpoint of the integration of the prosthesis into the body-image, before the pattern is set, it is critical that the child be equipped with a prosthesis early in life. . . . Children rapidly acquire a sense of possessiveness toward the prosthesis as if it were literally a part of themselves."

Reciprocity and Phantom Taming

During the 1970s and 1980s, the discourse on phantom-prosthetic relations changed once again, characterizing the relationship between ghost and machine as entirely reciprocal. Prostheses were certainly remarkable in that they facilitated phantom animation—inciting and renormalizing phantoms—and they were curative—alleviating, preventing, or minimizing phantom limb sensation and, more importantly, phantom pain. In fact, prostheses were deemed universally desired and unequivocally desirable. "Technology can provide a new amputee with sophisticated prosthetic devices which perform many functions as adequately as the original. . . . [T]he adjustment work an amputee faces may be ameliorated by successful use of a prosthesis. *Almost all recent amputees, regardless of age or state of health, want an artificial limb*" (Lundberg and Guggenheim 1986, 199, 206; emphasis added). At the same time, the phantom's presence was considered paramount to recovery; enormously useful to the amputee, the phantom was a marker of potential and of achievement (Sacks 1987). For instance, those amputees whose phantoms failed to "develop" were thought to have difficulty managing prosthetic devices. By the late 1980s, reporting that one felt naked without a prosthesis was considered a sign of apt execution, but more significantly, of meaningful integration, coupling, or embodiment (Lundberg and Guggenheim 1986). Indeed, by this time, phantom loss was overtly maligned. Sacks (1987, 67; emphasis added), for example, wrote, "The disappearance of a phantom may be disastrous, and its recovery, its reanimation, *a matter of urgency.*"

By slapping his stump, one of Sacks's patients resurrected his phantom each morning. "He must 'wake up' his phantom in the mornings: first he flexes the thigh-stump towards him, and then he slaps it sharply—'like a baby's bottom'—several times. On the fifth or sixth slap the phantom suddenly shoots forth, rekindled, *fulgurated,* by the peripheral stimulus. Only then can he put on his prosthesis and walk" (Sacks 1987, 67; original emphasis).

This ritual of phantom awakening and prosthetic animation or quickening demonstrated the kind of reciprocity that was indicative of phantom-prosthetic relations during this period. While the prosthesis was roused by the phantom, the phantom was tamed by its structure. As one amputee explained, "There's this *thing*, this ghost-foot, which sometimes hurts like hell—and the toes curl up, or go into spasm. . . . It goes away when I strap the prosthesis on and walk. I still feel the leg then, vividly, but it's a *good* phantom, different" (Sacks 1987, 69; original emphasis). Haunted limbs were envisioned as productive forces, capable of "fleshing out" prostheses (Saadah and Melzack 1994), while prostheses provided the kind of requisite structure necessary for ensuring phantom refinement. In other words, the phantom needed to be tamed or civilized if its animating properties were to be fully realized and if its very reality was to be heightened by prosthetization. For example, Melzack (1990, 89; emphasis added) wrote,

> The most astonishing feature of the phantom limb is its "reality" to the amputee, which is *enhanced by wearing an artificial arm or leg*; the prosthesis feels real, "fleshed." Amputees in whom the phantom leg has begun to "telescope" into the stump, so that the foot is felt to be above floor level, report that the phantom fills the artificial leg when it is strapped on and the phantom foot occupies the space of the artificial foot in its shoe.

Further, as phantom pain became epidemic, reaching its peak during the 1980s and 1990s, phantom limbs were regularly depicted as potentially quite dangerous, capable of pathologization, and therefore, researchers and clinicians emphasized the therapeutic properties of prostheses. They found that prosthetization was correlated with the prevention, reduction, and elimination of phantom limb pain (see for example Abramson and Feibel 1981). By contrast, the pathological phantom—the distorted, twisted, pained phantom—had its origins in disuse and neglect, in the failure to properly civilize embodied ghosts.

By the turn of the twenty-first century, researchers demonstrated that prosthesis use decreased cortical reorganization or remapping and that decreased or reversed reorganization was correlated with a decrease in pain (see for example Weiss, et al. 1999). They found that the extent of reorganization was directly related to daily prosthesis use (see for example Karl, et al. 2004) and to the presence and intensity of phantom limb pain (see for example Fraser, et al. 2001). However, it was not just prosthesis use alone that researchers considered most efficacious for ameliorating or even avoiding the onset of pain altogether. Functional prostheses were the key (see for example Abramson and Feibel 1981). For instance, the use of upper limb myoelectric prostheses rather than purely cosmetic alternatives permitted more extensive use of the residual limb, reduced phantom pain, and correlated with less cortical reorganization (see for example Lotze, et al. 1999; Weiss, et al. 1999). In other words, the curative power of prostheses was a consequent of habitual use, deep embodiment, and, importantly, prosthetic sophistication.

Advances in limb replacement technologies also appreciably contributed to the reconceptualization of amputation surgery as "constructive" rather than destructive or reconstructive. Although some clinicians had described the procedure as "reconstructive" as early as the mid-twentieth century, amputation was predominantly thought to represent a failure of medicine because it demarcated the limits of surgical promise (Smith 2001; Williamson 1992). Curtailing disease or minimizing trauma through the imposition of functional, psychological, and social losses had historically distinguished amputation from other surgical procedures. But by 2000, amputation surgery was fundamentally constructive; it built something from nothing and was the antithesis of disease or injury. Campbell argued, "Sometimes people, amputees and their friends and families, see it as a destructive surgery, but it is really a constructive surgery that allows people to get on with their lives" (Campbell 2005). Likewise, Dr. Burgess, orthopedic surgeon and founder of the Prosthetic Outreach Program, described it as "creating a new interface between the body and the world" (Smith 2001, 1).[16] Late-modern amputation surgery fashioned a new working interface between the body and its world, while prosthetization engendered a novel vision or version of embodiment. Together these constituted a profoundly reimagined way of being.

The prosthetized amputee has become the figurative and literal icon of late-modern malleability (Tofts 2002), a dominant representation of the realization of deep biomedical and techno-scientific body-optimization. The "pleasurably tight coupling" (Haraway 1985) indicative of late-modern techno-corporeality that purportedly enhances self-autonomy and self-control normalizes reassembly, while simultaneously subverting the pathetic vulnerability of flesh. By the end of the twentieth century, techno-corporeal mergers were commonplace and the malleability of the human body became central to the prosthetic imaginary.

> Western science and technology have arrived . . . at a new, postmodern imagination of human freedom from bodily determination. Gradually and surely, a technology that was first aimed at the replacement of malfunctioning parts has generated an industry and an ideology fueled by fantasies of rearranging, transforming, and correcting, an ideology of limitless improvement and change, defying the historicity, the mortality, and, indeed, the very materiality of the body. . . . In place of God the watchmaker, we now have ourselves, the master sculptors of the plastic. (Bordo 1997, 335)

Profound Coinciding and Deep Integration

By about 2000, prostheses were attributed with an influence that had in some respects supplanted that of phantoms. For example, Melzack (Melzack, et al. 1997, 1609; emphasis added) wrote of one of his patients that he "likens his prosthesis to a glove, which *envelops* his life-like PH [phantom] hand." In this article, the prosthesis was constructed as active, as "enveloping" the phantom. Compare this with Melzack's (1989, 2; emphasis added) description of the same phenomenon almost a decade earlier: "The amputee with a painless phantom, however, may find that the reality of the phantom is enhanced by wearing an artificial arm or leg; the phantom usually *fills* the prosthesis 'like a hand fits into a glove'; the prosthesis feels real, 'fleshed out.'" Here, the phantom was depicted as active, described as "filling" in or out the artificial limb.

Still, phantom limbs had hardly become superfluous; in fact, over the first decade of the twenty-first century, phantoms were constructed as a requisite means through which the curative, restorative, and transcendent properties of prostheses were had. Although the pained phantom could be unpredictable, could pathologize in horrible ways, the painless phantom was consistently lauded for its animating properties. And, successful integration, incorporation, and embodiment by way of animation were considered central to adaptation after limb loss (Kurzman 2004). Sobchack (2010, 631–32) described how the process of incorporation made her feel whole, seamless, "at once, *both new and renewed*"; she wrote,

> I primarily sense my leg as an active, quasi-absent "part" of my *whole body*. . . . I do not feel the object "place" where the flesh of my stump ends and the material of my prosthesis begins. Indeed, whether I am sitting or walking, there seems only the slightest difference, the merest "echo," between my two legs. Rather, their expressive reciprocity, their mirroring each of the other . . . is perceived as a general "seamlessness." . . . My diffused "phantom" both figuratively and functionally elongated and grew into the hollow of my prosthetic socket— occupying, thickening and substantiating it, finally "grasping" it so that it made sense to me and became corporeally integrated and lived as my own body.

At the ACA conference, prosthetists spoke of the animation process and its usefulness in allowing an amputee to become facile with a prosthesis quickly and to develop a more "natural"-looking gait. In fact, I was able to observe the process of animation that prosthetists and amputees seemed to negotiate. I found that unlike components (parts of prostheses) or the byproducts of construction (molds and impressions) that were readily discarded or even reemployed as tools, a completed artificial limb was treated with care. Check sockets (a clear impression of the stump), pylons, and other components or residues of prosthetization were divested of life, while prostheses that were "owned," embodied, and animated were vital.

Because of their animating properties, the productive aspects of phantom limbs continued to be emphasized despite the hype about the incredible transformative power of advanced prostheses. And, it was at this time that researchers' reports of phantom disappearance and phantom fading were interpreted as demonstrative both of the curative properties of prostheses and of the potential for phantoms to cause what was called *absolute synchronicity*. Because prostheses were thought to have the capacity to manage unruly phantoms as well as provoke phantoms into materializing, one would expect references to phantom disappearance—especially when a prosthesis was donned—to be relatively rare. In fact, they were not. Phantom fading and disappearance were commonly reported throughout the 1990s and 2000s, the period of peak interest in the phenomenon. Interest was certainly a consequent of increased anxiety concerning phantom loss because of the phantom's intrinsic utility, but it was also motivated by the need to explain why some phantoms were not persuasively "seduced" by the incredible sophistication, commanding power, and hybridized beauty of prostheses. In other words, why weren't all phantoms provoked or coaxed into animation by prostheses? The answer was quite simple: they were if only you knew where to "look."

References to phantom disappearance and fading during this period did not undermine the remarkability of prostheses (which did happen to some extent during the post-WWII period) because disappearance was offered up by some as irrefutable evidence of the therapeutic properties of artificial limbs (especially in cases of pain) and as demonstrative of their taming influence. Disappearance became the product of absolute synchronicity or the experiential merging of phantom and prosthesis. The absolute synchronicity argument had its roots in coinciding or coalescing, found frequently during the 1950s and 1960s. But, what differentiated coinciding from absolute synchronicity or "fusion"—as it was sometimes called—was that in the latter case ethereal and artificial appendages, ghosts and machines, literally "became one." They were experientially coupled such that neither was felt independently of the other. They were not simply sensed as superimposed on one another, coordinated in terms of posture and movement. Rather they fused, "disappearing" from consciousness, becoming of-the-body. For example Andre (2001, 195) and colleagues wrote,

Prosthetic devices could be incorporated or even fused with the phantom. Prosthetic devices and normal phantom limbs are confounded in use. . . . Phantoms tend to disappear in amputees who wear their prosthesis regularly, being replaced by the illusion of a normal body. Thus amputees may confound their prosthetic limbs with their normal primary limb as long as the prosthesis meets the mechanical and kinesthetic expectations of the lost limb and remains under control like a real limb.

It was because prostheses cured phantom pain and because absolute synchronicity could be achieved that phantoms disappeared altogether when a prosthesis was donned and almost magically reappeared the moment a prosthesis was doffed. This "disappearing act" was proof that artificial and phantom limbs were as much a part of the body as fleshy limbs had always been.

Cortical Reorganization and Phantom Utility

As a consequence of the potential for prosthetic animation to prevent phantom pain and enable facile prosthesis use, painless phantoms were constructed as productive, critical to the rehabilitation of amputees. They were the means through which prostheses were embodied, through which the brain adopted or accepted the new limb "as its own." From the 1980s onward, painless phantoms had an essential utility. Painful phantom limbs, on the other hand, which had no obvious purpose or physiologic advantage, should be curtailed and as it would turn out, could become a problem of the past. Importantly, this was because of the tendency for prosthetization to prevent cortical remapping, the source of phantoms both painful and benign. Dr. Mark P. Jensen, professor in the Department of Rehabilitation Medicine at the University of Washington in Seattle, stated, "My personal belief is that phantom limb pain is relatively easy to treat if your intervention reduces cortical reorganization" (Jensen 2005). Reorganization was thought to be reduced by the habitual use of advanced, functional prostheses, and in fact, the reported pain prevalence rate declined during the 2000s to as low as 50 percent from its historic high during the late 1980s and 1990s. Katz had "recognized" the potential for prostheses to ameliorate pain more than a decade before. He recounted,

> I predicted in a paper in 1992 that extensive use of the stump—and I think that is essentially what these new prostheses do is they generate use dependent change—would cause the reoccupation phenomenon that leads to decreased pain. I think old prostheses just were not adequate. Flor and others have shown the relationship between phantom pain and type of prosthesis; cosmetic prostheses did not result in a reduction in pain whereas the more modern ones that involve a use of the stump did. (Katz 2005)

It was also through the potential for phantom "exercise" to effect cortical reorganization (and the phantom pain associated with such remapping) that the fundamental utility of phantoms was widely appreciated. Unfortunately, this tendency also left healthy phantoms vulnerable. Because remapping could be prevented through phantom training and exercise (by keeping the would-be dormant or silent area of the homunculi active) and because painful and painless phantoms alike were the effect of that same phenomenon (the byproduct of cortical plasticity), the lauded painless phantom along with the maligned painful phantom became endangered, at least theoretically. If the phantom were kept fit and healthy, the area of the brain previously devoted to the amputated part would not lapse into silence or idleness, becoming vulnerable to encroachment by adjacent body parts of the sensory or motor homunculi (or other structures). The connection to the periphery kept active through phantom exercise (whether in the form of willed movements or virtual reality) was thought to prohibit "invasion." Still, most researchers agreed that phantoms materialized as a consequence of cortical reorganization despite contestation over the extent of remapping, the structures or areas of the brain involved, or the underlying mechanisms.

Perhaps more significant was the finding that although it was possible to prevent or reverse cortical reorganization through phantom exercise, amputees who wore functional prostheses accomplished this end without the need for visualization, phantom training, or virtual reality. Remapping was prevented by the replacement of sensation from the periphery as functional prostheses engaged residual nerves and musculature, sending "input" to the cortex, fooling the brain into "thinking" the limb was "alive and well." For example, the Sauerbruch prosthesis "is a mechanical device connected to one of the muscles of the arm by cables that operate a rod terminating at its proximal end in a surgically created tunnel in the muscle that operates it. Movement of the prostheses is produced by contraction and relaxation of that muscle" (Weiss, et al. 1999, 132). Deeply integrated or embodied prostheses, like the Sauerbruch, assertedly produced or ensured greater intimacy with the cerebral cortex, keeping the lines of communication between the periphery and the center open and active.

This became the model along which the mind-body connection was envisioned by many researchers. Appendages of any kind that provided proper sensorial input or feedback could trick the brain and become a part of "you" because the brain easily adopted parts like these as its own.

> The brain knows that it has an arm and a hand because it is connected to these things and gets feedback from them. The same could be true for robotic or virtual appendages. If you control a remote hand that senses objects and sends tactile sensations back to your brain, it behaves as if it's your own hand. It becomes part of you. Your body becomes extended beyond the surface of your skin. . . . New appendages . . . could be added to the body [and] the brain would eventually come to regard these as its own. In other words, the prosthetic limb would become a sensory add-on rather than an indication that something was missing. . . . [S]tudies of brain plasticity show that . . . future bodies may no longer be limited to two arms, two legs, two eyes, and two ears. (Geary 2002, 112–13)

Moreover, as pundits suggest, we may be tempted to go beyond the addition of a third eye that lets us see with greater clarity, maybe even behind our backs, or a third leg that enables a mean game of hopscotch or

Twister. We may, in fact, increasingly engage in the "once-unthinkable choice" of amputating limbs that are less than perfect (Okeowo 2012, 1) or, more disturbingly perhaps, amputating limbs that are relatively "limiting" when compared to, for example, legs that perform as if they were powered by a five-speed engine.

In 2007, an amputee sprinter was accused of "techno-doping" and (potentially and in "practice") of unfairly outperforming able-bodied competitors. His coach was quoted as saying, "He is like a five-speed engine with no second gear." He possessed the kind of enhanced-performance that Össur prosthetics—and many other of the manufacturers at the ACA conference—promised, the kind that could seduce those of us who are enthusiastically devoted to competition into the once unthinkable: "Will technological advantages cause athletes to do something as seemingly radical as having their healthy natural limbs replaced by artificial ones? . . . 'Is it self-mutilation when you're getting better limbs?'" (Longman 2007, 2, 1, 4).

Disease, defect, injury, even the inherent "weakness" of the flesh may provide the impetus or "opportunity" for acquiring better limbs, for "electively" amputating undeniably viable, "perfectly healthy" appendages. In fact, by about 2000, self-demand amputation was realized by some and a new late-modern disease surfaced that was termed "apotemnophilia."

All of this "potential" is only possible because of the inherent propensity for the human brain to accept virtual, artificial, ethereal, and other limbs as its own; it seems that a limb is a limb is a limb. The brain's underlying plasticity is what assertedly explains the indiscriminate adoption of parts. In fact, Ramachandran (2011, 38) intimated that we have recently evolved from *Homo sapien* to *Homo plasticus*. He wrote, "Without . . . plasticity we would still be naked savanna apes—without fire, without tools, without writing, lore, beliefs, or dreams. We really would be 'nothing but' apes, instead of aspiring angels" (Ramachandran 2011, 38). Life without beliefs or dreams would be like the fiery depths of hell. Lore and fire, on the other hand, is what angelic humans possess because their cortices are supple and characterized by dynamism.

Without plasticity, we would roam naked. Without plasticity, we would be nothing more than apes that are unable to write about being apes.

The Fate of Phantoms

By the turn of the twenty-first century, the ghost in the machine converted loss into gain, absence into presence, and unremarkable embodiment into late-modern malleability—the type of malleability indicative of "plastic" brains, augmented/able bodies, and shape-shifting phantoms. However, we cannot forget that the fate of phantoms rests on precisely how the future of phantom-prosthetic relations unfolds. The implications of this line of thinking should be made clear. Because phantom limbs are thought to materialize as the geography of the cortex reorganizes and because advanced prostheses that are deeply integrated or embodied prevent or reverse the process of reorganization, phantoms have became endangered, vulnerable to displacement by prostheses, vulnerable to extinction. As Taub explained in the case of phantom pain,

> You can manipulate the amount of cortical reorganization by increasing or decreasing the use of a body part. Functional prostheses expand the cortical representation into the dormant area. Now there is a flaw in the logic, but I'm not willing to say that it is wrong. What you are really doing is increasing the input in the stump, not increasing the input to the hand that is not there. Nevertheless, the phantom pain over a period of time decreases dramatically, down to zero in most people. (Taub 2005)

The sophistication of prosthetic technologies (e.g., temperature or pressure sensitivity), further physiologic incorporation (e.g., osseointegrated prostheses that attach directly to the bone, providing proprioceptive stimulation at the skeletal and deep tissue level, or neural integration), in conjunction with increased use (e.g., immediate postoperative fitting and early fitting for children), greater adaptability (e.g., prosthetic attachments like swimming fins, golf spikes, or climbing feet that are length adjustable), and biomechanical elaboration (e.g., the use of animal and mechanic models like the cheetah leg or the hydraulic knee) are implicated in the decline of the phantom limb prevalence rate. In fact, phantoms, it seems, are "disappearing." By around 2010, what once was considered a universal phenomenon became common, occurring in between 60 and 75 percent of the amputee population (see for example Ray, et al. 2009).

Phantom-prosthetic relations have since about 2010 been characterized by an uncomfortable tension. Phantoms animate and are integral to the successful embodiment of an artificial limb and hence, to efficacious prosthetization as well as to hastening healthy adjustment to limb loss. In fact, as prosthetic technologies have become increasingly sophisticated, the discourse on phantom-prosthetic relations has highlighted the importance of phantom health in enabling amputees to deeply embody and manage their prostheses. Through the potential of phantom exercise to reverse cortical reorganization and as a consequence of their capacity to animate, phantoms have developed a widely acknowledged intrinsic utility. Moreover, they have been central to tapping into the functional, the beneficial, and the adaptive aspects of cortical plasticity, and they have been an extraordinarily rich "resource" for researchers and practitioners. Nevertheless, phantoms are "disappearing" and the prevalence rate is expected to continue to decline as innovations in prosthetic science lead to greater levels of functional and sensorial recovery. As a consequence, phantoms have become vulnerable to being "theorized into extinction." Today, many amputees never experience phantoms, painful or otherwise, and prosthetic sophistication it seems is accountable. Ironically, the very process that assertedly brings embodied ghosts to life, cortical remapping, is the same one that phantoms have undermined because of their "natural" inclination toward, and friendly relations with, prostheses.

7

Conclusion

Authenticity and Extinction

How and why has the phantom become at once the Holy Grail of neuro-scientific investigation into subjective experience, the nature of the self, consciousness, and the mind-body connection at the same time that it has become "matter" or substance on the precipice of theoretical extinction? How did that which was characterized by trickery, deceit, spite, and the meaningless ways of a disturbed mind become characterized by exquisite pain, grotesque distortion, and the disordered/disordering brain and then ultimately by fundamental utility, neuronal remodeling, evolutionary purpose, and a natural proclivity for the technology that could mean its ruin? In short, how after the turn of the twenty-first century did phantom-prosthetic relations go so awry when ghosts and machines have never been more theoretically and practically, more conceptually and materially intimate?

Employing the concept of authenticity as a rhetorical frame through which biomedical knowledge on phantom limb syndrome and the biopolitics of phantom-prosthetic relations in the present-day context is revisited, I address the significance of phantoms becoming at once extraordinary and seemingly inconsequential, as well as show how phantom-prosthetic relations have transformed and been transformed by the modernization of amputation. Embedded in this neat framework are also some larger epistemological and ontological questions about embodiment in the contemporary context of technological fetishism, about the phantom-based biopolitical project of mastery, exploitation, and valuation, about the seductive appeal and import of the body-in-the-brain, about what counts as disability when bodies (impaired or not) are "brain-based," about the androcentric sexing/gendering of the biomedicalized body, about the unique aspects of techno-corporeal conjoin-ment in the case of amputation, and about the "accomplishment" of medical legitimacy.

First, I use the phenomenon of phantom penis to examine biomedical claims of scientific authenticity. What counts as legitimate knowledge about phantoms has defined the parameters of their existence and established their physiologic potential (even if ethereal appendages and other parts have not been wholly obliging). Past and present-day penile phantoms alike are touted as exceptional among embodied ghosts because, like the fleshy organs they at times emulate, phantom penises have distinctive properties; accordingly, they have much to teach us about both pleasure and pain. Second, I show how through the struggle to secure phantom authenticity, embodied fraudulence gave way to the epiphenomenal body, a conceptual move that reasserts a tired monist physicalism and, in the form of Melzack's neuromatrix, establishes the primordial body-in-the-brain as unequivocally male and masculine. Third, I show how novel populations have been enlisted in the debate over the experientially based versus hard-wired body-in-the-brain, effectively altering what counts as authentic amputation (as well as embodied wholeness and authentic disability). As a testimony to their profundity and amorphousness, phantoms found their way into the brains of both transsexuals and those "healthy-limbed" people who consider their digits and appendages to be vile and offending. Once brains (like bodies) developed the potential to be "amputated," who precisely counted as an amputee had to be reimagined and consequently, this ghost story is being rewritten once again. Fourth, the biomedical narrative about phantom origins incorporated the findings from research engaging two cutting-edge technologies, virtual reality and mirror neurons. As virtual reality is used to ameliorate pain and reawaken dead phantoms—those paralyzed by nonuse—and with the "discovery" of shiny mirror neurons that reflect the world of bodies "out there," the authentic origin of phantoms has once more been found outside of cortices. Phantoms are found in the very contexts in which they have always circulated, in the very bodies that they have always mimicked, and in the very technologies that they have always had such an affinity for. Fifth, reengaging the concept of prosthetic transcendence, I ask what counts as authentic transformation vis-à-vis prostheses and with what implications. Amputees have become icons of technologic liberation and central to our prosthetic imaginary. Still, phantoms undermine the naturalized relationship between prostheses and corporeal enhancement with implications for both phantom well-being and friendly phantom-prosthetic relations. Lastly, I use the case of the theoretical extinction of phantoms to address authentic death and to consider whether the question about phantom extinction is ultimately the right one to ask. The politics of life, after all, are always already the politics of death. Perhaps the right question to ask is, Who gets to decide?

The Authenticity of Science and Phantom Penis

Adding to a long line of scholarship that aims to intentionally demystify medical knowledges and claims of expertise, scientific-ness, and domain, a critical analysis of the psychological/psychiatric and (bio) medical constructions of phantom limb syndrome and phantom-prosthetic relations reveals the contingent nature of such knowledge systems, while also exposing the work involved in generating and legitimating biomedical and techno-scientific "facts." These knowledge systems are always a reflection of the social milieu in which they are engendered (Harding and Figueroa 2003), and authenticity in science and medicine is commonly achieved in precisely the same way as it is in other realms of social life—by borrowing from previously established knowledges and practices. Such is the case with phantom penis.

Although there are relatively few cases of penile/testicular amputation in the medical and psychological/psychiatric literature and although these references are often devoid of any real detailed or engaged analysis, male genitalia are referred to more often than any other phantom-ed body part aside from digits and limbs. One might conclude that the overrepresentation of male genitalia in the phantom literature is a consequent of curiosity or that it amounts to pure gratuitousness. However, the phantom penis has always been considered a noteworthy doppelganger of this fleshy appendage because of the distinctive qualities that the penis is thought to possess.

One of the first references to phantom penis can be found in a footnote in Mitchell's (1872) *Injuries of Nerves and Their Consequences*. This is a brief recounting of a case of phantom erection after amputation of the penis. However, it was not until 1950 when Heusner (1950, 128) detailed two cases of phantom penis and one of phantom testes that this "nonlimb ghost" was afforded any thorough consideration. The author told the story of a seventy-year-old man who awakened from a pneumonia-induced state of delirium to find that his penis had somehow been traumatized, necessitating complete amputation. Despite having been impotent prior to the incident, the man developed a life-like phantom penis felt as permanently erect. As Heusner (1950, 129) recounted,

> The reality, if you will, of this ghost was attested to by the patient's description of its size, shape and posture . . . by his sheepishly confessed practice of often peeping under the bed-clothes for visual assurance that the organ was, in truth, immaterial . . . [and by] a pressing desire to reach out into extrapersonal space and squeeze the apparition's tip for relief.

Tragically, a gunshot wound to the spine four years later left him paralyzed and consequently impoverished of his ethereal erection.

Although phantom penis and testes were regularly mentioned in the literature from the 1940s onward, it was not until the 1990s that interest in phantom penis, genitals, and testes would rival that of the 1950s. One of the most illustrative articles written on the subject was a review of twelve cases of penile amputation by Fisher (1999), who argued that penile ghosts were similar to other phantom-ed parts in that they were often accurate representations of the size, shape, and position of the intact penis prior to amputation. However, they were decidedly unlike other body parts in a significant respect: the penis had the capacity to become erect. Other phantoms, Fisher (1999, 55; emphasis added) contended, "may be influenced by mental concentration, emotional states, surprise, pain, wearing a prosthesis, etc., but show *no change comparable to that of the phantom erection.*" This argument echoed that of Heusner (1950, 132), who claimed that penile and testicular phantoms must have the same prevalence rate as limbs because they were truly "fantastic" organs. Male genitalia, he explained, had the requisite capacity to "move" (like all commonly or universally experienced phantom-ed parts such as limbs) and perhaps more importantly, were distinctive "spearheads" that penetrated the world:

> The testis, however, is unique among viscera in that its emergence from the abdomen induces the formation of visual and possibly other engrams which endow it with a phantom potential similar to that of limbs and axial protuberances. . . . A phantom is always a part which has been endowed with a measure of voluntary motion, that is, with motion which relates the individuals to the world about him. . . . [O]utjuttings of the body wall into the world about . . . are the spearheads of our conscious relations, not only *to* but *with* that world; that is, they are spearheads of our effective action upon the world. . . .The testicle and penis are endowed with only what may be called cremasteric motion of pulling up—a motion of a part of the body upon the body. . . . [They] are as fantastic as they are ribald. (Heusner 1950, 131–32; original emphasis)

Despite their ribald or obscene nature, out-jutting male genitalia initiated *man's* "effective action upon the world," his "conscious relations" with the "world about him" " (Heusner 1950, 131, 132). The protruding penis did so principally when it "moved," when it was erect. By way of contrast, phantom clitoris, labia, or ovary have never been reported in the American medical literature, and phantom breast has regularly been depicted as incidental and rare.[1] This is true despite Simmel's (1966b, 332) early and apparently ignored argument that the breast was equally as inimitable as the penis; it was

> the site of a variety of pressure experiences in addition to those common to the whole body surface. With position changes there are pressure changes in response to gravity. As the breast enlarges during pregnancy there are accompanying sensations of engorgement which in some individuals recur regularly just prior to or during menstruation. There are the tumescent changes of the nipple in response to light touch. There are

pressure sensations with lactation, and a variety of ever changing pressure sensations in the woman who is nursing an infant.

She also enlisted subjects in a series of swaying exercises that elicited reports of movement and other distinctive sensations. In a standing position, subjects were asked to brace themselves on a table, bend forward, and sway back and forth with their eyes closed. One patient replied, "It doesn't feel as if it is gone, isn't that funny, the other side [the phantom] is heavy, makes the bra too tight" (Simmel 1966b, 339). Breasts, she argued, were unique in that they "moved" in ways dissimilar from other body parts. They were, in fact, as remarkable as the exalted penis. One could also argue that at least some breasts jut out into the world to a greater extent than the flaccid penis and that all breasts do so more consistently than the erect penis. Nevertheless, phantom breasts remained far from "fantastic" or "special." The phantom penis was regarded as "a *very special syndrome* even within the field of phantom phenomenology" (Fisher 1999, 56; emphasis added).

A decade after Fisher's comprehensive study of the phenomenon, phantom penis was still touted as comparably fertile research material. For example, Wade and Finger (2010, 309) proposed that "important information may be gained by studying penile phantoms, especially because . . . they are less likely than limb amputations to be painful and are often reported as pleasurable and associated with erections." It seems that the phantom penis has remained uniquely positioned to provide the kind of information instrumental to understanding both pleasure and pain, a rare phantom to be sure.

Laqueur (1990, 241; emphasis added) aptly demonstrated in his *Making Sex*, that the "external *active* penis" has long been juxtaposed to the "internal *passive* vagina." Female genitalia have been constructed as derivative of or secondary to male genitalia, sometimes as comparatively rudimentary (Moore and Clarke 1995), as well as internal rather than "out-jutting," a contention that was and is reflected in assumptions about which organs and body parts persist in a phantom-ed state, with what regularity, and why. This is, of course, not the first time that the androcentric bias in science, medicine, or technology has been exposed (see for example Lederman and Bartsch 2001; Lerman, Oldenziel, and Mohun 2003; Wyer, et al. 2001). What is telling about the case of phantom penis is not the (arguably typical) denigration of the female body and the privileging of the male, but rather the obvious conflation of maleness and masculinity, the failure of researchers to modernize their androcentric worship of male genitalia (after over one hundred years), and the offensive reduction of masculine embodiment to a spearhead. In fact, the stump too is equatable to a *large* penis" (Ramachandran 2009, 775; emphasis added), presumably ready to assault and overtake the world like all mounted spearheads that threaten to wound, master, destroy, or own.

The particular hypotheses, theories, experiments, and experiences, and the particular suppositions, data, and knowledges that are deemed credible and justifiable are the ones that have constituted a framework through which phantom peculiarities were apprehended, phantom physiology was realized, and phantom authenticity was cultivated. The morphology of phantoms, their bizarre and idiosyncratic ways, their biomedical facticity and "realness," their very existence has always been at least partly dependent on which knowledge claims were deemed legitimate and why.

The history of phantoms, however, is about much more than how ghost stories are told and by whom. The study of phantoms is and has been a biopolitical project in mastering and exploiting embodied ghosts (taming, harnessing, and arousing "the absent"), in establishing the corporeality of apparitions (further validating and reifying corporeal ideology), in the valuation of bodies (especially active, productive, trustworthy, devoted, and augmented male bodies) and body parts (whether phantom-ed, homuncular, scheme-ed, virtual, artificial, or fleshy), in dissecting the "fractioned" body (central to biomedical and techno-scientific liberatory and transformative prosthetization), and in territorializing and commodifying "missing" body parts (painful, distorted, paralyzed, or uncivilized parts that necessitate biomedical intervention), all of which have been contingent upon establishing the authenticity of biomedical and techno-scientific claims.

The Authenticity of Phantoms and the Epiphenomenal Body

The ambiguity characteristic of embodied ghosts and phantom-prosthetic relations has at least partly been a consequence of contemporary attempts at re-visioning the field in an effort to explain why research has yielded such discrepant data and in an attempt to legitimate the work being done on this arguably obscure, illusive, and amorphous phenomenon. As a consequence of the biomedical legitimation of phantom limb syndrome, vulnerable populations multiplied, symptomatology elaborated, pain became epidemic, and phantom parts proliferated. And as phantoms resisted attempts at biomedical rationalization, researchers struggled to identify the "real McCoy," those that were analytically severed from painful stumps, far-fetched stories, and disturbed minds, those that could be causally accounted for, and those that followed the right rules.

In their early history, phantoms were thought to upset the overall economy of the male body and were conceived as emblematic of the physical and mental weaknesses that fractioned and feminized (O'Connor 2000). They were evidence that the body could be persuasively fraudulent. Today, amputation no longer feminizes the mind or emasculates the body. Rather, it demonstrates that the brain-based body, whether in the form of the homunculi or the neuromatrix, is primordially male (and undeniably masculine). The somatosensory homunculus has always been a strip of cortical tissue with massive hands, enormous lips, and an immense "out-jutting" penis. And, vis-à-vis Melzack's neuromatrix, phantoms demonstrate that the innate (and relatively invariant) body-in-the-brain reflects *man's* kinesthetic legacy in his quest for survival. Like the knife-fighter crouched and readied for action, man's natural position at rest is one poised on the brink of violence, one unambiguously offensive. Curiously, "man's" primordial position at rest is not the very posture regularly assumed by women all over the world when giving birth, one poised on the brink of genesis, one unambiguously protective.

Phantoms are no longer evidence of embodied fraudulence; they are regarded as neuroscientific proof that the body is epiphenomenal. Through brain imaging and other forays into the cortices of amputees, brain-based body parts have become authentic and fleshy ones superflu-ous, if not illusory. The sensorial quality of corporeality no longer resides in the body but rather within the three-pound organ that as contempo-rary neuroscientists argue is capable of generating, of creating, every-thing we feel. The implications of this line of reasoning are staggering. The body has been taken out of the equation just when social scientists of all stripes have made the loud and emphatic call to bring the body back in. Consequently, a massive body of research and theorizing is neglected that starts with the premise that we both *have a body* and *are a body*.

Moreover and critically speaking, we cannot simply manipulate or manufacture embodied sensorial (or other more complex) experiences both because bodies are agents with "wisdom . . . intentionality and pur-pose" (Scheper-Hughes and Lock 1991, 409) that wittingly and unwittingly join social and political projects of all kinds and because sensorial and other experiences occur *within contexts*. For example, when Melzack pro-poses that the brain can generate every sensation from excruciating pain to orgasm, he denies the role that language plays in framing our experience of pain (for example, "lancinating," "dreadful," and "wretched" pain that must be experienced as qualitatively different from "wrinkled," "raw," and "dry" pain), and he neglects the fact that orgasms are always—without excep-tion—contextualized. After Sem-Jacobsen (1968) stimulated the posterior frontal lobe of a man who trembled, flushed, and ejaculated, I imagine his patient might have described the "orgasm" as unlike any he had experi-enced before, and who knows what he might have said about the pleasures (or horrors) of brain-based "electrode-sex" in a laboratory setting.

Moreover, this line of logic constitutes an expression of physical monism that exemplifies many of the contemporary psychic/psychologi-cal and biologic/biomedical approaches to the "mind-body problem." The body—like the mind—is reduced to the brain, and in effect, sensory expe-rience, perception, consciousness, indeed our sense of self are all reduced to what neurons do and do not do, why, where, and under what conditions. Do not get me wrong. I share the assertion that neurons are agents that produce real effects. But, neurons can never be understood outside of or independent from the cortical tissue, the brains, the skulls, the bodies, the selves, and the contexts in which they are nested. And perhaps more to the point, we are not reducible to the neuron. In fact, on some days, I feel like *much more* than what my neurons are up to. Nevertheless, the phantom-ed and prosthetized body-in-the-brain underscores the growing import of the neurosciences and the seductive appeal of brain-based theorizing.

The "expansion of the imaging armamentarium . . . provides more visual artifacts for circulation, and this extensive and growing body of images fosters the idea that pictures are the appropriate medium for representing ourselves and our stories" (Joyce 2008, 164). Visualization technologies also allow for more and more forays into cortices of interest, with the effect of strategically conflating bodies and brains. As bodies are reduced to (visualized) neuronal activity (or inactivity), the biopolitical order will increasingly become a problem of critical importance with widespread implications that one can only speculate about. Will we want to see more, making the brain like the body ever more transparent while stimulating the impulse toward "perfectibility, modifiability, and control" (van Dijck 2005, 5)? Will we want to intervene, tricking the gullible brain in ever more imaginative and consequential ways?

The fate of phantoms is, of course, central to the way this future will unfold. From a neuroscientific perspective, the phantom is precious because it is the model along which the body-in-the-brain is understood and because it is a means through which intervention can be realized. From a biopolitical perspective, the phantom is precious because it is our proverbial canary in the mine, a "fowl" corpse readied for autopsy.

The Authenticity of Amputation and Transsexuality

As phantoms became proof that the body is superfluous, one could contend that ghosts would, by extension, be understood as pure simulacra—only a copy of a copy. If "*your own body* is a phantom, one that your brain has temporarily constructed purely for convenience" (Ramachandran and Blakeslee 1998, 58; original emphasis), then intact limbs are fabrications and phantom limbs only reproductions of those same fabrications. Instead, this line of thinking eventuated in phantoms becoming more real than real at least in part because today they are as unique as we are. By around 2009, they were regularly described as idiosyncratic, unique, and distinctive (Anderson-Barnes, et al. 2009; Weeks, Anderson-Barnes, and Tsao 2010). For instance, McAvinue and Robertson (2011, 2193) wrote,

> [It] is a highly unique condition, the experience of which varies consider-
> ably from person to person in terms of reason for amputation, the shape
> and form of the phantom limb, the quality of PLP [phanton limb pain]
> and PLS [phantom limb sensation], the frequency, duration and intensity
> of PLS and PLP episodes, the existence of exacerbating factors and the
> time course of the phantom limb experience.

Despite the asserted idiosyncratic nature of phantoms, however, some researchers have continued to insist that the pathogenesis of phantom sensation and phantom pain is rooted in the innately "hard-wired" body scheme, often in the form of Melzack's neuromatrix (the genetically deter-mined convoluted structure of the internal image of one's body). Not only is this position antithetical to the plasticity paradigm that was so widely accepted within the neurosciences by the 1990s, but the theory's validity has been criticized, with critics "emphasizing that while it may address vari-ous aspects of phantom phenomena, it cannot be tested on phantom sensa-tions that are pain-free. As a result, the theory is difficult to establish as the sole reason for the existence of phantom limbs" (Weeks, Anderson-Barnes, and Tsao 2010, 280). The neuromatrix is faulted for its inability to explain distorted, supernumerary, and many other phantoms because these speci-mens do not reflect "normal" physiology, the kind of primordial physiology that would expectedly be characteristic of the innate body-in-the-brain.

Nevertheless, some researchers continue to argue that congenital phantoms, ghostly appendages of limbs that never existed, testify to the innate quality of the neuromatrix, the homunculi, or the body scheme. This is assertedly evidenced by the lack of cortical reorganization or remapping in individuals born with foreshortened or missing limbs and/ or digits. The brains of congenital amputees are apparently not like those of traumatic or surgical amputees, but rather are like those of what are referred to as "healthy" people. And, as Dr. Taub argued, this is true of the vast majority of congenital amputees: "About 98–99 percent of . . . [those] who develop badly damaged extremities [in utero] do not have cortical reorganization" (Taub 2005). Others, however, found that movement of existing foreshortened limbs did produce cortical reorganization, and Dr. Katz elaborated on why this tendency continues to be so curious:

> I think it is very hard to explain. I think the idea that people with congenitally absent limbs can feel phantoms is fascinating because of what we know to date about plasticity. One would think that in utero if a limb is not developing, the areas of cortical tissue, spinal cord and thalamus subserved by a limb that is no longer developing would not develop (or would not be subserved to a limb that does not exist). It would be reoccupied earlier. (Katz 2005)

Congenital amputees have often been at the center of phantom controversies, but another population surfaced as a possible means of adjudicating between the innate and the experientially based body-in-the-brain. Ramachandran and McGeoch (2007) proposed that transsexuals offered a unique opportunity to assess the relationship between the body scheme/image and the birthed physical body. They found that male-to-female (MtF) transsexuals who had a penis amputated due to a "mismatch between their gender-based 'body image' and that of their body's actual physical form" had a lower incidence of phantom penis than those men who had penile amputations for other reasons because "men have an internal image of their penis as part of their body image, and women of their breasts" (Ramachandran and McGeoch 2007, 1002). In addition, female-to-male (FtM) transsexuals had penile phantoms despite having been born with female genitalia. The authors wrote, "More than half of the around 30 female-to-male transsexuals we have interviewed, claim to have experienced this, often since early childhood" (Ramachandran and McGeoch 2007, 1003).

This line of research purportedly demonstrates that dissemblances exist between the physical and the brain-based body and that by extension, congenital amputees can either experience or be impoverished of phantom sensation or awareness. More importantly, it also suggests that the gendered nature of the body scheme and, thus, the physical body is both found in the brain and expressed in the form of the penis and the breast (rather than the clitoris, labia, ovaries, etc.). Female genitalia are inconsequential to the body-in-the-brain and the fetishized breast is identified as the brain-based marker of both sex and gender, femaleness and femininity.

Further, "transsexual phantoms" reiterate the syndrome's import, solidifying the indispensability of embodied ghosts and elevating the value of the phantom's neuroscientific investigation. As Ramachandran and McGeoch (2007, 1002; emphasis added) proposed, "Phantom sensations offer a *unique window* into how nature and nurture interact to create one's body image." Perhaps most significantly, this line of reasoning demonstrates that whether in the form of the body scheme/image, the homunculi, or the neuromatrix, this highly contested and, as some have argued, purely theoretical structure escaped the laboratories and clinical spaces where "typical" amputees were found, as well as the cortices where "typical" phantoms dwelled. Moreover, despite the seemingly inevitable displacement or death of phantoms, these practiced transgressors once again began to proliferate and to lend themselves to "other" discourses of authenticity. But, this was not the first time that authenticity had spread.

When Authenticity Spreads and the Case of Apotemnophilia

The second he felt the bullet enter his body, George Boyer knew it was going to be a good day. Or maybe he had already known from the instant he woke up. On that early September morning in 1992, Boyer had risen to find the Florida sun suspending the world in amber. . . . "There are large, beautiful, long-leaf yellow pines, gently moving their fuzzy tops against the blue of the sky, the greenness made golden by the sunlight up there," he had written in his journal that afternoon. It was beneath those same pines that his landlord eventually found him, slumped over on the grass, his left leg severed just below the hip, disappearing into a puddle of blood and bone. A shotgun was lying by his side. Boyer himself had pulled the trigger. (Mearz 2006, 1)

At the turn of the twenty-first century, ABC News (2000) reported that two hundred people worldwide suffered from a disorder called "apotemnophilia," a disorder characterized by the desire to amputate healthy limbs and digits, those unaffected by disease or functional impairment.

> In May 1988 a seventy-nine-year-old man from New York traveled to Mexico and paid $10,000 for a black-market leg amputation; he died of gangrene in a motel. In October 1999 a mentally competent man in Milwaukee severed his arm with a homemade guillotine, and then threatened to sever it again if surgeons reattached it. That same month a legal investsigator for the California state bar, after being refused a hospital amputation, tied off her legs with tourniquets and began to pack them in ice, hoping that gangrene would set in, necessitating amputation. (Elliott 2003, 209)

ABC News had apparently grossly underestimated the number of people afflicted with apotemnophilia. Elliott (2000, 73) in his article "A New Way to Be Mad,"[2] suggested that on the internet alone there were "enough people interested in becoming amputees to support a minor industry."[3] Two years later, Furth and Smith (2002) argued that the disorder affected between 1 and 3 percent of the population, and in 2005, Bayne and Levy (2005) proposed that apotemnophiles numbered in the thousands.[4]

In January of 2000, a number of British papers ran a story about a Dr. Robert Smith, a Scottish surgeon at the National Health Service (NHS) District Royal Infirmary Medical Center, who performed two elective amputations, one in 1997 and another in 1999 (Dyer 2000).[5] Despite the fact that the infirmary's medical director, chief executive, and ethics committee were consulted prior to both surgeries, the NHS banned further amputations in 2000. The onslaught of negative media coverage and the public outcry against performing such amputations prompted infirmary personnel to make the decision to terminate the practice (Bayne and Levy 2005; Dotinga 2000).[6] Although Dyer (2000) described the two men as psychologically disturbed and other news reports suggested that these were cases of extreme body dysmorphic disorder (Elliott 2000),[7] extensive psychological testing prior to surgery reportedly demonstrated that the men were not incompetent, and in a public interview, both men said they were happier and had a better quality of life without their alien limbs (Bayne and Levy 2005; Elliott 2000; Fisher and Smith 2000); in Dr Smith's words, "They were delighted with their new state" (Berger, et al. 2005).[8] To his dismay, Smith had six healthy-limb removal candidates at the time the hospital banned the procedure (Dotinga 2000).[9]

John Money, professor emeritus at Johns Hopkins University, in 1977 termed the disorder "apotemnophilia," literally meaning "love of amputation" (Money, Jobaris, and Furth 1977).[10] Apotemnophiles—also referred to as "voluntary amputees," "self-demand amputees," "elective amputees," or "wannabes"—have been described as having a sexual fetish of an extreme nature, the desire to have sex as an amputee (Bensler and Paauw 2003; Dotinga 2000; Money, Jobaris, and Furth 1977). Money (1977) and his colleagues clearly differentiated between apotemnophiles and acrotomophiles. Apotemnophiles, or wannabes, were thought to desire amputation because they were aroused by the idea of having sex as an amputee, while acrotomophiles, or devotees, were sexually attracted to amputees and did not desire amputation for themselves.[11] The use of the suffix "philia" categorized both disorders as one of a set of psychosexual disorders called "paraphilias" or "perversions" (Money, Jobaris, and Furth 1977).[12]

Subsequent research purportedly demonstrated that there were two distinct groups previously subsumed under the label "apotemnophile": those who desired amputation for sexual reasons and those who did not express an underlying sexual component (Berger, et al. 2005). As Elliott (2000) suggested, despite the fact that Money had constructed these two categories on the basis of either attraction or fetish, in the end Money confused apotemnophiles and acrotomophiles and sexualized both (Elliott 2000, 74, in a letter from Dr. Robert Smith).

Researchers, clinicians, as well as wannabes themselves, have used two discursive frames in an effort to legitimate apotemnophilia and distance the disorder from sexual fetishization: an identity-based discourse and an amputated-brain discourse. First, researchers argued that apotemnophiles described their bodies as deficient (Fisher and Smith 2000; Furth and Smith 2002), incongruent (Phillips, et al. 2010), or incomplete (Berger, et al. 2005; Dyer 2000; Elliott 2000; First 2004) and their limbs intended for amputation as alien (Bayne and Levy 2005; Dotinga 2000), intrusive (Ramachandran 2009), or surplus (Elliott 2000; Fisher and Smith 2000). They commonly used the language of self-actualization in the form of both self-transformation and the true-self, similar to that of transsexualism (Lawrence 2006),[13] and they typically described their desire as lifelong (Bayne and Levy 2005; Bruno 1997; Cameron 2003; Dotinga 2000; Dyer 2000; First 2004; Fisher and Smith 2000).[14] For example, using the metaphor of pruning, Furth and Smith (2002) defined elective amputation as a source of renewal or self-transformation and stated that "actualized" apotemnophiles often report that they feel reborn, that they have aligned their ideal corporeal form with their true-self. First (2004, 922)[15] provided the following examples of imagined and actualized pruning:

> "After the amputation I would have the identity that I've always seen myself as." ... "At some moment, I saw an amputee and I understood that that's the way I should be." ... "Sounds paradoxical—I would feel whole without my leg." ... "I felt like I was in the wrong body; that I am only complete with both my arm and leg off on the right side."

In a case study detailed by Furth and Smith (2002, 42), they wrote,

> The client described his amputation as a "minor inconvenience," compared to the major "compelling drive" for amputation with which he had lived for so many years. ... His only regret was that he had not succeeded in obtaining an amputation earlier in life and that he had to wait until in his sixties to achieve such satisfaction.

Researchers have also invoked a discourse that borrowed conceptually from phantom limb syndrome in the form of homuncular amputation. Fisher and Smith (2000) proposed that apotemnophilia was analogous to phantom limb and that the disorder was best understood as neuro-physiological rather than psychological in origin. From this perspective, "if a particular body part . . . fails to be represented in the body image, then the result may be a desire to have it removed" (Ramachandran 2009, 776). Although they subsequently rejected its applicability, Bayne and Levy (2005, 76)[16] explained, "Whereas the body schema of individuals with phantom limbs includes body parts that they lack, other patients do not have the body schema of body parts they have."

The process of "borrowing" legitimacy from another disease, condition, disorder, or syndrome is arguably a strategy intended to manufacture credibility in the case of a highly contested or contestable illness— to, in Hacking's (1986, 1995, 6) terms, "make up people" as verifiable apotemnophiles and to demonstrate that authentic selves can be trapped in inauthentic bodies. The mechanism through which the public recognition of a condition, disease, or disorder contributes to the dispersion of both a disease discourse and the realized or materialized effects of the disease is what he terms "semantic contagion." Semantic contagion is the process through which emerging categories (diseases and their symptomology) are used to interpret present and future behavior, thoughts, feelings, and the like, as well as to retroactively reinterpret one's history.

At stake in the legitimation process is what amounts to and who gets to determine embodied wholeness. Embodied wholeness no longer implies living with the physical body that one was born with, nor does it necessitate that the body's composition be made up of "birthed" physical parts. The use of cadaveric (tissues derived from a dead body, especially human), mechanical (machines and inorganic "tissues" that replace the functionality or aesthetic of the body), biomechanical (tissue-machine hybridization), transplanted (organs or tissues transferred from one person to another or from one part of the body to another), and xenotransplanted (organs or tissues transferred from a member of one species to a member of another species) body parts, without question, marked a dramatic change in the lived experience of embodied wholeness.

Still, what actualized apotemnophiles demonstrate is that embodied wholeness or completeness can also be typified by "the partial." The body one is born with may be "overcomplete" (Ramachandran 2009, 775), necessitating (biomedical) "pruning." In fact, the tendency for wannabes to be sexually attracted to amputees or to have amputation-specific "love-maps"

(Lawrence 2006, 274) purportedly testifies to the deep and intense necessity underlying elective amputation and hence, the urgency and import of the matter. As Ramachandran (2009, 776) and his colleagues described it, one has a preference for "one's own body 'type.' . . . [O]striches prefer ostriches as mates . . . pigs prefer porcine shapes . . . [and] a donkey is attracted to donkey-like creature[s]." Vis-à-vis the body scheme, embodied wholeness—as it is manifest through both one's desired physical form and the "natural" object of one's desire—becomes overdetermined.

Moreover, some researchers argue that corporeal ideology in the form of overdetermined embodied wholeness has implications for what counts as authentic disability. For example, Mearz (2006, 4) asked, "Can you still consider a physical defect a handicap if it helps someone function on a higher level? And does the answer to that question ultimately redefine what disability means?" In a similar vein, Bayne and Levy (2005, 84) suggested,

> On the one hand, one can argue that wannabes have an overly rosy image of what life as an amputee involves. . . . [O]n the other hand, one could also argue that those of us who are able-bodied have an overly pessimistic image of the lives of the disabled. As able-bodied individuals, we might be tempted to dwell on the harm that accompanies amputations and minimize what is gained by way of identification.

It is important to note, however, that proposing that (some or all) disability is brain-based extracts from the equation political, economic, spatial/geographic, social/cultural, and relational/interpersonal contexts. Disability becomes nothing more than a mismatch between the body and the brain or, unlike the unproblematized abled body, something that "your brain has temporarily constructed purely for your [and others' in]convenience" (Ramachandran and Blakeslee 1998, 58). This is a conceptual and political move that is dangerous. The danger lies in denying the importance of context, potentially confounding once again disability (as a social process of exclusion, oppression, and discrimination) and impairment (as an ontological process of lack, excess, or "difference"). Even if impairment is made problematic by framing it in terms of that which it is not (i.e., amputation does not constitute impairment for some people because it is restorative), this does not necessarily translate into less pity, ostracization, or discrimination, into less disability.

There are also implications here for what is worth saving. As Scheper-Hughes (2005, 153,155) argued, the expansion of "medical citizenship" often translates into the commodification of bodies and their parts, such that "a divisible body with detached and demystified organs [are] seen as ordinary and 'plain things,' simple material for medical consumption" (see also Scheper-Hughes 2001, 2006). In the case of traumatic or surgical amputation, gone is the anxiety expressed in terms of the medical handling practices of amputated parts found predominantly during the 1950s and 1960s. "Spirit members" no longer haunt amputees from the grave, most often in the form of continued pain. Today, amputated parts are not invested with continued vitality such that amputees retain a sense of deep connection with the remainder and a deep care for how it is to be disposed of. In fact, ideas such as these have been reduced to pure myth (Mortimer, et al. 2002). That is, however, unless they are regarded as surplus; amputated limbs do have a vital spirit when they come from apotemnophiles, when they remedy a mismatch between body and brain for both the donor and the recipient, when they are a transplanted "gift." Indeed, Furth and Smith (2002) recognized the value of this rare commodity and proposed establishing a network between (elective) amputation surgeons and limb transplantation units.

Authentic Origins and Augmented Reality

Implicit in the notion of homuncular amputation is the contention that the brain is hard-wired with respect to body image and yet, the body-in-the-brain has been widely regarded as amenable to dramatic and massive reorganization. Since around 1990, whether in the form of neural sprouting or unmasking, phantom appendages and other parts were asserted to be a consequent of the reorganization of the human cortex; the geography of the brain remaps itself in response to the loss of sensory input, in response to cortical silence (as well as to "excessive input"). Still, brain-based parts situated in the somatosensory and motor homunculi (as well as other cortical structures) retain loyalty to the lost physical parts to which they were allied in the form of atrophied cortical islands of allegiance and consequently, researchers and clinicians use phantom exercise, increasingly sophisticated and deeply embodied prostheses, and even "immersive" virtual reality (see for example Giummarra and Moseley 2011; Giummarra, et al. 2011) in an attempt to control cortical reorganization by supporting established connections, preventing new ones, and/or upsetting others.

Virtual or augmented reality "presents the perceived phantom arm on a flat screen in 3D which is controlled via a wireless glove worn on the intact arm. As the intact arm moves so the avatar follows with realistic finger and hand movements" (Cole, et al. 2009, 847). Subjects who used the glove report a sense of agency over their phantoms, experience embodiment of their phantoms, and have pain relief. The Defense Advanced Research Projects Agency (DARPA) has also established a "virtual integration environment" at Walter Reed for the purpose of experimenting in methods of phantom pain reduction and "captur[ing] real-time surface EMG activity" from the exceptional brains of demobilized amputees (Zeher, et al. 2011, 730). Virtual reality is a means through which one of the military's most formidable agencies can access the brains and, by extension, the bodies and minds of dismembered soldiers. Moreover, mobility has once again assumed a curative role and, in fact, pain itself is constructed as the impetus for therapeutic movement because it provokes the body into action. "Pain might not be simply a sensation but be a need state, like thirst or hunger. Perhaps the need, in part, is for action" (Cole, et al. 2009, 853).

Entering into virtual reality allows amputees to feel the "realness" that phantoms inherently possess, especially in the case of phantom paralysis or learned nonuse. And, the haunted limbs that occupy virtual gloves are the model along which the brain and the body are envisioned to relate in both "fantasy" and "reality." Ironically, thanks to 3D screens and wireless gloves, the fictive and the real virtually became one.

More ironic, perhaps, is the newest origin story that made its way into the literature circa 2010 in the form of the mirror neuron (Giummarra and Moseley 2011; Hanling, et al. 2010). Weeks and Tsao (2010, 463) wrote,

Given that body image is therefore clearly plastic and malleable, it seems possible that an amputee could readily assimilate a limb-like object into his body image to provide the visual feedback that corresponds to the phantom sensations he experiences. This effect of ownership and pain relief is likely to be mediated by the mirror neuron system. This system, in which some of the same regions of motor neurons are active in both a person performing movements and one observing movements being performed, was first discovered in the macaque and later confirmed in humans.

Researchers argue that when an amputee or a wide-eyed macaque watches someone move, mirror neurons are activated and the brain "interprets" this action in much the same way that self-movement is interpreted. This, they surmise, leads to the incorporation of another person's limb into the amputee's body image. For example, Weeks and Tsao's (2010, 462) bilateral patient "discovered that an itch on either phantom leg . . . was relieved by scratching the leg of a compatriot's intact leg or by scratching his prosthesis in the corresponding location." Or Giummarra (2011, 695) and her colleagues wrote of one women who "reported that her phantom foot felt ticklish when her husband 'tickled' the prosthetic foot," and they concluded that 16 percent of amputees (and 30 percent of "healthy individuals") experience synaesthetic pain (Giummarra and Moseley 2011, 525). Mirror neurons could also, of course, lead an amputee who watched another amputee to incorporate limblessness into his or her body image, with all the concomitant "behavioral tendencies" that amputees adopt and exhibit.

One of the means through which authenticity is secured in medicine and science is by recycling old ideas, presenting them in a very new and, in this case, "shiny" package. The mirror neuron hypothesis—that viewing others' bodies in motion is registered in the brain in a similar way to self-movement—is reminiscent of the arguments made about *exposure phantoms* in postwar contexts. In the post-WWII years, for example, phantom pain was thought to be brought on by seeing an amputee or even having known another amputee prior to amputation. Most importantly, the mirror neuron is demonstrative of the fact that, despite being brain-based, phantoms can and did find their way back into social contexts.

The Authenticity of Corporeal Transformations

Change in biomedicine, neuroscience, pain medicine, amputation surgery, and prosthetic science has profoundly affected the lived consequences of congenital, traumatic, surgical, and elective amputation in
the modern context. Moreover, these changes have altered the meaning
of amputation and prosthetization in regard to what Scheper-Hughes and
Lock (1987, 7) called the "social-body," or "the representational uses of the
body as a natural symbol with which to think about nature, society, and
culture." The authors argued that the healthy body functions as a model
for conceptualizing social and societal wholeness and vigor, while the ill
or disabled body is representative of "social disharmony, conflict, and disintegration" (Scheper-Hughes and Lock 1987, 7). In a similar vein, Tich-
kosky (2007, 12) proposed that disability alone, as "a process of meaning
making," can tell us as much about vigor as it does about disharmony, as
much about societal wholeness as it does about disintegration, especially
if we look at "authoritative representations" (Titchkosky 2000, 198) like
those advanced by biomedicine. These, she contends, readily produce
"disability-knowledge" (Titchkosky 2000, 206) because after all, "meaning making takes place somewhere and is done by someone" (Titchkosky
2007, 12). Thus, it is necessary not only to examine the implications of the
modernization of amputation for amputees but also to ask how and to
what effect the social body has been modified; such representational and
symbolic perturbations are undeniably consequential for all of us.

As biomedicine has become ever more oriented toward transformation
rather than restoration, what the healthy social body connotes and evokes
has been deeply altered. In her seminal article on cyborgs, Clarke (1995a)
distinguished modern from postmodern approaches to biomedicine, arguing that postmodern approaches are characterized by the expansion, application, and increased legitimation of science in medical matters all kinds.
This transition has had weighty implications in terms of the nature of and
impetus for medical intervention. "Postmodern approaches are centered
on re/de/sign and *transformation*," and postmodern bodies are increasingly manipulated and augmented (Clarke 1995a, 140; original emphasis;

Clarke 2003). Prosthetic science has certainly been an exemplar of the postmodern approach in that design is no longer inspired by the desire to return bodies to "normal" states but rather by the desire to transcend the inadequacies of the human body. As one example of the instantiation of what is termed "the Biomedical TechnoService Complex," prosthetic science has contributed to a sociocultural milieu in which techno-corporeal hybridization has become increasingly normative (Clarke, et al. 2003, 2). Moreover, the rationalization of postmodern prosthetic transformations is indicative of a "post-human" epistemological shift that, as Hayles (1999, 2–3) critically argued, rests on the assumptions that biologic embodiment is purely incidental, the body is the "original prosthesis," and humanity is amenable to seamless articulations with technologies. We are living in a context in which the actualization and the moral and aesthetic acceptability of profound corporal transformation have converged. Indeed, prosthetized transformation *is* expressed authenticity.

Giddens (1991, 20), in his *Modernity and Self-Identity,* suggested that a core feature of late modernity is the undermining of certainty; what may have previously been considered fixed, whether social or natural, is necessarily thrown into radical doubt (Giddens 1994a). No-"thing" is spared reflexive (re)organization; even the natural and fundamental aspects of or knowledges about bodies are subject to debate.

> The body was a "given," the often inconvenient and inadequate seat of the self. With the increasing invasion of the body by abstract systems all this becomes altered. The body, like the self becomes a site of intersection, appropriation and reappropriation, linking reflexively organized processes and systematically ordered expert knowledge. The body itself has become emancipated—the condition for its reflexive restructuring. Once thought to be the locus of the soul, then the centre of dark, perverse needs, the body has become fully available to be "worked upon" by the influences of high modernity. (Giddens 1994b, 218)

Consequently, the body has increasingly been understood, and indeed lived, as plastic (Deitch 1992; Featherstone 1991; Gray, Mentor, and

Figueroa-Sarriera 1995), notational (Prasad 2005), fragmented (Wegenstein 2002), communal/interchangeable (Elshtain 2005; Hogle 1995; Synnott 1993; Williams 1997), or a work of art (Eckermann 1997). It has no essentiality, nor obdurate core, no obstinate ontological foundation and thus, the body is amenable to transformation and retransformation, to being "worked upon."[17] And, worked upon it has become. As Williams and Bendelow (1998, 68) suggested, this "sets up something of a paradox, namely: the greater our ability to control the human body, the more uncertain our sense of what precisely it is, what is 'natural' about it and, perhaps most worryingly of all, what it might become" (see also Shilling 2003). If Dr. Burgess, orthopedic surgeon and founder of the Prosthetic Outreach Program, is right that prosthetization "creat[es] a new interface between the body and the world" (Smith 2001:1), then prostheses not only modify the bodies of amputees and the social worlds they inhabit, but they also reposition the border between able-bodiedness and disability, blur the once-sharp edge between interiority and exteriority, and reposition the crossing point between the inert and the vital.

Authentic Disability and Cyborg Fantasies

Some scholars have argued that the people who necessarily interface with technology as a consistent and enduring way of life may help others to overcome the fear of being dependent upon technology (Kaufert and Locker 1990). Others too have advocated for the acceptance of technologically mediated embodiment (Haraway 1985, 1992) or prosthetically enabled disability (Betcher 2001), and some have suggested that we should fully embrace the fact that we may be the last of the "pure" humans (see for example Deitch 1992) in part because we are all only temporarily able-bodied (Hughes 2007). Beautiful examples of "successful" enhancement are truly abundant, regularly peppering our literary and image-oriented landscapes. For example, Jamie Goldman, who appeared in *Women's' Sports Illustrated, Sports and Fitness Magazine, USA Today,* the *Los Angeles Times, CNN, Time, O* (Oprah Winfrey's magazine), and a nationally televised Adidas commercial (Goldman and Cagan 2001), is a widely known Paralympic athlete. After bilateral amputation, Jamie made herself five inches taller and uncritically marveled at the new cyborg body that made her stronger and more capable:

> I jumped up and down on my "cheetah legs," my carbon flex sprinting prosthetics. . . . When I wear them, especially when I run, they make me feel more like a robot than a human being. . . . These carbon flex legs were a force to be reckoned with, it was hard to stand still on them, and when I wanted to stop moving, I had to grab on to someone or catch myself against a wall. . . . They really put that speed underneath me. . . . I marvel at them still, at how carbon fiber and metal has changed my life so dramatically and given me a new way to challenge myself and become a stronger and more capable human being. (Goldman and Cagan 2001, 5,153,166)

Other scholars are interested in how these techno-corporeal couplings are accomplished and with what implications. For example, Kurzman (2003, 5) acknowledged the increased intimacy with which American amputees have come to embody prostheses, but cautioned against abstracting the prosthetized-amputee out of lived contexts. More importantly, though, Kurzman (2003, 5) asked us to reflexively consider the implications of conceptualizing prostheses as "enabling agents." Bordo (1993, 246) too outlines what she calls the elements of the "paradigm of plasticity" and exposes a series of "effacements," including the homogenizing, normalizing, and disciplining effects of these kinds of couplings. Likewise, Shildrick (1999) warned that the rhetoric of technologization conflates the normal and the normative, and argued that body modification is not a practice of transgression but rather an attempt at normalization vis-à-vis chasing a denaturalized ideal.

Nevertheless, I will suggest that prosthetization is an inevitability for most amputees[18] and as a result, positions them as central to the prosthetic imaginary. Amputees in the contemporary context are constructed as a "superior category on an unspoken continuum of disabled bodies" (Serlin 2004, 35), as icons of military-inspired, technologically induced liberation, as enabled cyborgs.[19] This is true despite the fact that

the cyborgs who inhabit popular discourses and who circulate as powerful icons of our posthuman future are far from "statistically" normative.
The typical prosthetized amputee is likely to be a male,[20] below-knee
(BK) amputee,[21] who is older,[22] African American,[23] and has lost his leg
to vascular disease.[24] Regardless of how unrepresentative of the "statistically normative" amputee the cyborg may be, it nonetheless commands
a particular power because of its primacy as a popular icon. At the risk
of dismissing the work accomplished by disability theorists and activists who have argued against the reification of the pitiful child–super-
crip dichotomy (Linton 2006), neutralizing disability though decon-
textualization (Jeffreys 2002), or neglecting the fact that there is always
something unsaid underlying popular (or unpopular) narratives of the
disabled (Frank 2000), I suggest that amputees inhabit a unique position relative to our understanding of disability and embodiment because
cyborgs decenter able-bodiedness. Even as pure fantasy, they represent
what becomes of those who join "the revolution" and as such, they pre-
figure the future of lived techno-corporeal conjoin-ment.

Authentic Death and Phantom Extinction

To be sure, prostheses are distinctively transformative; they have transformed the social body and the prosthetic imaginary as well as the bodies, minds, and brains of amputees. Still, we cannot forget the role that
phantoms have played in engendering such transformations. When
phantom-prosthetic relations are properly historicized, they effectively
undermine the naturalized association between prostheses and corporeal enhancement. Prostheses have never had an unmediated relationship with bodies, minds, brains, or publics. It has only been by way of
phantoms that prostheses turned idle, dependent, emasculated bodies into powerful extensions of a newly industrialized and militarized
nation. It has only been through phantoms that prostheses salvaged feminized minds, those severed from the psychic robustness only secured
though physical wholeness. It has only been via phantoms that neuronal
connections in the brains of amputees were either fortified or lost. It

has only been through phantoms that prostheses have been amenable to facilitating corporeal transgression.

Phantoms have allowed techno-corporeal coupling to feel intimate, cozy, deep, and natural. The awe-inspiring quality of prostheses was never just because wood, rubber, plastic, steel, carbon, and the like could be molded into uncanny copy-cats or even futuristic alternatives. The greatness of prostheses was always a consequent of what could be done with them because they were embodied, because they were animated, because they were lived.

Dissecting phantoms, dismantling prostheses, and denuding the "cultural filaments" (Casper 1998a, 24) that connect ghosts and machines certainly renders visible (1) the work done, the assumptions made, and the biopolitics behind generating and legitimating biomedical knowledge; (2) the weighty and far-reaching implications of the circulation and spread of that knowledge; (3) and the lived consequences of the widespread adoption (or even debate about the veracity and authenticity) of biomedical knowledge for those invested in, affected by, and "implicated" in (Clarke and Montini 1993, 46) its form, features, and fate. Dissecting, dismantling, and denuding also reveal something fundamental about "affiliative objects" (Suchman 2005), those objects that are promiscuous or at least highly sociable; prostheses and phantoms have been at any one time both original and replica, both old and new, iterations of both pasts and futures. Prostheses that were meant for the kinds of intimacies that forge transcendent and revelatory transformations and phantoms that had a natural inclination toward, and in fact a steadfast desire for, technologic coupling and even absolute synchronicity were always in Frank's (2007, 523) terms destined to be "overwritten by 'newer and newer versions.'"

Given these tendencies, should amputees, clinicians, neuroscientists, apotemnophiles, transsexuals, as well as prostheses, neuromatrices, mirror neurons, and others be concerned with keeping phantoms safe, with staving off their theoretical extinction, with urgent and intensive conservation practices? Maybe, but phantoms have always been liable to recall, reawakening, or resurrection because they are devoted to technologic quickening and because they stir so easily in their graves. Virtual reality in the form of thought or embedded experiments, an electrode strategically placed on the cortex, another amputee living with admiration or dependency, a provocative dream of wholeness or fragmentation, or even a simple mirror positioned to trick the gullible brain can bring dead phantoms back to life with evident ease. It seems that phantom death is rarely authentic because embodied ghosts are not bound by the notions of conceptual, material, or temporal permanence. It seems that it is difficult to kill a ghost.

Perhaps in the end the question about phantom displacement, endangerment, or extinction is misguided. Instead of wondering what a biomedically based theory of extinction can tell us about phantoms or prostheses, should we ponder what a phantom-based theory of life (animation), death (extinction), and afterlife (reawakening) can tell us about biomedicine and biopower? Instead of mourning the possible loss of phantoms, maybe we should wait to see how they might shape-shift, escape their biomedical confines once again, "infect" new populations, or occupy new vital, inert, conceptual, or virtual body parts. Maybe we should wait to see how commanding a presence the Holy Grail will have among neuroscientists and what other transformations the "misbehavior ghost" might engender. Perhaps too we should exploit the "phantom window" not just to peer into the cortices, psyches, and brain-based bodies of amputees but also to see more clearly the effects of the often uncontested knowledges, mystified practices, and claims of authenticity that characterize biomedicine and the biopolitical order in the twenty-first century.

Notes to Chapter 1

1. Observation has been used extensively in the social sciences and is an ideal method for recording interactions or events that unfold naturally. In addition, observation allows a complex process, such as gait training, to be broken down into its constitutive components, revealing how it is accomplished and how variations emerge. I observed at the annual Amputee Coalition of America Conference in Dallas, Texas, in August of 2006, where I also conducted both formal and informal interviews. I attended all of the conference sessions, panels, "networking rooms," and workshops, and when events were not scheduled, I observed at the gait analysis clinic or in a large exhibit hall where prosthetic manufacturers and service providers could be found.

2. Grounded theory operates under the assumption that action occurs within material interactional spaces and thus embraces an understanding of social phenomena as emergent. Grounded theorists are interested in action and the "built nature" of social phenomena and are sensitive to the indigenous quality of meaning. In practice, conceptual discovery and ordering of in vivo relations allows researchers to identify continuities between data elements, as well as variations between emerging categories and meaning systems. But, more importantly, conceptual "discovery" as opposed to "application" allows the data to tell the story. Grounded theory, developed by Glaser, Strauss, and Corbin (see for example Glaser and Strauss 1967; Strauss 1987; Strauss and Corbin 1998), is a mode of analysis and a comprehensive tool predicated on data analysis as ongoing, as opposed to a strict data collection/data analysis split, and is integral for projects that use a technique of recursive analysis or "constant comparison." This type of analysis allows researchers to trace and detail new or emerging directions, patterns, or themes; solidify connections; generate categories or codes for data organization; and expound on these codes in ways that amplify their depth, strength, and analytic value (Strauss and Corbin 1998). Situational analysis, as Clarke (2005) argued, revitalized traditional grounded theory by bringing it around the postmodern turn and displacing its positivistic inclinations. Using a cartographic approach to data analysis and interpretation, situational mapping is a means through which

various data are read together and a means through which the major actors and elements of the research are identified and situationally related. My project takes seriously the role of discourses and the nonhuman in the construction of such "things" as bodies, technologies, and biopolitics. It is precisely because situational analysis provides an approach that "simultaneously address[es] voice and discourse, text and the consequential materialities and symbolisms of the nonhuman, the dynamics of historical change, and, last but far from least, power in both its more solid and fluid forms" that it is an ideal analytic approach (Clarke 2005, xxii).

3. Content analysis appreciates artifacts that exist for consumptive, instructive, practical, or other purposes as also communicative of aspects of sociocultural arrangements; things and texts always tell a story. What is particularly productive about this type of analysis is that it captures the taken-for-granted, "naturalistic, 'found' quality" of artifacts (Reinharz 1992, 147), and the coupling of "found" and "produced" data in a single study acts as a means of increasing analytic robustness (Bouma and Atkinson 1995; Reinharz 1992). However, traditional content analysis is typically considered a quantitative method with a number of essential features, including the formation of a hypothesis and the establishment a list of a priori codes or categories. In stark contrast, my approach to content analysis was inspired by grounded theory and was an interpretive, inductive process characterized predominantly by revision, and thus, was more amenable to the qualitative tendency to "read" various kinds of data together, and to allow data to emerge from texts. Eight hundred and five articles and texts published between 1870 and 2011 were analyzed.

4. Qualitative, in-depth, semistructured interviewing is a particularly apt method of data collection when the research question cannot be answered simply. Complex narratives that reconstruct events, fill in historical blanks, and detail personal experiences are uncovered through the set of techniques specific to this type of interviewing. I conducted ten interviews with key American and Canadian scientists and clinical researchers investigating some aspect of phantom limb syndrome who were selected by reviewing the scholarship on phantom phenomena. Each interview was tailored to the particular respondent, his or her work, and his or her contributions to the published literature but remained open and dynamic—a process consistent with the flexible, iterative nature of semistructured interviewing (Rubin and Rubin 1995). When possible, the interviews were conducted in person; otherwise they were conducted via telephone.

I have chosen not to engage amputees' narratives or accounts aside from those provided by experts in the field—stories filtered through biomedical logics and lenses. This research strategy, often referred to as studying "up" rather than "down," is not meant to privilege biomedical over lay discourses, but rather to undermine knowledge claims based on the supposition of rigor, expertise, and scientific-ness.

5. Why, over the last two or three decades, has the body become an overt object and site of intellectual inquiry? Many structural and ideological factors have contributed: (1) the defacement of the Cartesian mechanistic body (in at least some circles) and the erosion of durable binaries, including mind/body; (2) feminist engagements with the issue of embodied difference and the body as a site of patriarchal control (Shilling 2005); the emergence of biopolitical issues of demographic change such as the graying of the population (Turner 1991; Williams and Bendelow 1998); shifts in the nature of governmentality that emphasizes the physical body as an object of control (Lupton 1999; Shilling 2005); the cultural contradictions of capitalism and the amplification of consumer culture (Falk 1994; Featherstone 1991); the proliferation of risk-pervasive environments (Armstrong 1995; Beck 1992; Giddens 1991); reflexive late-modernization and the proliferation of uncertainty (Frank 1991; Shilling 2003, 2005; Turner 1991; Webster 2002; Williams 1997); and the emergence and elaboration of the health regime (Crawford 1987,1994, 2004).

6. Neural interfacing involves harnessing "naturally occurring" neuronal activity via computer chips implanted in the brain (Andersen, et al. 2004; de Peralta Menendez, et al. 2005; Musallam, et al. 2004). As Naam (2005, 181) reported, considerable interest in neural integration has developed, and "more than a dozen universities and at least three private companies are now working to develop the brain-computer interface." This technology is purportedly the most significant breakthrough in prosthetic technologies to date, one that has implications far beyond limb replacement. For example, "the effort [is seen] as part of an impending revolution that could eventually make [neural interfacing] as commonplace as Palm Pilots and spawn a whole new industry centered around the brain" (Regalado 2001, 1). "Whatever the date, this technology will eventually become a common enabling option for the disabled, and at that point, people will surely start talking about using the same technology for elective human augmentation" (Branwyn 1993, 5).

7. As Sharon Betcher (2001, 49) remarks,

> Unlike the able bodied, who may imagine the technologically endowed body as somehow bionic or indestructible, the disabled person becomes even more acutely aware of the need to take up what Iragaray calls "the like-death-watch." Disabled persons must physically wrestle with the exquisite loveliness of and frustration with one's own transient tissues at the same time as s/he wrestles with the physical and psychic cumbersomeness, the severe rigidity, if also acquired grace, of the technologically endowed body.

Notes to Chapter 2

1. Epidural anesthesia became contraindicated for female lower limb amputees (Mackenzie 1983) because of its association with the reoccurrence of phantom limb pain (Uncles, Glynn, and Carrie 1996) despite the fact that the incidence rate was only 5 percent (Tessler, Angle, and Kleiman 1992).

Notes to Chapter 3

1. An exception is Melzack's (1989, 2) reference in the late 1980s to phantoms some-times feeling more real than the intact limb "because it has a tingling or 'pins-and-needles' quality that, initially at least, makes it highly salient."

2. In a study of seventy-six upper limb amputees, 50 percent said they would prefer not to have their phantoms, 41 percent did not mind them, and 9 percent would prefer to keep them (Fraser, et al. 2001).

3. Recognition that the distal parts of phantoms are sensed as the most vivid and are often the source of the most persistent sensations has been documented every decade since the 1930s. Researchers have at times suggested that amputees are more "attached" to these parts or that as phantoms "naturally" fade and disappear, these are simply the "last parts to go." Since the turn of the twenty-first century, researchers have proposed that distal vividness reflects the fact that these parts occupy larger neuronal areas in the somatosensory and motor cortices.

4. Incidence and prevalence are hopelessly conflated in the literature. When it was impossible to distinguish between the two, I treated the reported figure as a prevalence rate.

5. There are exceptions within the literature. See for example, Jankovic and Glass (1985, 433), Jacobson and Chabal (1989, 984), and Rybarczyk, Edwards, and Behel (2004, 949).

6. Baszenger (1998a) argued that pattern theory existed alongside specificity theory, which proposed that certain noxious inputs accumulate to produce pain. She wrote, "Particular patterns of nerve impulses generating pain are produced by summation of the skin sensory input at the dorsal horn cells. Pain results when the total output of the cells exceeds a critical level" (Baszanger 1998a, 51). In addition, affect theory is identified as a "third protagonist . . . [that] follow[ed] the Aristotelian tradition, according to which pain was a property of the soul" (Baszanger 1998a, 53).

7. Kolb (1950a) identified one case study in which the patient was subjected to twenty-seven different surgical procedures, including multiple reamputations.

8. Sherman's 1997 survey of the literature, investigating the breadth and effectiveness of available treatment options for phantom pain, uncovered very little success. He found that six patients were reportedly cured by existing treatment modes: one was cured by drinking alcohol; two via increased use of their prosthesis; one through injection of an unspecified substance; and one through nerve strangu-lation. Of those who obtained a significant permanent reduction in pain, two found relief with analgesics, and electrical stimulation of the stump was effective for one. The following were also reported as alleviating pain in a single case: local anesthetics; massage of the stump end; unspecified nerve block; stump desensi-tization; and ultrasound of the stump. In another study, 49 of 590 veterans were told by their physicians that there was no treatment available (Wartan, et al. 1997).

9. Katz (1998, 595) gave the following reply: "In their haste to declare this 'dodo' extinct and to abandon research in this area, McQuay and colleagues would

deprive those individuals undergoing amputation of the possibility of a future with less pain. We must continue to investigate methods to reduce the frequency and intensity of this very real and difficult pain problem."

Notes to Chapter 4

1. Ambrose Paré (1510–1590), the "towering father of French surgery" (Engstrom and Van de Ven 1985, 1; Porter 2002), was the first known to use linen ligation without cautery in amputation surgery, prior to the advent of the tourniquet (Vitali 1978), and to perform an elbow disarticulation (Rang and Thompson 1981). In addition, he introduced the practice of amputation site selection based on postoperative prosthetic fitting, a modern surgical doctrine (Rang and Thompson 1981). He also invented both upper and lower extremity prosthetics (Engstrom and Van der Ven 1985; Rang and Thompson 1981).

2. As Finger and Hustwit (2003, 675) argued, the assumption that phantom limb was absent from scholarly and literary writings until Paré's reference is an "historical shortcoming [that] still dominate[s] the literature." For references to the phenom-enon's obscuration see, for example, Frederiks 1963. Lamarier published work on the pathophysiology of sensation from separated parts in 1778, suggesting that this inter-val is probably much more narrow (Olry and Haines 2002). Other significant refer-ences to phantoms include Rene Descartes' seventeenth-century public writings and private correspondences (Finger and Hustwit 2003), William Porterfield's self-report in his *Treatise on the Eye* in 1759 (Wade and Finger 2003), John Hunter's description of two cases of phantom penis in 1786 (Wade 2003), Erasmus Darwin's interpreta-tion of phantoms within empiricist philosophy in 1794 (Wade 2003), Albrecht von Haller's comment in a book published in 1762 (Finger and Hustwit 2003), Aaron Lemos's volume on *The Continuing Pain of an Amputated Limb,* published in 1798 (Frederiks 1963), and Johannes Muller's elaboration of thirteen causes of sensa-tion after amputation in 1826 (Wade 2003). For both a comprehensive overview of eighteenth- and nineteenth-century references to phantom limb and a detailed presentation of early descriptions from Ambrose Paré, Rene Descartes (Wade 2003), Aaron Lemos, Charles Bell (Furukawa 1990), and Silas Weir Mitchell, see Finger and Hustwit 2003. Also see Price and Twombly's (1972) published manuscript on case study, short description, and classification references of phantoms from 1610 to 1798.

3. Goler (2004, 163–64) detailed the war-hastened practice of recording battlefield wounds and conditions that resulted in the collection of severed limbs. The parts were processed by the curator of the Army Medical Museum in Washington, who preserved them in alcohol or salt water. See Goler (2004) for a description of the museum, its collection practices, and its specimens.

4. "The stump hospital" was the common name for the United States Army Hospital for Injuries and Diseases of the Nervous System, located outside Philadelphia in 1866 (Goler 2004).

5. The terms "body image" and "body scheme" (also spelled "schema") were used interchangeably within the literature. Some authors used the term to denote a

single structure, *the* body scheme, while others refer to a set of representations, *multiple* schemata. Further, the terms were often poorly defined (Van Wirdum 1965). This was true despite a few attempts to maintain conceptual clarity within the field. For example, Hoffman (1954a, 147) advocated differentiating between (1) the body image, or the sense of body position derived via proprioceptive senses; (2) the body scheme, or the basic recognition of the body; and (3) the bodily ego, or an amalgamation of the body image and scheme. Omer (1981, 754) advocated differentiating between (1) the body ideal, or the idealized image of the body; (2) the body percept, or the model of body movement and appearance; (3) the body concept, or the thoughts, memories, and attitudes about the body derived interpersonally; and (4) the body ego, or that aspect of the personality that concerns itself with the body image.

6. Phantom breast was first acknowledged by Ambrose Paré circa 1551 (Bressler, Cohen, and Magnusson 1956, 181) and was mentioned in a footnote in Mitchell's (1872) unprecedented volume, *Injuries of Nerves and Their Consequences* several centuries later.

7. Gerber (1994) suggested that two sets of solutions were advanced to address the reintegration problem: public welfare actualized in, for example, the G.I. Bill of Rights, and public education in the form of literature instructing women to do their part in restoring traditional roles in American households.

8. Krane and Heller (1995, 23) found that in children ages five to nineteen who had experienced amputation, whether attributed to congenital absence, trauma/infection, or cancer, 100 percent experienced phantoms, and that pain was a symptom in the overwhelming majority. Still, reports given by children remained suspect because they were often deemed not credible (see for example Flor, Elbert, and Muhlnickel 1998).

9. Scholars who have been interested in the relationship between power and discourse as it relates to medicine, science, technology, and the body in the modern and late-modern contexts have critically examined the role that medical discourses, knowledges, and practices have played in the naturalization of disease; the division between mind and body (Gordon 1988; Leder 1984); the reduction of disease and illness to the biological and the simplification of the body, its processes, and its structures to the biophysical machine (Weitz 1996); the surveillance of the ill and the temporary-well or at-risk (Armstrong 2002; Foucault 1973); the monopolization of the position of legitimate arbiters of normality and pathology (Conrad and Schneider 1980); the expansion of the scope of the medical gaze (Zola 1972); the shift from cure to prevention (Hughes 2000); the individualization of the responsibility for health and wellness (Turner 1996); and the instantiation of disease, wellness, and disability metaphors as legitimizing world views (Douglas 1966, 2003).

10. Causal mechanisms included central biasing, wind-up, hyperexcitability, sensitization, irritation, reverberating circuit, vicious circle, gate control, and other pattern-generating mechanisms.

11. Sherman (1989, 1994, 1997) wrote prolifically on the subject of the psychology of U.S. veterans and argued against the use of psychoanalysis for the treatment of phantom limb or phantom pain.

12. The term "engram" can be found in the phantom literature as early as the 1950s.

13. These experiments precipitated a fear among researchers that phantoms could actually be invoked or exacerbated in amputees by anesthesia, particularly in women. In fact, epidural anesthesia became contraindicated for lower limb amputees (Mackenzie 1983; Uncles, Glynn, and Carrie 1996) even though the reported incidence rate was only 5 percent (Tessler, Angle, and Kleiman 1992).

14. Other researchers have continued to employ the concept, though typically as an abstraction, a conceptual corollary of the cortical regions of the brain known as the homunculi.

15. Melzack (1990) theorized that these three circuits simultaneously process information internal to the neuromatrix. The information is then distributed to other parts of the brain, producing an output termed the "neurosignature," which purportedly generates conscious awareness.

Notes to Chapter 5

1. Researchers used Magnetic Resonance Imaging (MRI), including Functional Magnetic Resonance Imaging (fMRI) and Structural Magnetic Resonance Imaging (sMRI), Magnetoencephalographic (MEG) recordings, Magnetic Source Imaging (MSI), Positron Emission Tomography (PET) scans, Computed Tomography (CT) scans, Neuroelectric Source Imaging (ESI), electromyograms (EMGs), and Stereotactic Mapping (SM) among other techniques.

2. "Phantoms in the Brain" has also has been the subject of a PBS special and featured on the BBC. In *Newsweek*'s annually published *Century Club*, Ramachandran was named "one of the hundred most prominent people to watch in the next century." See the following site for details: http://psy.ucsd.edu/chip/ramabio.html.

3. For a comprehensive overview of the work of Wilder Penfield see the compilation of articles entitled "Wilder Penfield: His Legacy to Neurology" in the *Canadian Medical Association Journal*, June 1977.

4. As Wood (2002, xv–xvi) explains,

    Corneluis Agrippa believed . . . that humans could be grown from mandrake roots. His contemporary, Paracelsus published instructions on the manufacture of a "homunculus," or miniature man. Human semen, Paracelsus suggested, should be put into an airtight jar and buried in horse manure for forty days. After this, it was to be "magnetized," then preserved at the temperature of a mare's womb and fed human blood for forty weeks. A small, fully formed person was thought to emerge after this procedure.

5. Instructions can be found on the Woodrow Wilson Biology Institute website on mapping your own homunculus. Complete with a materials list, procedure, and examples of analyses, the instructions explain that the shape of your homunculus can be determined with the help of two assistants. The process involves a

blindfold and pricking yourself with toothpicks. See the following site for details: http://www.woodrow.org/teachers/bi/1991/homunculus.html.

6. The work of Henderson and Smyth (1948) is an exception; they not only referenced the work of Penfield and Boldrey but also argued that the "anatomical substrate is in the sensori-motor cortex."

7. Pons's work is often considered an elaboration of that begun in the mid-1980s by Dr. Michael Merzenich, a neuroscientist at the University of California–San Francisco (Merzenich, et al. 1983; Merzenich, et al. 1984). Merzenich and his colleagues conducted a series of experiments in which they amputated the middle fingers of several adult owl monkeys and stimulated the remaining fingers. Using neural imaging, Merzenich found that the area of the brain previously corresponding to the amputated finger responded to stimulation of the adjacent fingers. In *Discover* (Shreeve 1993, 3), Merzenich was quoted as saying, "There had always been a countercurrent to the mainstream that suspected the brain could make such adjustments. . . . We witnessed them happening."

8. The details of the case of the Silver Springs monkeys vary by source according to the number of monkeys involved, the number of postdeafferentation years, and the number of monkeys euthanized. A disturbing video detailing the specifics of the abuse produced by People for the Ethical Treatment of Animals (PETA) can be found at the following site: http://www.petatv.com/tvpopup/Prefs.asp?video=silver-spring-monkeys.

9. Dr. Taub was eventually convicted of providing inadequate veterinary care, but the Maryland appeals court overturned the conviction in 1984 (Green 2005).

10. The monkeys had mutilated their own arms; a spokesperson at the NIH attributed their behavior to unrelenting phantom limb pain (Holden 1989).

11. The "hard-wired brain" is associated with the work of David Hubel and Torsten Wiesel at Harvard University. The two were awarded the Nobel Prize for their work in 1981 (Barinaga 1992; Shreeve 1993).

12. These were later referred to as reference zones (RZ) (Moore, et al. 2000), trigger points (Fraser, et al. 2001), and misallocation points (Condes-Lara, et al. 2000).

13. There are a few earlier references to trigger zones found on the contralateral limb. See for example Dernham 1986.

14. Ramachandran and Blakeslee (1998) speculate that foot fetishes might result from the normal boundary crossing of the homuncular feet and genitalia.

15. The two parts of the body found at the "end" of the map would only be adjacent to a single other homuncular body part.

16. In addition, there has long been a connection between phantom formation and sexual intercourse. Kolb (1950b, 469–70) gives one of the first accounts:

> A married man 58 years of age came to the clinic complaining of pain in a phantom left hand. He declared that two years and nine months previously, while working alone on a neighbor's farm his left hand was caught in a corn picker. He stated that he was unable to extricate himself and watched the hand and arm slowly being mangled over a period of ninety minutes. He was

taken to the hospital immediately after being released where amputation was performed at the junction of the upper and middle third of the forearm. The patient felt well until after he returned home. He was aware of the existence of [a] phantom extremity but it was not then painful. Later, after attempting sexual intercourse, the sensation of pain in the phantom hand was experienced for the first time. This pain recurred repeatedly when attempting the sexual act.

Others have reported the disappearance or withdrawal of the phantom after orgasm, especially after masturbation (Miles 1956).

17. Additional areas of the brain that have been shown to reorganize are the supplementary motor or sensory areas, the thalamus, and other subcortical regions.

18. Some researchers suggested that telescoping was a product of use-dependent reorganization and thus, was an adaptive phenomenon associated with less phantom limb pain (Katz 1992b; Ramachandran, Stewart, and Rogers-Ramachandran 1992).

19. Two exceptions are the work of Condes-Lara, et al. (2000) and Schwenkreis, et al. (2001). Condes-Lara (2000) and colleagues argued that nonpainful sensations were positively correlated with reorganization of the thalamic and the somatosensory and motor regions of the cortex, while Schwenkreis (2001) and colleagues showed that phantom pain intensity was not correlated with reorganization. Others found different activation patterns in the same structures for phantom limb and phantom pain (Willoch, et al. 2000). For example, when an amputee imagined painful finger movements and nonpainful finger movements, different parts of the cortex were activated (Rosen, et al. 2001).

20. Others have hypothesized that both sprouting and unmasking are simultaneously at work (Aglioti, Bonazzi, and Cortese 1994; Darian-Smith and Gilbert 1994; Das and Gilbert 1995; Doetsch 1997; Elbert, et al. 1997; Flor, et al. 1995; Florence and Kaas 1995; Merzenich and Kass 1982). In my interview with Taub (2005), he suggested that

[t]here are demonstrations that this or that mechanism operates at some times but as to what is going on at any one specific time, one doesn't know. What was generally believed to be the case was—that is, after the Pons et al. study—was that there was a combination of axonal sprouting from neurons that are intact in the vicinity of the debris of the neurons that have died. There was also the consideration of unmasking of previously silent neurons. Those are both not only excellent hypotheses but you can demonstrate that they occur. And, an increase in the excitability of the remaining neurons possibly associated with something called "deafferentation supersensitivity." . . . There is a disinhibition of the small diameter fibers in the thalamus which would give rise, obviously, to an increase in excitability of the areas that they project to. What I really believe is that there are a number of mechanisms that no one has thought of that may be more important than anything that anyone has been talking about recently.

Notes to Chapter 6

1. A study of nine Paris hospitals published in 1842 reported an overall mortality rate of 39 percent, 52 percent for major amputations and 62 percent for thigh amputations (Wangensteen, Smith, and Wangensteen 1967).

2. Between 1851 and 1873, eighteen patents were granted for artificial upper limbs, 76 for artificial legs, and a total of 133 for amputation-related technologies (Figg and Farrell-Beck 1993).

3. The Civil War was depicted by historians as the first modern war characterized by exceptional brutality (Cervetti 2003) and a more faithful representation in the media (Goler 2004).

4. Although modern surgical technique improved postoperative survival rates, the procedure remained extremely risky. Fernie (1981) reported that two-thirds of amputees died within the first five years. In another study published four years later, fifty-eight patients who had undergone amputation for peripheral vascular disease were contacted for a follow-up after two years; researchers found that 41 percent of the original sample had died (Jensen, et al. 1984). A study the subsequent year investigated both vascular and traumatic amputations performed between 1970 and 1977. During this period, 624 amputations were performed, and at the time of investigation, only ninety-five patients were still alive, a 15 percent survival rate (Krebs, et al. 1985). Van der Schans and Geertzen (2002) reported the survival rate for amputation due to end-stage vascular disease as 15–33 percent. The five-year survival rate for lower extremity amputees is less than 50 percent, 40 percent for diabetes-related amputations, the most common cause of amputation today (Bloomquist 2001a). And, of the diabetic amputees who survive, approximately half will lose the second leg within five years (Bloomquist 2001a). The data available on amputation incidence and prevalence in the United States are extremely ambiguous. The United States does not maintain a national database (Sherman and Sherman 1985) and the structure of the health care delivery system has precluded researchers from conducting an accurate census (Wilson 1998). Reports of incidence have ranged from 75,000 in 1945 (Thomas and Haddan 1945), to 40,000 in 1947 (CPD 1947), 30,000 in 1986 (Dernham 1986), an average of 133,235 annually between 1988 and 1996 (Dillingham, Pezzin, and MacKenzie 2002a), 47,300 in 1992 (Rounseville 1992), 185,000 in 1996 (Bloomquist 2001b) and 203,000 in 2001 (Bloomquist 2001b). Reports of prevalence have ranged from 925,000 in 1945 (Thomas and Haddan 1945) to 275,000 in 1977 (Shurr and Cook 1990), 450,000 in 1982 (Stein and Warfield 1982) 1,285,000 in 1996 (ACA 2002), and 413,000 in 1998 (Wilson 1998).

5. The establishment of the National Security Council, the National Security Agency, the Pentagon, the Strategic Air Command, the Central Intelligence Agency, the Defense Department, the Army Special Forces Group, and the Green Berets, along with the arms race and the stationing of millions of soldiers abroad, testifies to the predominance of the American war culture during this period (Farber 1994).

6. Historically in rural areas, the barber or pharmacist typically functioned as the prosthetist. After measuring, taking a casted-impression of the stump, and obtaining a shoe, the barber would prepare a box to be mailed to a limb company and instruct the amputee to toughen his stump skin (Pike and Nattress 1991).

7. Initially, financial support for the CPD came from the Office of Scientific Research and Development through its committee on Medical Research and the Office of the Surgeon General of the Army. After 1946, this obligation was fulfilled by the army and the VA (CPD 1946).

8. The U.S. Department of Veterans Affairs (VA) was created in 1930 to organize the activities of the government on behalf of U.S. veterans and was established as a Cabinet-level position in 1989 (VA 2002a). The Veterans Health Administration (VHA) is one of twenty-one organizations that exist within the VA (VA 2002a). The VHA manages the largest health care system in the nation, is one of the largest providers of graduate medical education, and is one of the nation's largest medical research organizations (VA 2002b)

9. The impetus for this meeting was the fervent public outcry that prosthetic provision, guaranteed to all amputee veterans since the post–Civil War period, was wholly inadequate (Kurzman 2003).

10. Subsequently, these and other campuses began offering coursework and, later, credentials in the field. These programs were formalized under the National Association of Prosthetic-Orthotic Educators (NAPOE), an educational organization representing the academic programs credentialed by the National Commission on Orthotic and Prosthetic Education (NCOPE), which assures the continuity of orthotic and prosthetic education (AAOP 2013). The American Board for the Certification in Orthotics Prosthetics and Pedorthics (ABC) was created in 1949 and is recognized as the preeminent national accreditation and certification body responsible for the competency of orthotists and prosthetists (ABC 2013).

11. The OWI's Office of Censorship was given the authority to review all international communications not reviewed by the military, as well as domestic communications from military installations and some industrial plants. This included review of photographs taken by military photographers (working in combat zones where access was denied to nonmilitary photographers), as well as personal photographs taken by soldiers.

12. A number of authors have argue that disability emasculates, for example Robert Murphy (1990) in the case of paraplegia, or that male disability, also in the case of paraplegia, represents a kind of double consciousness and that masculinity must be either reformulated, relied upon, or rejected (Gerschick and Miller 1994).

13. Congress allocated funds to support the manufacture of ten thousand of this model to be circulated to needy veterans in September of 1946 (Scrlin 2002).

14. The term "cyborg" typically refers to a "cybernetic organism," a human-technological hybrid or coupling (Gray, Mentor, and Figueroa-Sarriera 1995b), a "merging of the evolved and the developed, . . . [an] integration of the constructor and

the constructed, . . . systems of dying flesh and undead circuits, and of living and artificial cells" (Gray, et al. 1995, 2).

15. Incidence of amputation was 2 percent in WWI, 5.3 percent in WWII, and 13 percent in the Korean and Vietnam wars (Kirkup 1995).

16. Dr. Burgess also established, in collaboration with the U.S. Veterans Administration, the Prosthetics Research Study (PRS), considered one of the leading centers in the world for developing postoperative innovations, including immediate post-operative fitting (IPOF) of a prosthesis; the Seattle Foot, with an internal spring for active amputees; and the Seattle ShapeMaker software, used to design check sockets (POF 2005).

Notes to Chapter 7

1. The one exception in the literature is the reference to phantom menstrual cramps following hysterectomy (Dyer 2000).

2. Professor of philosophy and author in the history of psychiatry Carl Elliott investigates how "little-known psychiatric disorders spread, sometimes even reaching epidemic proportions, for reasons that nobody seems fully to understand" (Elliott 2000, 74).

3. A brief internet search demonstrates that hundreds of websites are devoted to elective or voluntary amputation. Some of the most frequented include secret-garden.com, paraamps.com, super-hosting.com/fascination, d-links.com, and ampworld.com. These sites include support groups, chat rooms, success stories, photo galleries, dating services, devotee paraphernalia for purchase, and advice on amputation. One listserve, for example, had fourteen hundred subscribers in 2000 (Elliott 2000) and by 2003, the number had grown to nearly thirty-seven hundred (Cameron 2003).

4. Once a rare and unheard of disorder, apotemnophilia has recently become a topic of interest within medical literature, as well as in the popular media. The disorder has been featured in the *Atlantic Monthly*, the *New York Times, Penthouse,* and *Hustler,* as well as on *Nip/Tuck* (shown in episode 3.07 in 2006), *CSI:NY* (shown in November 2004), *Untold Stories of the ER* (shown in November 2005), *Primetime* (shown in April 2006), the BBC documentary *Complete Obsession* (shown in winter of 1999), Melody Gilbert's *Whole,* a Sundance Documentary (shown in May 2003), and others.

5. The hospital charged forty-eight hundred dollars for each amputation (Dyer 2000).

6. Denis Canavan, a representative from the region where the two procedures were conducted, demanded an investigation by health officials and was quoted as saying, "The whole thing is repugnant and legislation needs to be brought in now to outlaw this"(Dotinga 2000, 1).

7. Considered the "poster boy" for the disorder (Dotinga 2000, 2), apotemnophile Dr. Gregg Furth (2002) wrote one of the first books on the subject with his coauthor Dr. Robert Smith. The authors proposed the term "Amputee Identity Disorder" (AID) as an alternative to "Body Dysmorphic Disorder" (BDD). Those

with BDD are preoccupied with the delusion of the exceedingly ugly or defective/ diseased nature of their bodies. Apotemnophiles, on the other hand, reportedly do not imagine their bodies as defective or ugly, but as deficient (Fisher and Smith 2000; Furth and Smith 2002). Apotemnophilia has also been related to Munchhausen syndrome (Bensler and Paauw 2003), masochism (Bensler and Paauw 2003), Gender Identity Disorder (First 2004), and Factitious Disability Disorder (FDD) (Bruno 1997). Others have suggested the terms "Body Identity Transfer" (Dotinga 2000) and "Body Integrity Identity Disorder" (BIID) (First 2004).

8. In defense of himself, Dr. Smith argued, "They are really quite a desperate bunch," and he warned that apotemnophiles will take action on their own when denied medical intervention (Bayne and Levy 2005), attempting self-amputation or even suicide. In fact, attempts have included lying on a train track (Dyer 2000; Elliott 2000), use of a chainsaw (Elliott 2000), use of a shotgun (Dyer 2000; Elliott 2000, 2003), use of dry ice (Elliott 2000, 2003), use of a guillotine (Elliott 2000), and use of a tourniquet (Bensler and Paauw 2003). Because of attempts like these, Dr. Smith described the two operations as "the most satisfying" surgeries he had ever performed (Elliott 2000, 73). However, Dr. Smith did advocate for amputation as a treatment for apotemnophilia only under a certain set of conditions, including psychological examination and a year living as closely to an amputee as possible (Furth and Smith 2002).

9. Dr. Gregg Furth, coauthor of Dr. Money's 1977 paper, approached Dr. Smith about an amputation, to which Smith agreed. Ultimately, he was unable to fulfill the request (Henig 2005).

10. References to the syndrome first appeared more than a century ago (Everaed 1983).

11. Devotees are thought to desire amputation as part of sexual arousal, the fantasy of which fades after climax and changes over time in terms of amputation type (which limb, how many, etc.). Conversely, wannabes reportedly envision themselves as living as amputees and the amputation type/level remains constant. A third category, pretenders, feign disability in order to attract devotees (Bruno 1997). However, some wannabes are also pretenders. In a study of fifty-two subjects, First (2004) found that 92 percent reported pretending by bending their leg back and tying it up, using crutches or a wheelchair, hiding a limb in clothing, wrapping the limb in bandages, or using a prosthesis. Although "true" wannabes are not primarily motivated by sexual desire, they often suggest that their sex life would probably improve because they would feel more secure with their bodies. Bruno (1997) reported that 61 percent of devotees are also pretenders and 51percent of devotees are also wannabes.

12. Richard von Krafft-Ebing in 1886 catalogued paraphilias in *Psychopathia Sexualis*. Included in this text were necrophilia, bestiality, and a number of fetishes, including those for disturbed body parts (Elliott 2000).

13. Many investigators have equated apotemnophilia with transsexuality or Gender Identity Disorder (Bayne and Levy 2005; Elliott 2000; First 2004; Fisher and

Smith 2000; Furth and Smith 2002; Mearz 2006). Apotemnophilia is thought to parallel transsexuality in that (1) both are characterized by pretending, actively imagining oneself in another corporeal form, as well as acting out some approximation of that form; (2) both are characterized by reports of an inability to live with the birthed body, often manifesting in attempts to alter the "look" and "feel" of the body; and (3) both are characterized by the use of a certain language that identifies an incongruity of body image and self-concept or identity (First 2004). Furth and Smith (2002, 10) qualified this comparison by suggesting that

> the difficulty many will perceive in the removal of healthy limbs to relieve the apotemnophiliac's psychic pain is that the final status of being an amputee does not receive the positive endorsement of the final status which a transgendered person achieves by an operation. Being male or being female is regarded as a positive outcome. Being an amputee is not regarded as a favorable outcome. It is only better than being dead, not better than having healthy limbs.

14. In a series of fifty-two in-depth interviews conducted by First (2004), he found that the most common reason for desiring amputation was to resolve a mismatch between the body and the self.
15. Dr. Michael First is a psychiatrist at Columbia University and editor of the *Diagnostic and Statistical Manual*, fourth edition (DSM-4). His study was undertaken to assist in determining whether apotemnophilia should be included in the DSM-5 (First 2004).
16. Bayne and Levy (2005) suggested that this explanation was unlikely because wannabes did not exhibit impairment in body control and because realized apotemnophiles use prostheses. The authors subsequently endorsed the label BIID, suggesting that the disorder was probably rooted in a body image–physical body mismatch. Bayne and Levy (2005) also offered First's study of fifty-two apotemnophiles as evidentiary. First reported that 37 percent of respondents felt that their limb was "different" in some way, 13 percent felt that their limb was not their own, 5 percent reported less intense sensation in the alien limb, and 5 percent reported more intense sensation.
17. Blum (2003, 42) uses the term "body landscape" to emphasize surface and to suggest that the body is lived as "transformative topography." Thus, we each have an embodied landscape that is bounded (we have an understanding of where our bodies end and where they begin), hierarchicized (we differentially invest in and value parts of our bodies), and transformable/transformed (we each have an appreciation of our bodies as amenable to alterations of different kinds, a threshold of transformation). In other words, "Our bodies are held together with the residues of everything they have been, should have been, were not, could be, are not" (Blum 2003, 43).
18. Diane DeVries in Gelya Frank's (2000) *Venus on Wheels* represents a departure from this normative tendency.
19. One study found that 61 percent of amputees forgot they were amputees "most of the time" (Silber and Silverman 1958). Almost half of the respondents said that they could do "as much" as nonamputees, and 14 percent reported that they were

able to do "somewhat more." In another study, 156 amputees were asked, "Do you feel handicapped?" Seventy-two percent of below-knee, 62 percent of above-knee, and 40 percent of bilateral amputees reported that they did not (Kegel, et al. 1977). In another study of 45 amputees, Sherman (1999) found that six respondents did not consider themselves disabled, fifteen considered themselves mildly disabled, four felt quite disabled, and none felt very disabled. Furst and Humphrey (1983) found that able-bodied people often overemphasized the degree and role of disability in amputees' lives; able-bodied respondents rated amputees as highly unfortunate, while amputees rated themselves as only marginally less fortunate after amputation (see also Horgan and MacLachlan 2004). Other scholars have also written about the process, implications, or tendency for amputees to reject the "disabled" label (Kurzman 2003; Watson 2002).

20. Fernie (1981) suggested that the ratio of male to female amputees is approximately nine to one.

21. In 1986, 85 percent of amputees were lower limb (Dernham 1986). In 1990, 90 percent of amputations were lower limb, 50 percent of which were below-knee (BK), 40 percent of which were above-knee (AK), and 10 percent of which were hip disarticulation (Winchell 1995). In 1992, 85 percent of amputations were lower-limb (Rounseville 1992). That same year, Williamson (1992) reported that 8.3 percent of all amputations were upper-limb, 91.7 percent were lower-limb, 2 percent were hip disarticulations, 32.6 percent were above-knee, 0.7 percent were knee disarticulations, 53.8 percent were below-knee, and 2.6 percent were ankle or Symes disarticulations. In 1989, the international standards organization adopted terms applicable to amputation levels, congenital limb deficiencies, and prostheses. Terms describing the amputation level of acquired amputees (commonly referred to as "AK," "BK," "AE," and "BE") were replaced by "trans" (across axis of long bone), "disarticulation" (through center of joint), and "partial" (hands and feet below the ankle and wrist). The terms used for congenital amputees include "transverse" (normal development beyond deficiency) or "longitudinal" (absence of skeletal anatomy within the long axis of the limb) (Schuch and Pritham 2002).

22. Davidson (2002) reported that in the United States, amputees were typically between the ages of fifteen and thirty. However, one of the most comprehensive public health surveys of the amputee population conducted by Glattly in 1964 and updated by Kay and Newman in 1975 (Fernie 1981) demonstrated a distribution highest for those ages fifty-one through eighty (Wilson 1998).

23. The risk of amputation increases with age, particularly among African Americans. For example, in 1996, African Americans represented 12 percent of the United States population, but they accounted for one-quarter of vascular amputations (Dillingham, Pezzin, and MacKenzie 2002a). Around the year 2000, among persons with diabetes, African Americans, Hispanics, and Native Americans were at a higher risk for lower-limb loss than whites, and vascular amputation rates for African Americans were twice those of other races (Dillingham, Pezzin, and Mackenzie 2002b).

24. The vast majority of amputations are related to vascular disease, estimated by Dernham (1986) at 85 percent, by Bohne (1987) at 80 percent, by Shurr and Cook (1990) at 70 percent, by Rounseville (1992) at 80 percent, and by Williamson (1992) at 74 percent. Dillingham, Pezzin, and MacKenzie (2002a) found that vascular amputations between 1988 and 1996 increased 3 percent annually (an overall increase of 27 percent), while the amputation rate attributable to trauma declined 5.6 percent annually, and malignancy-related amputations declined 4.7 percent annually. Congenital amputations, which accounted for less than 1 percent of amputations, remained stable. Comparably, in 1938, 28 percent of a study including 42 amputations resulted from trauma, 36 percent from vascular disease, 16 percent from infection, 8 percent from tumor, and 12 percent from miscellaneous causes (Livingston 1938).

REFERENCES

AAOP. 2013. "History." *American Association of Orthotists and Prosthetists*: http://www. oandp.org/about/history.

ABC. 2002. "About the ABC." *American Board for Certification in Orthotics, Prosthetics, and Pedorthics*: www.abcop.org.

ABC News. 2000. "Surgical questions: Questions raised over amputations of two healthy legs." *ABC*: www.abcnews.go.com.

Abramson, A. S., and A. Feibel. 1981. "The phantom phenomenon: Its use and disuse." *Bulletin of the New York Academy of Medicine* 57:99–112.

ACA. 2013. "Prosthetics FAQs for the new amputee." *Amputee Coalition of America*: www.amputee-coalition.org.

Acerra, Nicole E., Tina Souvlis, and G. Lorimer Moseley. 2007. "Stroke, complex regional pain syndrome, and phantom limb pain: Can commonalities direct future management?" *Journal of Rehabilitation Medicine* 39:109–14.

Adler, Patricia A., and Peter Adler. 2011. *The tender cut: Inside the hidden world of self-injury*. New York: New York University Press.

Aglioti, Salvatore, Andrea Bonazzi, and Feliciana Cortese. 1994. "Phantom lower limb as a perceptual marker of neural plasticity in the mature human brain." *Proceedings of the Royal Society of London B: Biological Sciences* 255:273–78.

Aglioti, Salvatore, Feliciana Cortese, and Cristina Franchini. 1994. "Rapid sensory remapping in the adult human brain as inferred from phantom breast perception." *Neuroreport* 5:473–76.

Akrich, Madeleine. 1995. "User representations: Practices, methods, and sociology," in *The approach of constructive technology assessment*, edited by A. Rip, T. J. Misa, and J. Schot. New York: St. Martin's Press.

Alessandria, Maria, Roberto Vetrugno, Pietro Cortelli, and Pasquale Montagna. 2011. "Normal body scheme and absent phantom limb experience in amputees while dreaming." *Consciousness and Cognition* 20:1831–34.

Ament, Philip, James T. Grace, John T. Phelan, and Aaron Ament. 1964. "Removal of phantom pain after hemipelvectomy." *New York State Journal of Medicine* 64:2907–8.

Andersen, R. A., J. W. Burdick, S. Musallam, B. Pesaran, and J .G. Cham. 2004. "Cognitive neural prosthetics." *Trends in Cognitive Science* 8:486–93.

Anderson-Barnes, Victoria C., Caitlin McAuliffe, Kelley M. Swanberg, and Jack W. Tsao. 2009. "Phantom limb pain: A phenomenon of proprioceptive memory." *Medical Hypotheses* 73:555–58.

Andre, J. M., N. Martinet, J. Paysant, J. M. Beis, and L. Le Chapelain. 2001. "Temporary phantom limbs evoked by vistibular caloric stimulation in amputees." *Neuropsychiatry, Neuropsychology, and Behavioral Neurology* 14:190–96.

Appenzeller, O., and J. M. Bicknell. 1969. "Effects of nervous system lesions on phantom experiences in amputees." *Neurology* 19:141–46.

Arena, John G., Richard A. Sherman, Glenda M. Bruno, and James D. Smith. 1990. "The relationship between situational stress and phantom limb pain: Cross-lagged correlational data from six month pain logs." *Journal of Psychosomatic Research* 34:71–77.

Armstrong, David. 1995. "The rise of surveillance medicine." *Sociology of Health and Illness* 17:393–404.

———. 2002. "The rise of surveillance medicine," in *The sociology of health and illness reader,* edited by S. Nettleton and U. Gustaffson. Cambridge,UK: Polity.

Arnheim, Rudolf. 1986. "The two faces of gestalt psychology." *American Psychologist* 41:820–24.

Bailey, A. A., and F. P. Moersch. 1941. "Phantom limb." *Canadian Medical Association Journal* 45:37–42.

Bakheit, A. M., and S. Roundhill. 2005. "Supernumerary phantom limb after stroke." *Postgraduate Medical Journal* 81:1–2.

Balsamo, Anne. 1995. "Forms of technological embodiment: Reading the body in contemporary culture." *Body and Society* 1:215–37.

———. 1996. *Technologies of the gendered body: Reading cyborg women.* Durham, NC: Duke University Press.

Barad, Karen. 1999. "Agential realism: Feminist interventions in understanding scientific practice," in *The science studies reader,* edited by M. Biagioli. New York: Routledge.

Barinaga, M. 1992. "The brain remaps its own contours." *Science* 258:216–18.

Baszanger, Isabelle. 1989. "Pain: Its experience and treatments." *Social Science and Medicine* 29:425–34.

———. 1992. "Deciphering chronic pain." *Sociology of Health and Illness* 14:181–215.

———. 1998a. *Inventing pain medicine: From the laboratory to the clinic.* New Brunswick, NJ: Rutgers University Press.

———. 1998b. "Pain physicians: All alike, all different," in *Differences in medicine: Unraveling practices, techniques, and bodies,* edited by M. Berg and A. Mol. Durham, NC: Duke University Press.

Bayne, T., and N. Levy. 2005. "Amputees by choice: Body integrity identity disorder and the ethics of amputation." *Journal of Applied Philosophy* 22:75–86.

Beaulieu, Anne. 2002. "Images are not the (only) truth: Brain mapping, visual knowledge, and Iconoclasm." *Science, Technology, and Human Values* 27:53–86.

Beck, Ulrich. 1992. *Risk society: Towards a new modernity.* London: Sage.

Beller, A. J., and E. Peyser. 1951. "Prefrontal lobotomy for phantom limb and phantom pain." *Journal of the International College of Surgeons* 16:432–35.

Bendelow, Gillian A. 2006. "Pain, suffering, and risk." *Health, Risk, and Society* 8:59–70.

Bensler, J. M., and D. S. Paauw. 2003. "Apotemnophilia masquerading as medical morbidity." *Southern Medical Journal* 96:674–76.

Berger, B. D., J. A. Lehrmann, G. Larson, L. Alverno, and C. I. Tsao. 2005. "Nonpsychotic, nonparaphilic self-amputation and the internet." *Comprehensive Psychiatry* 46:380–83.

Berger, S. M. 1980. "Conservative management of phantom-limb and amputation-stump pain." *Annals of the Royal College of Surgeons of England* 62:102–5.

Bergmans, Lonneke, Dirk G. Snijdelaar, Joel Katz, and Ben J. P. Crul. 2002. "Methadone for phantom limb pain." *Clinical Journal of Pain* 18:203–5.

Betcher, Sharon. 2001. "Putting my foot (prosthesis, crutches, phantom) down: Considering technology as transcendence in the writings of Donna Haraway." *Women's Studies Quarterly* 3 and 4:35–53.

Blakeslee, Sandra. 2006. "Out-of-body-experience? Your brain is to blame." *New York Times* D6.

Bloomquist, Thom. 2001a. "Amputation and phantom limb pain: A pain-prevention model." *Aana Journal* 69:211–17.

———. 2001b. "Prevention: The next chapter on phantom limb pain." *InMotion* 11:1–3.

Blum, John Morton. 1976. *V was for victory: Politics and American culture during World War II*. New York: Harcourt Brace Jovanovich.

Blum, Virginia L. 2003. *Flesh wounds: The culture of cosmetic surgery*. Berkeley: University of California Press.

Bohne, Walther H. O. 1987. *Atlas of amputation surgery*. New York: Thieme Medical Publishers.

Bolderly, E., and W. Penfield. 1937. "Somatic motor and sensory representation in the cerebral cortex of man as studied by electrical stimulation." *Brain* 60:389–443.

Bordo, Susan. 1993. *Unbearable weight: Feminism, western culture, and the body*. Berkeley: University of California Press.

———. 1997. "'Material girls': The effacements of postmodern culture," in *The gender and sexuality reader: Culture, history, political economy*, edited by R. N. Lancaster and M. di Leonardo. New York: Routledge.

Bors, E. 1951. "Phantom limbs of patients with spinal cord injury." *Archives of Neurology and Psychiatry* 66:610–31.

Bouma, Gary, and G. B. J. Atkinson. 1995. *A handbook of social science research: A comprehensive and practical guide for students*. Oxford: Oxford University Press.

Bourdieu, Pierre. 1997. *Outline of a theory of practice*. Cambridge: Cambridge University Press.

Bourke, Joanna. 1996. *Dismembering the male: Men's bodies, Britain, and the Great War*. Chicago: University of Chicago Press.

Bowring, Finn. 2003. *Science, seeds, and cyborgs: Biotechnology and the appropriation of life*. London: Verso.

Branwyn, Gareth. 1993. "The desire to be wired: Will we live to see our brains wired to gadgets?" *Wired Magazine* 1.04: www.wired.com/wired/archives.

Braverman, D. L., and B. C. Root. 1997. "'Phantom' carpal tunnel syndrome." *Archives of Physical Medicine and Rehabilitation* 78:1157–59.

Bressler, Bernard, Sanford I. Cohen, and Finn Magnussen. 1956. "The problem of phantom breast and phantom pain." *Journal of Nervous and Mental Disease* 123:181–87.

Brodie, Eric E., Anne Whyte, and Bridget Waller. 2003. "Increased motor control of a phantom leg in humans results from the visual feedback of a virtual leg." *Neuroscience Letters* 341:167–69.

Brodwin, Paul E. 1992. "Symptoms and social performances: The case of Diane Reden," in *Pain as human experience: An anthropological perspective,* edited by M. J. D. Good, P. E. Brodwin, B. J. Good, and A. Kleinman. Berkeley: University of California Press.

Bromage, P. R., and R. Melzack. 1974. "Phantom limbs and the body schema." *Canadian Anaesthesia Society Journal* 21:267–74.

Browder, J., and J. P. Gallagher. 1948. "Dorsal cordotomy for painful phantom limb." *Annals of Surgery* 128:456–69.

Brown, Elspeth. 2002. "The prosthetics of management: Motion study, photography, and the industrialized body in World War I America," in *Artificial parts, practical lives: Modern histories of prosthetics,* edited by K. Ott, D. Serline, and S. Mihm. New York: New York University Press.

Brown, Nik, and Andrew Webster. 2004. *New medical technologies: Reordering life.* Cambridge, UK: Polity.

Brown, Walter A. 1968. "Post amputation phantom limb pain." *Diseases of the Nervous System* 29:301–6.

Bruno, Richard L. 1997. "Devotees, pretenders, and wannabes." *Journal of Sexuality and Disability* 15:243–60.

Butler, Judith. 1993. *Bodies that matter: On the discursive limits of "sex."* New York: Routledge.

Buxton, S. D. 1957. "Phantom limb." *Practitioner* 178:500–502.

Callon, Michel. 1986. "Some elements of a sociology of translation: Domestication of the scallops and the fishermen of St. Brieuc Bay," in *Power, action, and belief: A new sociology of knowledge?* edited by J. Law. London: Routledge.

———. 1999. "Actor-network theory: The market test," in *Actor network theory and after,* edited by J. Law and J. Hassard. Malden, MA: Blackwell.

Cameron, Kirk. 2003. "Cutting off arms and legs for 'mental health: Family research report.'" *Free Republic!:* http://www.freerepublic.com/focus/f-news/1056008/posts .

Campbell, Kellye M. 2005. *Interview by author.* Seattle, WA, July 19.

Carlen, P. L., P. D. Wall, H. Nadvorna, and T. Steinbach. 1978. "Phantom limbs and related phenomena in recent traumatic amputations." *Neurology* 28:211–17.

Casale, R., L. Alaa, M. Mallick, and H. Ring. 2009. "Phantom limb related phenomena and their rehabilitation after lower limb amputation." *European Journal of Physical and Rehabilitation Medicine* 45:1–8.

Casale, Roberto, Francesco Ceccherelli, Alaa Abd Elaziz Mohamed Labeeb, and Gabriele E. M. Biella. 2009. "Phantom limb pain relief by contralateral myofascial injection with local anasthetic in placebo-controlled study: Preliminary results." *Journal of Rehabilitation Medicine* 41:418–22.

Casper, Monica J. 1995. "Fetal cyborgs and technomoms on the reproductive frontier: Which way to the carnival," in *The cyborg handbook*, edited by C. H. Gray, H. J. Figueroa-Sarriera, and S. Mentor. New York: Routledge.

———. 1998a. *The making of the unborn patient: A social anatomy of fetal surgery.* New Brunswick, NJ: Rutgers University Press.

———. 1998b. "Working on and around human fetuses: The contested domain of fetal surgery," in *Differences in medicine: Unraveling practices, techniques, and bodies*, edited by M. Berg and A. Mol. Durham, NC: Duke University Press.

Casper, Monica J., and Lisa Jean Moore. 2009. *Missing bodies: The politics of visibility.* New York: New York University Press.

Casper, Monica J., and Heather Laine Talley. 2005. "Special issue: Ethnography and disability." *Journal of Contemporary Ethnography* 34:115–20.

Cervetti, Nancy. 2003. "S. Weir Mitchell: The early years." *American Pain Society Bulletin* 13:1–6.

Chadderton, H. C. 1978. "Prostheses, pain, and sequelae of amputation, as seen by the amputee." *Prosthetics and Orthotics International* 2:12–14.

Chong-cheng, Xue. 1986. "Acupuncture-induced phantom limb and meridian phenomenon in acquired and congenital amputees: A suggestion of the use of acupuncture as a method for investigation of phantom limb." *Chinese Medical Journal* 99:247–52.

Clarke, Adele E. 1995a. "Mommy, where do cyborgs come from anyway?" in *The cyborg handbook*, edited by C. H. Gray, H. J. Figueroa-Sarriera, and S. Mentor. New York: Routledge.

———. 1995. "Research materials and reproductive science in the United States, 1910–1940," in *Ecologies of knowledge: Work and politics in science and technology*, edited by S. L. Star. Albany: State University of New York Press.

———. 2003. "The more things change, the more they [also] remain the same." *Feminism and Psychology* 13:34–39.

———. 2005. *Situational analysis: Grounded theory after the postmodern turn.* Thousand Oaks, CA: Sage.

Clarke, Adele E., and Theresa Montini. 1993. "The many faces of RU486: Tales of situated knowledges and technological contestations." *Science, Technology, and Human Values* 18:42–78.

Clarke, Adele E., and Virginia L. Olesen. 1999. "Revising, Diffracting, Acting," in *Revisioning women, health, and healing: Feminist, cultural, and technoscience perspectives*, edited by A. E. Clarke and V. L. Olesen. New York: Routledge.

Clarke, Adele E., Janet Shim, Laura Mamo, Jennifer Ruth Fosket, and Jennifer Fishman. 2003. "Biomedicalization: Technoscientific transformations of health, illness, and U.S. biomedicine." *American Sociological Review* 68:161–94.

Clynes, Manfred E., and Nathan S. Kline. 1995. "Cyborgs in space," in *The cyborg handbook*, edited by C. H. Gray, H. J. Figueroa-Sarriera, and S. Mentor. New York: Routledge.

Cohen, Henry, and H. Wallace Jones. 1942. "The reference of cardiac pain to a phantom left arm." *British Heart Journal* 5:67–71.

Cole, Jonathan, Simon Crowle, Greg Austwick, and David Henderson Slater. 2009. "Exploratory findings with virtual reality for phantom limb pain: From stump motion to agency and analgesia." *Disability and Rehabilitation* 31:846–54.

Condes-Lara, M., F. A. Barrios, J. R. Romo, R. Rojas, P. Salgado, and J. Sanchez-Cortazar. 2000. "Brain somatic representation of phantom and intact limb: A fMRI study case report." *European Journal of Pain* 4:239–45.

Connell, Bob. 1995. "Masculinity, violence, and war," in *Men's lives,* edited by M. S. Kimmel and M. A. Messner. Boston: Allyn and Bacon.

Conrad, Peter. 1975. "The discovery of hyperkinesis: Note on the medicalization of deviant behavior." *Social Problems* 23:12–21.

———. 2007. *The medicalization of society: On the transformation of human conditions into treatable disorders.* Baltimore, MD: Johns Hopkins University Press.

Conrad, Peter, and Joseph W. Schneider. 1980. *Deviance and medicalization: From badness to sickness.* St. Louis, MO: Mosby.

Cook, Albert W., and William H. Druckemiller. 1952. "Phantom limb in paraplegic patients: Report of two cases and an analysis of its mechanism." *Journal of Neurosurgery* 9:508–16.

CPD. 1946. "Research reports on artificial limb." Washington, DC: National Research Council Committee on Prosthetic Devices.

———. 1947. "Terminal research reports on artificial limbs." Washington, DC: National Research Council Committee on Artificial Limbs.

CPI. 2004. "Yourability: A guide for every step of your life." Fraser, MI: College Park Industries.

Crawford, Cassandra S. 2005. "Actor network theory," in *Encyclopedia of Social Theory,* vol. 1, edited by G. Ritzer. Thousand Oaks, CA: Sage.

———. 2009a. "From pleasure to pain: The role of the MPQ in the language of phantom limb pain." *Social Science and Medicine* 69:655–61.

———. 2009b. "The inarticulacy/indescribability of pain: A rejoinder to Mowat." *Social Science and Medicine* 69:666–669.

———. 2009c. "Overdetermination." *Encyclopedia of case study research,* edited by A. Mills. Thousand Oaks, CA: Sage.

———. 2013. "'You don't need a body to feel a body': Phantom limb syndrome and corporeal transgression." *Sociology of Health and Illness* 1:15.

Crawford, Robert. 1984. "'A cultural account of health': Control, release, and the social body," in *Issues in the political economy of health care,* edited by J. McKinlay. London: Travistock.

———. 1987. "Cultural influences on prevention and the emergence of a new health consciousness," in *Issues in the political economy of health care,* edited by J. McKinlay. London: Tavistock.

———. 1994. "The boundaries of the self and the unhealthy other: Reflections on health, culture, and AIDS." *Social Science and Medicine* 38:1347–65.

———. 2004. "Risk ritual and the management of control and anxiety in medical culture." *Health* 8:505–28.

Cronholm, B. 1951. "Phantom limbs in amputees." *Acta psychiatrica Neurologica Scandinavica Supplementum* 72:1–310.

Czerniecki, Joseph. 2005. Interview by author. Seattle, WA, July 21.

Dallenbach, K. M. 1939. "Somesthesis," in *Introduction to psychology*, edited by E. G. Boring, H. S. Langfeld, and H. P. Weld. New York: Wiley.

Daniel, E. Valentine. 1994. "The individual in terror," in *Beyond the body proper*, edited by M. Lock and J. Farquhar. Durham, NC: Duke University Press.

Darian-Smith, C., and C. D. Gilbert. 1994. "Axonal sprouting accompanies functional reorganization in adult cat striate cortex." *Nature* 368:737–40.

Das, A., and C. D. Gilbert. 1995. "Long-range horizontal connections and their role in cortical reorganization revealed by optical recording of cat primary visual cortex." *Nature* 375:780–84.

Davis, R. W. 1993. "Phantom sensation, phantom pain, and stump pain." *Archives of Physical Medicine and Rehabilitation* 74:79–91.

de Peralta Menendez, Rolando Grave, Sara Gonzalez Andino, Lucas Perez, Pierre W. Ferrez, and Jose del R. Millan. 2005. "Non-invasive estimation of local field potentials for neuroprosthesis." *Cognitive Processing* 6:59–64.

Deitch, Jeffrey. 1992. *Post Human*. Amsterdam: Idea Books.

Dernham, P. 1986. "Phantom limb pain." *Geriatric Nursing* 7:34–37.

Dettmers, C., T. Adler, R. Rzanny, R. van Schaych, C. Gaser, T. Weiss, W. H. Miltner, L. Bruckner, and C. Weiller. 2001. "Increased excitability in the primary motor cortex and supplementary motor area in patients with phantom limb pain after upper limb amputation." *Neuroscience Letters* 307:109–12.

Deuchar, R. 1981. "Minor amputee problems." *Australian Family Physician* 10:114–17.

Dhillon, G. S., T. B. Kruger, J. S. Sandhu, and K. W. Horch. 2005. "Effects of short-term training on sensory and motor function in severed nerves of long-term human amputees." *Journal of Neurophysiology* 93:2625–33.

Dillingham, T. R., L. E. Pezzin, and E. J. MacKenzie. 2002a. "Limb amputation and limb deficiency: Epidemiology and recent trends in the United States." *Southern Medical Journal* 95:875–83.

———. 2002b. "Racial differences in the incidence of limb loss secondary to peripheral vascular disease: A population-based study." *Archives of Physical Medicine and Rehabilitation* 83:1252–57.

DiMartino, Christina. 2000. "Capturing the Phantom." *InMotion* 10:1–5.

Doetsch, G. S. 1997. "Progressive changes in cutaneous trigger zones for sensation referred to a phantom hand: A case report and review with implications for cortical reorganization." *Somatosensory and Motor Research* 14:6–16.

Donald, David. 2002. "The Confederate as a fighting man," in *The Civil War soldier: A historical reader*, edited by M. Barton and L. M. Logue. New York: New York University Press.

Dorpat, T. L. 1971. "Phantom sensation of internal organs." *Comprehensive Psychiatry* 12:27–35.

Dotinga, Randy. 2000. "Out on a limb." *Salon*: www.Salon.com.

Douglas, Mary. 1966. *Purity and danger: An analysis of the concept of pollution and taboo.* New York: Routledge.

———. 2003. *Natural symbols: Explorations in cosmology.* New York: Routledge.

Dumit, Joseph. 2004. *Picturing personhood: Brain scans and biomedical identity.* Princeton, NJ: Princeton University Press.

Dyer, C. 2000. "Surgeon amputated healthy legs." *British Medical Journal* 320:332.

Easson, William M. 1961. "Body image and self-image in children: Phantom phenomenon in a 3-year-old child." *Archives of General Psychiatry* 4:619–21.

Eckermann, Liz. 1997. "Foucault, embodiment, and gendered subjectivities: The case of voluntary self-starvation," in *Foucault, health, and medicine*, edited by A. Petersen and R. Bunton. New York: Routledge.

Elbert, T., and B. Rockstroh. 2004. "Reorganization of human cerebral cortex: The range of changes following use and injury." *Neuroscientist* 10:129–41.

Elbert, T., A. Sterr, H. Flor, B. Rockstroh, S. Knecht, C. Pantev, C. Wienbruch, and E. Taub. 1997. "Input-increase and input-decrease types of cortical reorganization after upper extremity amputation in humans." *Experimental Brain Research* 117:161–64.

Elliott, Carl. 2000. "A new way to be mad." *Atlantic Monthly* 283:72–84.

———. 2003. *Better than well: American medicine meets the American dream.* New York: Norton.

Elshtain, Jean Bethke. 2005. "The body and the quest for control," in *Is human nature obsolete? Genetics, bioengineering, and the future of the human condition*, edited by H. W. Baillie and T. Casey. Cambridge, MA: MIT Press.

Engelhardt, Tom. 1995. *The end of the victory culture: Cold War America and the disillusioning of a generation.* New York: Basic Books.

Engstrom, Barbara, and Catherine Van de Ven. 1985. *Physiotherapy for amputees: The Roehampton approach.* Edinburgh: Churchill Livingstone.

Ertl, Jan. 2000. "Prosthetic primer: Pain and inactive residual extremity syndrome." *InMotion* 10:1–2.

Everaerd, W. 1983. "A case of apotemnophilia: A handicap as sexual preference." *American Journal of Psychotherapy* 37:285–93.

Fairley, Miki. 2004. "Phantom pain: Unlocking a mystery." *The O and P Edge*: www.oandp.com.

Falconer, Murray A. 1953. "Surgical treatment of intractable phantom-limb pain." *British Medical Journal* 1:299–304.

Falk, Pasi. 1994. *The consuming body.* New York: Sage.

Farber, David. 1994. *The age of great dreams: America in the 1960s.* New York: Hill and Wang.

Farrell, John. 1996. *Freud's paranoid quest: Psychoanalysis and modern suspicion.* New York: New York University Press.

Featherstone, Mike. 1991. "The body in consumer culture," in *The body: Social process and cultural theory*, edited by M. Featherstone, M. Hepworth, and B. S. Turner. Thousand Oaks, CA: Sage.

———. 1999. "Body modification: An introduction." *Body and Society* 5:1–13.

Fein, Elizabeth. 2011. "Innocent machines: Asperger's syndrome and the neurostruc-
tural self," in *Sociological reflections on the neurosciences*, edited by M. Pickersgill
and I. Van Keulen. Bingley, UK: Emerald.

Feindel, William. 1977. "To praise an absent friend." *Canadian Medical Association
Journal* 116:1365–67.

Fernie, Geoffrey R. 1981. "The epidemiology of amputation," in *Amputation surgery and
rehabilitation: The Toronto experience*, edited by J. P. Kostuik and R. Gillespie. New
York: Churchill Livingstone.

FI. 2005. "Revolution series: A revolution in motion." *Irvine: Freedom Innovations* 1–4.

Figg, Laurann, and Jane Farrell-Beck. 1993. "Amputation in the Civil War: Physical and
social dimensions." *Journal of the History of Medicine and Allied Sciences* 48:454–75.

Finger, Stanley. 1994. *Origins of neuroscience: A history of explorations into brain function*. New York: Oxford University Press.

Finger, Stanley, and Meredith P. Hustwit. 2003. "Five early accounts of phantom limb
in context: Pare, Descartes, Lemos, Bell, and Mitchell." *Neurosurgery* 52:675–86.

First, Michael B. 2004. "Desire for amputation of a limb: Paraphilia, psychosis, or a
new type of identity disorder." *Psychological Medicine* 35:919–28.

Fisher, A., and Y. Meller. 1991. "Continuous postoperative regional analgesia by nerve sheath
block for amputation surgery: A pilot study." *Anesthesia and Analgesia* 72:300–303.

Fisher, C. M. 1999. "Phantom erection after amputation of penis: Case description and
review of the relevant literature on phantoms." *Canadian Journal of Neurological
Sciences* 26:53–56.

Fisher, K., and R. Smith. 2000. "More work is needed to explain why patients ask for
amputation of healthy limbs." *British Medical Journal* 320:1147.

Flavin, Jeanee. 2009. *Our bodies, our crimes: The policing of women's reproduction in
America*. New York: New York University Press.

Flor, Herta. 2002a. "The modification of cortical reorganization and chronic pain by
sensory feedback." *Applied Psychophysiology and Biofeedback* 27:215–27.

———. 2002b. "Phantom-limb pain: Characteristics, causes, and treatments." *Lancet
Neurology* 1:182–89.

———. 2003. "Cortical reorganisation and chronic pain: Implications for rehabilitation." *Journal of Rehabilitative Medicine* 41:66–72.

Flor, Herta, T. Elbert, S. Knecht, C. Wienbruch, C. Pantev, N. Birbaumer, W. Larbig,
and E. Taub. 1995. "Phantom-limb pain as a perceptual correlate of cortical reorganization following arm amputation." *Nature* 375:482–84.

Flor, Herta, T. Elbert, and W. Muhlnickel. 1998. "Cortical reorganization and phantom
phenomena in congenital and traumatic upper-extremity amputees." *Experimental
Brain Research* 119:205–12.

Flor, Herta, W. Muhlnickel, A. Karl, C. Denke, S. Grusser, R. Kurth, and E. Taub. 2000. "A
neural substrate for nonpainful phantom limb phenomena." *Neuroreport* 11:1407–11.

Florence, S. L., and J. H. Kaas. 1995. "Large-scale reorganization at multiple levels of
the somatosensory pathway follows therapeutic amputation of the hand in monkeys." *Journal of Neuroscience* 15:8080–95.

Foucault, Michel. 1965. *Madness and civilization: A history of insanity in the age of reason.* Translated by R. Howard. New York: Vintage.

———. 1973. *The birth of the clinic: An archaeology of medical perception.* Translated by A. M. S. Smith. New York: Vintage.

———. 1978. *The history of sexuality: An introduction,* vol. 1. Translated by R. Hurley. New York: Vintage.

———. 1995. *Discipline and punish: The birth of the prison.* Translated by A. Sheridan. New York: Vintage.

Frank, Adam. 2007. "Phantoms limn: Silvan Tomkins and affective prosthetics." *Theory and Psychology* 17:515–28.

Frank, B., and E. Lorenzoni. 1989. "Experiences of phantom limb sensations in dreams." *Psychopathology* 22:182–87.

Frank, Gelya. 2000. *Venus on wheels: Two decades of dialogue on disability, biography, and being female in America.* Berkeley: University of California Press.

Fraser, C. M., P. W. Halligan, I. H. Robertson, and S. G. Kirker. 2001. "Characterising phantom limb phenomena in upper limb amputees." *Prosthetics and Orthotics International* 25:235–42.

Frazier, Shervert H. 1966. "Psychiatric aspects of causalgia, the phantom limb, and phantom pain." *Diseases of the nervous system* 27:441–50.

Frazier, Shervert H., and L. C. Kolb. 1970. "Psychiatric aspects of pain and the phantom limb." *Orthopedic Clinics of North America* 1:481–95.

Frederiks, J. A. M. 1963. "Occurrence and nature of phantom limb phenomena following amputation of body parts and following lesions of the central and peripheral nervous system." *Psychiatria Neurologia Neurochirurgia* 66:73–97.

Freund, Peter E. S., Meredith B. McGuire, and Linda S. Podhurst. 2003. *Health, illness, and the social body: A critical sociology.* 4th ed. Upper Saddle River, NJ: Prentice Hall.

Friedman, Lester D. 2004. "Introduction: Through the looking glass," in *Cultural sutures: Medicine and media,* edited by L. D. Friedman. Durham, NC: Duke University Press.

Fujimura, Joan H. 1986. "Bandwagons in science: Doable problems and transportable packages as factors in the development of the molecular genetic bandwagon in cancer research." Ph.D. dissertation, Sociology, University of California–Berkeley.

———. 1987. "Constructing doable problems in cancer research: Articulating alignment." *Social Studies of Science* 17:257–93.

Funakawa, I., Y. Mano, and T. Takayanagi. 1987. "Painful hand and moving fingers: A case report." *Journal of Neurology* 234:342–43.

Furst, L., and M. Humphrey. 1983. "Coping with the loss of a leg." *Prosthetics and Orthotics International* 7:152–56.

Furth, Gregg M., and Robert Smith. 2002. "Amputee identity disorder: Information, questions, answers, and recommendations about self-demand amputation." Bloomington, IN: Authorhouse Books.

Furukawa, T. 1990. "Charles Bell's description of the phantom phenomenon in 1830." *Neurology* 40:1830.

Gallinek, A. 1939. "The phantom limb: Its origin and relation to the hallucinations of psychotic state." *American Journal of Psychiatry* 6:1939.

Gangale, John P. 1968. "A review of the phantom sensation phenomenon." *Virginia Medical Monthly* 95:425–29.

Geary, James. 2002. *The body electric: An anatomy of the new bionic senses.* New Brunswick, NJ: Rutgers University Press.

Gerber, David A. 1994. "Heroes and misfits: The troubled social reintegration of disabled veterans in *The Best Years of Our Lives.*" *American Quarterly* 46:545–74.

Gerschick, Thomas J., and Adam Stephen Miller. 1994. "Coming to terms: Masculinity and physical disability," in *Men's lives,* edited by M. S. Kimmel and M. A. Messner. Boston: Allyn and Bacon.

Giddens, Anthony. 1991. *Modernity and self identity: Self and society in the late modern age.* Cambridge, UK: Polity.

———. 1994a. *Beyond left and right.* Cambridge, UK: Polity.

———. 1994b. "Living in a post-traditional society," in *Reflexive modernization: Politics, tradition, and aesthetics in the modern social order,* edited by U. Beck, A. Giddens, and S. Lash. Stanford, CA: Stanford University Press.

Gillis, L. C. 1964. "The management of painful amputation stump and a new theory for the phantom phenomenon." *British Journal of Surgery* 51:87–95.

Gilman, Sander L. 1998. *Creating beauty to cure the sole: Race and psychology in the shaping of aesthetic surgery.* Durham, NC: Duke University Press.

Giraux, P., and A. Sirigu. 2003. "Illusory movements of the paralyzed limb restore motor cortex activity." *NeuroImage* 20:S107–11.

Giuffrida, Orazio, Lyn Simpson, and Peter W. Halligan. 2010. "Contralateral stimulation, using TENS, of phantom limb pain: Two confirmatory cases." *Pain Medicine* 11:133–41.

Giummarra, Melita Joy, Nellie Georgiou-Karistianis, Michael E. R. Nicholls, Stephen J. Gibson, Michael Chou, and John L. Bradshaw. 2011. "Imprinting of past experiences onto phantom limb schemata." *Clinical Journal of Pain* 27(8):691–98.

Giummarra, Melita Joy, Stephen J. Gibson, Nellie Georgiou-Karistianis, and John L. Bradshaw. 2007. "Central mechanisms in phantom limb perception: The past, present, and future." *Brain Research Reviews* 54:219–32.

Giummarra, Melita, and G. Lorimer Moseley. 2011. "Phantom limb pain and bodily awareness: Current concepts and future directions." *Current Opinion in Anesthesiology* 24:524–31.

Glaser, Barry, and Anselm Strauss. 1967. *The discovery of grounded theory: Strategies for qualitative research.* Piscataway, NJ: Aldine Transaction.

Glassner, Barry. 1988. *Bodies: Why we look the way we do (and how we feel about it).* New York: Putnam.

———. 1995. "In the name of health," in *The sociology of health promotion: Critical analysis of consumption, lifestyle, and risk,* edited by R. Bunton, S. Nettleton, and R. Burrows. New York: Routledge.

Gleyse, Jacques. 1998. "Instrumental rationalization of human movement: An archeological approach," in *Sport and postmodern times,* edited by R. Bunton, S. Nettleton, and R. Burrows. New York: Routledge.

Glucklick, Ariel. 2001. *Sacred pain: Hurting the body for the sake of the soul.* New York: Oxford University Press.

Goldman, Jami, and Andrea Cagan. 2001. *Up and Running: The Jami Goldman story.* New York: Simon & Schuster.

Goler, Robert I. 2004. "Loss and the Persistence of Memory: 'The case of George Dedlow' and disabled Civil War veterans." *Literature and Medicine* 23:160–83.

Good, Byron J. 1994. "A Body in pain: The making of a world of chronic pain," in *Pain as human experience: An anthropological perspective,* edited by M.-J. D. Good, P. E. Brodwin, B. J. Good, and A. Kleinman. Berkeley: University of California Press.

Goodman, Jordon, Anthony McElligott, and Lara Marks. 2003. "Making human bodies useful: Historicizing medical experiments in the twentieth century," in *The cyborg handbook,* edited by C. H. Gray, H. J. Figueroa-Sarriera, and S. Mentor. New York: Routledge.

Gordon, Deorah. 1988. "Tenacious assumptions in Western medicine," in *Biomedicine examined,* edited by M. Lock and D. R. Gordon. Dordrecht, Netherlands: Kluwer.

Gray, Chris Hables. 2002. *Cyborg citizen.* New York: Routledge.

Gray, Chris Hables, and Steve Mentor. 1995. "Science fiction becomes military fact," in *The cyborg handbook,* edited by C. H. Gray, H. J. Figueroa-Sarriera, and S. Mentor. New York: Routledge.

Gray, Chris Hables, Steven Mentor, and Heidi J. Figueroa-Sarriera. 1995. "Cyborgology: Constructing the knowledge of cybernetic organisms," in *The cyborg handbook,* edited by C. H. Gray, H. J. Figueroa-Sarriera, and S. Mentor. New York: Routledge.

Green, Christopher D. 2000. *Introduction to "perception": An introduction to the Gestalt-Theorie by Kurk Koffka:* http: psychclassics.yorku.ca/Koffka/Perceptions/intro.htm.

Green, Erin. 2005. "A brighter day for Edward Taub." *Science Magazine* 276:1.

Grenville, Bruce. 2001. *The uncanny: Experiment in cyborg culture.* Vancouver: Arsenal Pulp Press.

Gross, Sky. 2011. "A stone in a spaghetti bowl: The biological and metaphorical brain in neuro-oncology," in *Sociological reflections on the neurosciences,* edited by M. Pickersgill and I. Van Keulen. Bingley, UK: Emerald.

Grossi, D., G. Di Cesare, and R. P. Tamburro. 2002. "On the syndrome of the 'spare limb': One case." *Perceptual and Motor Skills* 94:476–78.

Grosz, Elizabeth. 1994. *Volatile bodies: Toward a corporeal feminism.* Bloomington: Indiana University Press.

Gueniot, M. 1861. "D'une hallucination du toucher partieuliere a certains amputes." *Journal of Physiologie* 4:416.

Gutierrez-Mahoney, C. G. 1944. "The treatment of painful phantom limb by removal of the postcentral cortex." *Journal of Neurosurgery* 1:156–62.

Hacking, Ian. 1986. "Making up people," in *Autonomy, individuality, and the self in Western thought*, edited by T. C. Heller, M. Sosna, and D. E. Wellbery. Stanford, CA: Stanford University Press.

———. 1995. *Rewriting the soul: Multiple personality and the sciences of memory.* Princeton,NJ: Princeton University Press.

Haiken, Elizabeth. 1997. *Venus envy: A history of cosmetic surgery.* Baltimore, MD: Johns Hopkins University Press.

Halligan, Peter W., John C. Marshall, and Derick T. Wade. 1993. "Three arms: A case study of supernumerary phantom limb after right hemisphere stroke." *Journal of Neurology, Neurosurgery, and Psychiatry* 56:159–66.

———. 1994. "Sensory disorganization and perceptual plasticity after limb amputation: A follow-up study." *Neuroreport* 5:1341–45.

Hanling, Steven R., Scott C. Wallace, Kerry J. Hollenbeck, Brian D. Belnap, and Mathew R. Tulis. 2010. "Preamputation mirror therapy may prevent development of phantom limb pain: A case series." *Anesthesia and Analgesia* 110:611–14.

Hanna, Philip, Sanjeev Kumar, and Arthur S. Walters. 2004. "Restless legs symptoms in a patient with above knee amputations: A case of phantom restless legs." *Clinical Neuropharmacology* 27:87–89.

Haraway, Donna. 1985. "A manifesto for cyborgs: Science, technology, and socialist feminism in the 1980s." *Socialist Review* 80:65–108.

———. 1991. *Simians, cyborgs, and women: The reinvention of nature.* London: Free Association Books.

———. 1992. "The promise of monsters: A regenerative politics for inappropriate/d others," in *Cultural studies*, edited by L. Grossberg, C. Nelson, and P. A. Treichler. New York: Routledge.

Harber, William B. 1956. "Observations on phantom limb phenomena." *Archives of Neurology and Psychiatry* 75:624–36.

———. 1958. "Reactions to loss of limb: Physiological and psychological aspects." *Annals of the New York Academy of Sciences* 74:14–24.

Harding, Sandra, and Robert Figueroa. 2003. "Introduction," in *Science and other cultures: Issues in philosophies of science and technology*, edited by R. Figueroa and S. Harding. New York: Routledge.

Harré, Rom. 2002. "Material objects in social worlds." *Theory, Culture, and Society* 19:23–33.

Harrison, Gwendolen. 1951. "'Phantom limb' pain occurring during spinal analgesia." *Anaesthesia* 6:115–16.

Hartmann, Susan. 1978. "Prescriptions for Penelope: Literature on women's obligations to returning World War Two veterans." *Women's Studies: An Interdisciplinary Journal* 5:224.

Hayes, C., A. Armstrong-Brown, and R. Burstal. 2004. "Perioperative intravenous ketamine infusion for the prevention of persistent post-amputation pain: A randomized, controlled trial." *Anaesthesia and Intensive Care* 32:330–38.

Hayles, Katherine. 1999. *How we became posthuman: Virtual bodies in cybernetics, literature, and informatics.* Chicago: University of Chicago Press.

Hazelgrove, Jane F., and Peter D. Rogers. 2002. "Phantom limb pain: A complication of lower extremity wound management." *Lower Extremity Wounds* 1:112–24.

Head, H., and G. Holmes. 1911. "Sensory disturbances from cerebral lesions." *Brain* 34:102–254.

Helling, Thomas S., and W. Kendall. 2000. "The role of amputation in the management of battlefield casualties: A history of two millennia." *Journal of Trauma* 49:930–39.

Henderson, W. R., and G. E. Smyth. 1948. "Phantom limbs." *Journal of Neurology and Psychiatry* 11:88–112.

Henig, Robin Marantz. 2005. "At war with their bodies, they seek to sever limbs." *New York Times* D6, D10.

Herman, J. 1998. "Phantom limb: From medical knowledge to folk wisdom and back." *Annals of Internal Medicine* 128:76–78.

Hermes, Lisa M. 2002. "Military lower extremity amputee rehabilitation." *Physical Medicine and Rehabilitation Clinics of North America* 13:45–66.

Herrmann, L. B., and E. W. Gibbs. 1945. "Phantom limb pain: Its relation to the treatment of large nerves at the time of amputation." *American Journal of Surgery* 67:168–80.

Herschbach, Lisa. 1997. "Prosthetic reconstructions: Making the industry, re-making the body, modeling the nation." *History Workshop Journal* 44:23–57.

Heusner, A. P. 1950. "Phantom genitalia." *Transactions of the American Neurological Association* 75:128–31.

Hevey, David. 1992. *The creatures that time forgot: Photography and disability imagery.* New York: Routlege,

Hewitt, Kim. 1997. *Mutilating the body: Identity in blood and ink.* Bowling Green, OH: Bowling Green State University Popular Press.

Hilbert, Richard A. 1984. "The acultural dimensions of chronic pain: Flawed reality construction and the problem of meaning." *Social Problems* 31:365–78.

Hill, A. 1999. "Phantom limb pain: A review of the literature on attributes and potential mechanisms." *Journal of Pain Symptom Management* 17:125–42.

Hocky, Jenny, and Janet Draper. 2005. "Beyond the womb and the tomb: Identity, (dis) embodiment, and the life course." *Body and Society* 11:41–57.

Hoffman, Julius. 1954a. "Facial phantom phenomenon." *Journal of Nervous and Mental Disease* 122:143–51.

———. 1954b. "Phantom limb syndrome: A critical review of literature." *Journal of Nervous and Mental Disease* 119:261–70.

Hogle, Linda F. 1995. "Tales from the cryptic: Technology meets organism in the living cadaver," in *The cyborg handbook,* edited by C. H. Gray, H. J. Figueroa-Sarriera, and S. Mentor. New York: Routledge.

Holden, Constance. 1989. "Monkey euthanasia stalled by activists." *Science* 244:1437.

Holmes, Martha Stoddard. 2009. *Fictions of affliction: Physical disability in Victorian culture.* Ann Arbor: University of Michigan Press.

Hoover, Roy M. 1964. "Problems and complications of amputees." *Clinical Orthopaedics and Related Research* 37:47–52.

Hopton, John. 2003. "The state and military masculinity," in *Military masculinities: Identity and the state*, edited by P. R. Higate. Bel Air, CA: Praeger.

Horgan, Olga, and Malcolm MacLachlan. 2004. "Psychosocial adjustment to lower-limb amputation: A review." *Disability and Rehabilitation* 26:837–50.

Higate, Paul, and John Hopkins. 2005. "War, militarism, and masculinities," in *Handbook of studies on men and masculinities*, edited by M. S. Kimmel, J. R. Hearn, and R. W. Connell. Thousand Oaks, CA: Sage.

Hrbek, V. 1976. "New pathophysiological interpretation of the so-called phantom limb and phantom pain syndromes." *Acta Universitatis Palackianae Olomucensis Facultatis Medicae* 80:79–90.

Hsu, C., and J. A. Sliwa. 2004. "Phantom breast pain as a source of functional loss." *American Journal of Physical Medicine and Rehabilitation* 83:659–62.

Hughes, Bill. 2000. "Medicalized bodies," in *The body, culture, and society: An introduction*, edited by P. Hancock. Philadelphia: Open University.

———. 2007. "Being disabled: Towards a critical social ontology for disabilities studies." *Disability and Society* 22:673–84.

Hughes, J. 1996. "Biomechanics and prosthetics," in *Amputation: Surgical practice and patient management*, edited by G. Murdoch and A. B. Wilson. Oxford: Butterworth-Heinemann.

Hunter, J. P., J. Katz, and K. D. Davis. 2003. "The effect of tactile and visual sensory inputs on phantom limb awareness." *Brain* 126:579–89.

———. 2005. "Dissociation of phantom limb phenomena from stump tactile spatial acuity and sensory thresholds." *Brain* 128:308–20.

Huse, Ellena, Wolfgang Larbig, Herta Flor, and Niels Birbaumer. 2001. "The effect of opioids on phantom limb pain and cortical reorganization." *Pain* 90:47–55.

Hyden, Lars-Christer, and Michael Peolsson. 2002. "Pain gestures: The orchestration of speech and body gestures." *Health: An Interdisciplinary Journal for the Social Study of Health, Illness, and Medicine* 6:325–45.

In Der Beeck, Manford. 1953. "The phantom limb feeling and the body scheme: A study on the regression of the phantom." *Arquivos De Neuro-Psiquiatria* 11:223–28.

Jackson, Marni. 2002. *Pain: The fifth vital sign.* New York: Crown.

Jacobson, L., and C. Chabal. 1989. "Prolonged relief of acute postamputation phantom limb pain with intrathecal fentanyl and epidural morphine." *Anesthesiology* 71:984–85.

Jahangiri, M., A. P. Jayatunga, J. W. Bradley, and C. H. Dark. 1994. "Prevention of phantom pain after major lower limb amputation by epidural infusion of diamorphine, clonidine, and bupivacaine." *Annals of the Royal College of Surgeons of England* 76:324–26.

Jalavisto, Eeva. 1950. "Adaptation in the phantom limb phenomenon as influenced by the age of amputees." *Journal of Gerontology* 5:339–42.

————. 1954. "Patterns in perceptual constancy experiments and the phantom limb phenomenon in amputees." *Acta Physiologica Scandinavica* 31:167–82.

Jankovic, J., and J. P. Glass. 1985. "Metoclopramide-induced phantom dyskinesia." *Neurology* 35:432–35.

Jarvis, J. H. 1967. "Post-mastectomy breast phantoms." *Journal of Nervous and Mental Disease* 144:266–72.

Jeffreys, Mark. 2002. "The visible cripple (scars and other disfiguring displays included)," in *Disability studies: Enabling the humanities,* edited by S. L. Snyder, B. J. Brueggemann, and G.-T. Rosemarie. New York: Modern Language Association of America.

Jensen, Mark. 2005. Interview by author. Seattle, WA, July 20.

Jensen, Troels Staehelin, B. Krebs, J. Nielsen, and P. Rasmussen. 1983. "Phantom limb, phantom pain, and stump pain in amputees during the first 6 months following limb amputation." *Pain* 17:243–56.

————. 1984. "Non-painful phantom limb phenomena in amputees: Incidence, clinical characteristics, and temporal course." *Acta Neurologica Scandinaica* 70:407–14.

Jensen, Troels Staehelin, and Lone Nikolajsen. 2000. "Pre-emptive analgesia in postamputation pain: An update." *Progress in Brain Research* 129:493–503.

Joyce, Kelly A. 2006. "From numbers to pictures: The development of magnetic resonance imaging and the visual turn in medicine." *Science as Culture* 15:1–22.

————. 2008. *Magnetic appeal: MRI and the myth of transparency.* New York: Cornell University Press.

Kallio, K. E. 1952. "Phantom limb of forearm stump cleft by kineplastic surgery." *Journal International De Chirurgie* 12:110–19.

Karl, Anke, Niels Birbaumer, Werner Lutzenberger, Leonardo G. Cohen, and Herta Flor. 2001. "Reorganization of motor and somatosensory cortex in upper extremity amputees with phantom limb pain." *Journal of Neuroscience* 21:3609–18.

Karl, Anke, Werner Muhlnickel, Ralf Kurth, and Herta Flor. 2004. "Neuroelectric source imaging of steady-state movement-related cortical potentials in human upper extremity amputees with and without phantom limb pain." *Pain* 110:90–102.

Katz, J. 1992a. "Psychophysical correlates of phantom limb experience." *Journal of Neurology, Neurosurgery, and Psychiatry* 55:811–21.

————. 1992b. "Psychophysiological contributions to phantom limbs." *Canadian Journal of Psychiatry* 37:282–98.

————. 1998. "Phantom-limb pain: Author's reply." *Lancet* 351:595.

————. 2005. Phone interview by author. July 25.

Katz, J., and R. Melzack. 1987. "Referred sensations in chronic pain patients." *Pain* 28:51–59.

————. 1990. "Pain 'memories' in phantom limbs: Review and clinical observations." *Pain* 43:319–36.

Kaufert, Joseph, and David Locker. 1990. "Rehabilitation ideology and respiratory support technology." *Social Science and Medicine* 30:867–77.

Kegel, Bernice, Margaret L. Carpenter, and Ernest M. Burgess. 1977. "A survey of lower-limb amputees: Prostheses, phantom sensations, and psychosocial aspects." *Bulletin of Prosthetics Research* 10:43–60.

Keller, Evelyn Fox. 1996. "The biological gaze," in *FutureNatural: Nature, science, culture*, edited by G. Robertson, M. Mash, L. Tickner, J. Bird, B. Curtis, and T. Putnam. New York: Routledge.

Kessel, C., and R. Worz. 1987. "Immediate response of phantom limb pain to calcitonin." *Pain* 30:79–87.

Kevles, B. 1997. *Naked to the bone: Medical imaging in the twentieth century.* New Brunswick, NJ: Rutgers University Press.

Kimbrell, Andrew. 1993. *The human body shop: The engineering and marketing of life.* San Francisco: HarperSanFrancisco.

Kirkup, John. 1995. "Perceptions of amputation before and after gunpowder." *Vesalius* 1:51–58.

Klepinger, Linda L. 1980. "The evolution of human disease: New findings and problems." *Journal of Biological and Social Sciences* 12:481–86.

Knecht, S., H. Henningsen, T. Elbert, H. Flor, C. Hohling, C. Pantev, and E. Taub. 1996. "Reorganizational and perceptional changes after amputation." *Brain* 119:1213–19.

Knorr-Cetina, Karin. 1997. "Sociality with objects: Social relations in postsocial knowledge societies." *Theory, Culture, and Society* 14:1–30.

Knox, D. J., B. J. McLeod, and C. R. Goucke. 1995. "Acute phantom limb pain controlled by ketamine." *Anaesthesia and Intensive Care* 23:620–22.

Kolb, Lawrence C. 1950a. "Psychiatric aspects of treatment of the painful phantom limb." *Medical Clinics of North America* 34:129–41.

———. 1950b. "Psychiatric aspects of treatment of the painful phantom limb." *Mayo Clinic Proceedings* 25:467–71.

———. 1952. "Treatment of the acute painful phantom limb." *Mayo Clinic Proceedings* 27:110–18.

———. 1954. *The painful phantom: Psychology, physiology, and treatment.* Springfield, IL: Thomas.

Kosut, Mary, and Lisa Jean Moore. 2010. "Introduction: Not just the reflexive reflex," in *The body reader: Essential social and cultural readings*, edited by L. J. Moore and M. Kosut. New York: New York University Press.

Koven, Seth. 1994. "Remembering and dismemberment: Crippled children, wounded soldiers, and the Great War in Great Britain." *American Historical Review* 99:1167–1202.

Krane, Elliot J., and Lori B. Heller. 1995. "The prevalence of phantom sensation and pain in pediatric amputees." *Journal of Pain and Symptom Management* 10:21–29.

Krebs, Borge, Troels Staehelin Jensen, Karsten Kroner, Jorn Nielsen, and Has Stodkile Jorgensen. 1985. "Phantom limb phenomena in amputees." *Acta Orthopaedica Scandinavica* 56:179.

Kroll-Smith, Steve, and H. Hugh Floyd. 1997. *Bodies in Protest: Environmental illness and the struggle over medical knowledge.* New York: New York University Press.

Kugelmann, Robert. 1997. "The psychology and management of pain: Gate control as theory and symbol." *Theory and Psychology* 7:43–65.

Kuhn, Thomas. S. 1962. *The structure of scientific revolutions.* Chicago: University of Chicago Press.

Kurzman, Steve. 2003. "Performing able-bodiedness: Amputees and prosthetics in America." Dissertation, Anthropology, University of California–Santa Cruz.

———. 2004. "'There is no language for this': Communication and alignment in contemporary prosthetics," in *Artificial parts, practical lives: Modern history of prosthetics,* edited by K. Ott, D. Serlin, and S. Mihm. New York: New York University Press.

Kyllonen, R. R. 1964. "Body image and reaction to amputations." *Connecticut Medicine* 28:19–23.

Lacroix, R., R. Melzack, D. Smith, and N. Mitchell. 1992. "Multiple phantom limbs in a child." *Cortex* 28:503–7.

Lampland, Martha, and Susan Leigh Star. 2009. *Standards and their stories: How quantifying, classifying, and formalizing practices shape everyday life.* Ithaca, NY: Cornell University Press.

Laqueur, Thomas Walter. 1990. *Making sex: Body and gender from the Greeks to Freud.* Cambridge, MA: Harvard University Press.

Latour, Bruno. 1987. *Science in action: How to follow scientists and engineers through society.* Cambridge, MA: Harvard University Press.

———. 1991. "Technology is society made durable," in *A Sociology of monsters: Essays on power, technology, and domination,* edited by J. Law. London: Routledge.

Law, John. 1992. "Notes on the theory of actor-network: Ordering, strategy, and heterogeneity." *Systems Practice* 5:379–93.

———. 1997. *Traduction/Trahison: Notes on ANT.* Lancaster, UK: Centre for Science Studies, Lancaster University.

Lawrence, Anne A. 2006. "Clinical and theoretical parallels between desire for limb amputation and gender identity disorder." *Archives of Sexual Behavior* 35:263–78.

Lawton, Julia. 1998. "Contemporary hospice care: The sequestration of the unbounded body and 'dirty dying.'" *Sociology of Health and Illness* 20:121–43.

Leder, Drew. 1984. "Medicine and paradigms of embodiment." *Journal of Medicine and Philosophy* 9:29–43.

———. 1990. *The absent body.* Chicago: University of Chicago Press.

Lederman, Muriel, and Ingrid Bartsch. 2001. *The gender and science reader.* New York: Routledge.

Lemke, Thomas. 2011. *Bio-politics: An advanced introduction.* New York: New York University Press.

Lerman, Nina E., Ruth Oldenziel, and Arwen Mohun. 2003. *Gender and technology: A reader.* Baltimore, MD: Johns Hopkins University Press.

Li, Choh-Luh. 1951. "Observations on phantom limb in a paraplegic patient." *Journal of Neurosurgery* 8:524–27.

Linton, Simi. 2006. *My body politic: A memoir*. Ann Arbor: University of Michigan Press.

Livingston, W. K. 1938. "Fantom limb pain." *Archives of Surgery* 37:353–70.

Lock, Margaret. 2001. "Living cadavers and the calculation of death." *Body and Society* 10:135–52.

Long, Lisa. 2004. *Rehabilitating bodies: Health, history, and the American Civil War*. Philadelphia: University of Pennsylvania Press.

Longman, Jere. 2007. "An amputee sprinter: Is he disabled or too-abled?" *New York Times*: www.nytimes.com.

Lotze, M., W. Grodd, N. Birbaumer, M. Erb, E. Huse, and H. Flor. 1999. "Does use of a myoelectric prosthesis prevent cortical reorganization and phantom limb pain?" *Nature Neuroscience* 2:501–2.

Luke, Timothy W. 1996. "Liberal society and cyborg subjectivity: The politics of environments, bodies, and nature." *Alternatives* 21:1–30.

Lundberg, S. G., and F. G. Guggenheim. 1986. "Sequelae of limb amputation." *Advances in Psychosomatic Medicine* 15:199–210.

Lupton, Deborah. 1999. *Risk and sociocultural theory: New directions and perspectives*. New York: Cambridge University Press.

Lynch, Michael, and H. M. Collins. 1998. "Introduction: Humans, animals, and machines." *Science, Technology, and Human Values* 23:371–83.

Lynch, Michael, and Steve Woolgar. 1990. *Representations in scientific practice*. Cambridge, MA: MIT Press.

Mackenzie, N. 1983. "Phantom limb pain during spinal anaesthesia." *Anaesthesia* 38:886–87.

Mackert, Bruno-Marcel, Tanja Sappok, Sabine Grusser, Herta Flor, and Gabriel Curio. 2003. "The eloquence of silent cortex: Analysis of afferent input to deafferented cortex in arm amputees." *Neuroreport* 14:409–12.

Martin, Emily. 1999. "The woman in the flexible body," in *Revisioning women, health, and healing*, edited by A. E. Clarke and V. L. Olesen. New York: Routledge.

Mascia-Lees, Francis E. 2011. "Aesthetics: aesthetic embodiment and commodity capitalism," in *A companion to the anthropology of the body and embodiment*, edited by F. E. Mascia-Lees. Malden, MA: Wiley-Blackwell.

Mauss, Marcel. 1934. "Techniques of the human body." *Economy and Society* 2:70–88.

Mayeux, R., and D. F. Benson. 1979. "Phantom limb and multiple sclerosis." *Neurology* 29:724–26.

McAvinue, Laura P., and Ian H. Robertson. 2011. "Individual differences in response to phantom limb movement therapy." *Disability and Rehabilitation* 33:2186–95.

McDaid, Jennifer Davis. 2002. "'How a one-legged rebel lives': Confederate veterans and artificial limbs in Virginia," in *Artificial parts, practical lives: Modern histories of prosthetics*, edited by K. Ott, D. Serline, and S. Mihm. New York: New York University Press.

McGrath, P. A., and L. M. Hiller. 1992. "Phantom limb sensations in adolescents: A case study to illustrate the utility of sensation and pain logs in pediatric clinical practice." *Journal of Pain and Symptom Management* 7:46–53.

McNaughton, Francis L. 1977. "Impact on medical neurology." *Canadian Medical Association Journal* 116:1370.

McQuay, H. J., R. A. Moore, and E. Kalso. 1998. "Phantom-limb pain." *Lancet* 351:595.

Mead, George Herbert, and Charles W. Morris. 1934. *Mind, self, and society from the standpoint of a social behaviorist.* Chicago: University of Chicago Press.

Mearz, Melissa. 2006. "Final cut pro with 'whole': Twin cities–based filmmaker Melody Gilbert discovers less is more." *City Pages* 24.

Meier, Robert H. 2004. "History of arm amputation, prosthetic restoration, and arm amputation rehabilitation," in *Functional restoration of adults and children with upper extremity amputation*, edited by R. H. Meier and D. J. Atkins. New York: Demos Medical Publishing.

Mellström, Ulf. 2002. "Patriarchal machines and masculine embodiment." *Sociology of Health and Illness* 27:460–78.

Melzack, Ronald. 1973. *The puzzle of pain.* New York: Basic Books.

———. 1975. "The McGill Pain Questionnaire: Major properties and scoring methods." *Pain* 1:277–99.

———. 1976. "Pain: Past, present, future," in *Pain: New perspectives in therapy and research*, edited by M. Weisenberg and B. Tursk. New York: Plenum.

———. 1987. "The short-form McGill Pain Questionnaire." *Pain* 30:191–97.

———. 1989. "Phantom limb, the self, and the brain." *Canadian Psychology* 30:1–16.

———. 1990. "Phantom limbs and the concept of a neuromatrix." *Trends in Neurosciences* 13:88–92.

———. 1993. "Pain: Past, present, and future." *Canadian Journal of Experimental Psychology* 47:615–29.

———. 1995. "Phantom-limb pain and the brain," in *Pain and the brain: From nociception to cognition*, edited by B. Bromm and J. E. Desmedt. New York: Raven.

———. 2005. "The McGill Pain Questionnaire: From description to measurement." *Anesthesiology* 103:199–202.

———. 2006. Phone interview by author. July 22.

Melzack, Ronald, and P. R. Bromage. 1973. "Experimental phantom limbs." *Experimental Neurology* 39:261–69.

Melzack, Ronald, T. J. Coderre, J. Katz, and A. L. Vaccarino. 2001. "Central neuroplasticity and pathological pain." *New York Academy of Sciences* 933:157–74.

Melzack, Ronald, R. Israel, R. Lacroix, and G. Schultz. 1997. "Phantom limbs in people with congenital limb deficiency or amputation in early childhood." *Brain* 120:1603–20.

Melzack, Ronald, and Warren S. Torgerson. 1971. "On the language of pain." *Anesthesiology* 34:50–59.

Melzack, Ronald, and P. D. Wall. 1965. "Pain mechanisms: A new theory." *Science* 150:171–79.

Mercier, C., K. T. Reilly, C. D. Vargas, A. Aballea, and A. Sirqu. 2006. "Mapping phantom movement representations in the motor cortex of amputees." *Brain* 129:2202–10.

Merleau-Ponty, Maurice. 1962. *Phenomenology of perception.* New York: Routledge.

Merzenich, M., and J. H. Kass. 1982. "Reorganization of mammalian somatosensory cortex following peripheral nerve injury." *Trends in Neurosciences* 5:434–36.

Merzenich, M. M., J. H. Kaas, J. Wall, R. J. Nelson, M. Sur, and D. Felleman. 1983. "Topographic reorganization of somatosensory cortical areas 3b and 1 in adult monkeys following restricted deafferentation." *Neuroscience* 8:33–55.

Merzenich, M. M., R. J. Nelson, M. P. Stryker, M. S. Cynader, A. Schoppmann, and J. M. Zook. 1984. "Somatosensory cortical map changes following digit amputation in adult monkeys." *Journal of Comparative Neurology* 224:591–605.

Metman, Leo Verhagen, Jacqueline S. Bellevich, Seth M. Jones, Matt D. Barber, and Leopold J. Streletz. 2005. "Topographic mapping of human motor cortex with transcranial magnetic stimulation: Homunculus revisited." *Brain Topography* 6:13–19.

Michael, John W., and John H. Bowker. 1994. "Prosthetics/orthotics research for the twenty-first century: Summary 1992 conference proceedings." *Journal of Prosthetic and Orthotics* 6:100–107.

Mihm, Stephen. 2002. "'A limb which shall be presentable in polite society': Prosthetic technologies in the nineteenth century," in *Artificial parts, practical lives: Modern histories of prosthetics*, edited by K. Ott, D. Serline, and S. Mihm. New York: New York University Press.

Miles, James English. 1956. "Psychosis with phantom limb pain treated by chlorpromazine." *American Journal of Psychiatry* 112:1027–1028.

Miller, Jonathan. 1978. *The body in question*. New York: Random House.

Mitchell, David T. 2002. "Narrative prosthesis and the materiality of metaphor," in *Disability studies: Enabling the humanities*, edited by S. L. Snyder, B. J. Brueggemann, and R. Garland-Thomson. New York: Modern Language Association of America.

Mitchell, David T., and Sharon L. Snyder. 2000. *Narrative prosthesis: Disability and the dependencies of discourse*. Ann Arbor: University of Michigan Press.

Mitchell, Silas Weir. 1866. "The case of George Dedlow." *Atlantic Monthly* 18:1–11.

———. 1871. "Phantom limbs." *Lippincott's Magazine of Popular Literature and Science* 7:563–69.

———. 1872. *Injuries of nerves and their consequences*. Philadelphia: Lippincott.

Molotkoff, A. G. 1935. "The source of pain in amputation stumps in relation to the rational treatment." *Journal of Bone and Joint Surgery* 17:419–23.

Monaghan, Lee F. 2001. "Looking good, feeling good: The embodied pleasures of vibrant physicality." *Sociology of Health and Illness* 23:330–56.

Money, John, R. Jobaris, and Gregg M. Furth. 1977. "Apotemnophilia: Two cases of self-demand amputation as a paraphilia." *Journal of Sex Research* 13:115–25.

Moore, C. I., C. E. Stern, C. Dunbar, S. K. Kostyk, A. Gehi, and S. Corkin. 2000. "Referred phantom sensations and cortical reorganization after spinal cord injury in humans." *Proceedings of the National Academy of Sciences* 97:14703–8.

Moore, Lisa Jean, and Monica J. Casper. 2009. *Missing bodies: The politics of visibility*. New York: New York University Press.

Moore, Lisa Jean, and Adele E. Clarke. 1995. "Clitoral conventions and transgressions: Graphic representations in anatomy texts, c. 1900–1991." *Feminist Studies* 21:255–301.

————. 2001. "The traffic in cyberanatomies: Sex/gender/sexualities in local and global formations." *Body and Society* 7:57–96.

Morgenstern, F. S. 1964. "The effects of sensory input and concentration on post-amputation phantom limb pain." *Journal of Neurology* 27:58–65.

Morris, David B. 1991. *The culture of pain.* Berkeley: University of California Press.

————. 1998. *Illness and culture in the postmodern age.* Berkeley: University of California Press.

Mortimer, Clare M., Roderick J. M. MacDonald, Denis J. Martin, Ian R. McMillan, John Ravey, and Wilma M. Steedman. 2004. "A focus group study of health professionals' views on phantom sensation, phantom pain, and the need for patient information." *Pain and Headache* 54:221–26.

Mortimer, C. M., W. M. Steedman, I. R. McMillan, D. J. Martin, and J. Ravey. 2002. "Patient information on phantom limb pain: A focus group study of patient experiences, perceptions, and opinions." *Health Education Research* 17:291–304.

Mowat, Ryan. 2009. "Indescribable pain in literature: A commentary on Crawford." *Social Science and Medicine* 69 (5):662–65.

Murphy, Robert. 1990. *The silent body.* New York: Norton.

Murphy, William F. 1957. "Some clinical aspects of the body ego: With especial reference to phantom limb phenomena." *Psychoanalytic Review* 44:462.

Murray, Craig D., Stephen Pettifer, Toby Howard, Emma L. Patchick, Fabrice Caillette, Jai Kulkarni, and Candy Bamford. 2007. "The treatment of phantom limb pain using immersive virtual reality: Three case studies." *Disability and Rehabilitation* 29:1465–69.

Musallam, S., B. D. Corneil, B. Greger, H. Scherberger, and R. A. Andersen. 2004. "Cognitive control signals for neural prosthetics." *Science* 305:258–62.

Naam, Ramez. 2005. *More than human: Embracing the promise of biological enhancement.* New York: Broadway Books.

Nashold, B. S., Jr. 1969. "Stereotaxic midbrain lesions for central dysesthesia and phantom pain: Preliminary report." *Journal of Neurosurgery* 30:116–26.

Nathanson, M. 1988. "Phantom limbs as reported by S. Weir Mitchell." *Neurology* 38:504–5.

NCOPE. 2013. "About NCOPE." *National Commission on Orthotics and Prosthetics Education*: www.ncope.org.

Nikolajsen, L., S. Ilkjaer, K. Kroner, J. H. Christensen, and T. S. Jensen. 1997. "The influence of preamputation pain on postamputation stump and phantom pain." *Pain* 72:393–405.

Noritaka, Kawashima, and Tomoki Mita. 2009. "Metal bar prevents phantom limb motion: Case study of an amputation patient who showed a profound change in the awareness of his phantom limb." *Neurocase* 15:478–84.

Northwestern. 1995. "From craft to science: 50 years of prosthetics/orthotics research started with a meeting at Northwestern University." *Capabilities* 4:1–8.

————. 2002. "Prosthetics history page." *Northwestern University*: www.nupoc.northwestern.edu.

O'Connor, Erin. 2000. *Raw material: Producing pathology in Victorian culture.* Durham, NC: Duke University Press.

Okeowo, Alexis. 2012. "A once-unthinkable choice for amputees." *New York Times*: www.nytimes.com.

Olesen, Virginia L. 1992. "Extraordinary events and mundane ailments: The contextual dialectics of the embodied self," in *Investigating subjectivity: Research on lived experience*, edited by C. Ellis and M. Flaherty. Newbury Park, CA: Sage.

Olry, R., and D. E. Haines. 2002. "Phantom limb: Haunted body?" *Journal of the History of Neuroscience* 11:67–68.

Omer, G. E., Jr. 1981. "Nerve, neuroma, and pain problems related to upper limb amputations." *Orthopedic Clinics of North America* 12:751–62.

O'Neill, Kieran, Annraoi dePaor, and Malcolm Mac Lachlan. 1997. "An investigation into the performance of augmented reality for use in the treatment of phantom limb pain in amputees." Dublin: National University of Ireland–Dublin.

Össur. 2005. "Reaching out to make a difference." Aliso Viejo: Össur 1–2.

———. 2010. "Mauch knee plus." Össur: www.ossur.com.

Osterweis, Marian, Arthur Kleinman, and David Mechanic. 1987. *Pain and disability: Clinical, behavioral, and public policy perspectives*. Washington, DC: National Academy Press.

Ott, Katherine. 2002. "The sum of its parts: An introduction to modern histories of prosthetics," in *Artificial parts and practical lives: Modern histories of prosthetics*, edited by K. Ott, D. Serlin, and S. Mihm. New York: New York University Press.

Oudshoorn, Nancy Everdina, and Trevor Pinch. 2005. *How users matter: The co-construction of users and technology*. Cambridge, MA: MIT Press.

Paré, Ambrose. 1649. *The works of that famous chirurgeon Ambrose Parey*. Translated by T. Johnson. London: M. Clark.

Parks, C. M. 1973. "Factors determining the persistence of phantom pain in the amputee." *Journal of Psychosomatic Research* 17:97–108.

Pasveer, B. 1989. "Knowledge of shadows: The introduction of X-ray images in medicine." *Sociology of Health and Illness* 11:360–81.

Penfield, Wilder. 1958. *The excitable cortex in conscious man*. Liverpool, UK: Liverpool University Press.

Penfield, Wilder, and Edwin Boldrey. 1937. "Somatic motor and sensory representation in cerebral cortex of man as studied by electrical stimulation." *Brain* 60:389–443.

Penfield, Wilder, and T. Rasmussen. 1951. *The cerebral cortex of man*. New York: Macmillan.

Peniston-Bird, Corinna. 2003. "Classifying the body in the Second World War: British men in and out of uniform." *Body and Society* 9:31–48.

Pereira, Jose Carlos, and Rosana Cardoso Alves. 2011. "The labeled-lines principle of the somatosensory physiology might explain the phantom limb phenomenon." *Medical Hypotheses* 77:853–56.

Phillips, Katherine A., Sabine Wilhelm, Lorrin M. Koran, Elizabeth R. Didie, Brrain A. Fallon, Jamie Feusner, and Dan J. Stein. 2010. "Body Dysmorphic Disorder: Some key issues for DSM-V." *Depression and Anxiety* 27:573–91.

Pickering, Andrew. 1995. "Cyborg history and the World War II regime." *Perspectives on Science* 3:1–48.

Pickersgill, Martyn, and Ira Van Keulen. 2011. *Sociological reflections on the neurosciences.* Bingley, UK: Emerald.

Pike, Alvin C., and LeRoy W. Nattress. 1991. "The changing role of the amputee in the rehabilitation process." *Physical Medicine and Rehabilitation Clinics of North America* 2:405–14.

Pisetsky, J. E. 1946. "Disappearance of painful phantom limbs after electric shock treatment." *American Journal of Psychiatry* 102:599–601.

Poeck, K. 1964. "Phantoms following amputation in early childhood and in congenital absence of limbs." *Cortex* 1:269–75.

POF. 2013. "History." *Prosthetic Outreach Foundation*: http://pofsea.org/about-us/history.

Pollock, Lewis J., Benjamin Boshes, Alex J. Arieff, Isidore Finkelman, Meyer Brown, Norman B. Dobin, Benjamin H. Kesert, Stanley W. Pyzik, John R. Finkle, Eli L. Tigay, and Israel Zivin. 1957. "Phantom limb in patients with injuries to the spinal cord and cauda equina." *Surgery, Gynecology, and Obstetrics* 104:407–15.

Pons, T. P., P. E. Garraghty, A. K. Ommaya, J. H. Kaas, E. Taub, and M. Mishkin. 1991. "Massive cortical reorganization after sensory deafferentation in adult macaques." *Science* 252:1857–60.

Pontius, Anneliese, A. 1964. "Comparison of phantoms and atavistic body schema experiences in a schizophrenic: A contribution to the study of hallucinations." *Perceptual and Motor Skills* 19:695–700.

Porter, Roy. 1997. *The greatest benefit to mankind: A medical history of humanity.* New York: Norton.

———. 2002. *Blood and guts: A short history of medicine.* New York: Norton.

Postone, Norman. 1987. "Phantom limb pain: A review." *International Journal of Psychiatry in Medicine* 17:57–70.

Potter, Benjamin K., and Charles R. Scoville. 2006. "Amputation is not isolated: An overview of the US Army Amputee Patient Care Program and associated amputee injuries." *Journal of the American Academy of Orthopaedic Surgeons* 14:S188–90.

Prasad, Amit. 2005. "Making images/making bodies: Visibilizing and disciplining through Magnetic Resonance Imaging (MRI)." *Science, Technology, and Human Values* 30:291–316.

Prasad, P., and N. L. Das. 1982. "Phantom limb: Its properties and mechanism of pain." *Journal of Postgraduate Medicine* 28:30–33.

Price, Douglas B. 1976. "Phantom limb phenomenon in patients with leprosy." *Journal of Nervous and Mental Disease* 163:108–16.

———. 1998. "Phantom limb phenomenon after limb reattachment or cross-transfer: Three patient histories." *Psychosomatics* 39:384–87.

Price, Douglas B., and Neil J. Twombly. 1972. *The phantom limb phenomenon: A medical, folkloric, and historical study.* Translated by M. C. Osborne. Washington, DC: Georgetown University Press.

Probstner, Danielle, Luiz Claudio Santos Thuler, Neli Muraki Ishikawa, and Regina Maria Papais Alvarenga. 2010. "Phantom limb phenomena in cancer amputees." *Pain Practice* 10:249–56.

Rabinbach, Anson. 1990. *The human motor: Energy, fatigue, and the origins of modernity.* Berkeley: University of California Press.

Rabinow, Paul. 1996. *Essays on the anthropology of reason.* Princeton, NJ: Princeton University Press.

Ramachandran, V. S. 1994. "Phantom limbs, neglect syndromes, repressed memories, and Freudian psychology." *International Review of Neurobiology* 37:291–333, 369–72.

———. 1996. "What neurological syndromes can tell us about human nature: Some lessons from phantom limbs, capgras syndrome, and anosognosia." *Cold Spring Harbor Symposia on Quantitative Biology* 61:115–34.

———. 1998. "Consciousness and body image: Lessons from phantom limbs, capgras syndrome, and pain asymbolia." *Philosophical Transactions of the Royal Society of London. Series B, Biological Sciences* 353:1851–59.

———. 2005. "Plasticity and functional recovery in neurology." *Clinical Medicine* 5:368–73.

———. 2009. "Sexual and food preference in apotemnophilia and anorexia: Interactions between 'beliefs' and 'needs' regulated by two-way connections between body image and limbic structures." *Perception* 38:775–77.

———. 2011. *The tell-tale brain: A neuroscientist's quest for what makes us human.* New York: Norton.

Ramachandran, V. S., and Sandra Blakeslee. 1998. *Phantoms in the brain: Probing the mysteries of the human mind.* New York: William Morrow.

Ramachandran, V. S., David Brang, Paul D. McGeoch, and Willliam Rosar. 2009. "Sexual and food preference in Apotemnophilia and anorexia: Interactions between 'beliefs' and 'needs' regulated by two-way connections between body image and limbic structures." *Perception* 38:775–77.

Ramachandran, V. S., and W. Hirstein. 1998. "The perception of phantom limbs: The D. O. Hebb lecture." *Brain* 121:1603–30.

Ramachandran, V. S., and Paul D. McGeoch. 2007. "Occurrence of phantom genitalia after gender reassignment surgery." *Medical Hypotheses* 69:1001–3.

Ramachandran, V. S., and D. Rogers-Ramachandran. 1996. "Synaesthesia in phantom limbs induced with mirrors." *Proceedings of the Royal Society B: Biological Sciences* 263:377–86.

———. 2000. "Phantom limbs and neural plasticity." *Archives of Neurology* 57:317–20.

Ramachandran, V. S., M. Stewart, and D. C. Rogers-Ramachandran. 1992. "Perceptual correlates of massive cortical reorganization." *Neuroreport* 3:583–86.

Randall, G. C., J. R. Ewalt, and H. Blair. 1945. "Psychiatric reaction to amputation." *Journal of the American Medical Association* 128:645–52.

Rang, Mercer, and George H. Thompson. 1981. "History of amputations and prostheses," in *Amputation surgery and rehabilitation: The Toronto experience*, edited by J. P.
Kostuik and R. Gillespie. New York: Churchill Livingstone.

Ray, N. J., N. Jenkinson, M. L. Kringelbach, P. C. Hansen, E. A. Pereira, J. S. Brittain,
P. Holland, I. E. Holliday, S. Owen, J. Stein, and T. Aziz. 2009. "Abnormal thalo-
mocortical dynamics may be altered by deep brain stimulation: Using magneto-
encephalography to study phantom limb pain." *Journal of Clinical Neuroscience*
16:32–36.

Regalado, Antonio. 2001. "Brain-machine interface." *MIT Technology Review:* http://
www2.technologyreview.com/news/400879/brain-machine-interface.

Reilly, Karen T., and Angela Sirigu. 2008. "The motor cortex and its role in phantom
limb phenomena." *Neuroscientist* 14:195–202.

Reinharz, Shulamit. 1992. *Feminist methods in social research.* New York: Oxford University Press.

Reschke, K. 1934. "Lumbar ramisection for causalgia in an amputation." *International
Journal of Abstracts of Surgery* 59:504–5.

Restak, Richard. 1984. *The brain.* Toronto: Bantam.

Rey, Roselyne. 1993. *The history of pain.* Translated by L. E. Wallace, J. A. Cadden, and
S. W. Cadden. Cambridge, MA: Harvard University Press.

Ribbers, G., T. Mulder, and R. Rijken. 1989. "The phantom phenomenon: A critical
review." *International Journal of Rehabilitation Research* 12:175–86.

Riddoch, G. 1941. "Phantom limbs and body shape." *Brain* 64:197–222.

Riscalla, Louise Mead. 1977. "Is the phantom limb really a phantom?" *Journal of the
American Society of Psychosomatic Dentistry and Medicine* 24:76–81.

Rivera-Fuentes, Consuelo, and Lynda Birke. 2001. "Talking with/in pain: Reflections
on bodies under torture." *Women's Studies International Forum* 24:653 68.

Rodgers, Diane M. 2008. *Debugging the link between social theory and social insects.*
Baton Rouge: Louisiana State University.

Roeder, George H. 1996. "Censoring disorder: American visual imagery of World War
II," in *The war in American culture: Society and consciousness during World War II,*
edited by L. A. Erenberg and S. E. Hirsch. Chicago: University of Chicago Press.

Rose, Nikolas. 2003. "The neurochemical selves." *Society* 41:46–59.

———. 2007. *The politics of life itself: Biomedicine, power, and subjectivity in the twenty-
first century.* Princeton, NJ: Princeton University Press.

Rosen, G., K. Hugdahl, L. Ersland, A. Lundervold, A. I. Smievoll, R. Barndon, H.
Sundberg, T. Thomsen, B. E. Roscher, A. Tjolsen, and B. Engelsen. 2001. "Different
brain areas activated during imagery of painful and non-painful 'finger movements'
in a subject with an amputated arm." *Neurocase* 7:255–60.

Rosenberg, Charles E. 1989. "Disease in history: Frames and framers." *Milbank Quarterly* 6:1–15.

———. 1992. *Explaining epidemics and other studies in the history of medicine.* Cambridge: Cambridge University Press.

———. 2007. *Our present complaint: American medicine, past and present.* Baltimore, MD: Johns Hopkins University Press.

Roth, Wolff-Michael. 2005. "Making classifications (at) work: Ordering practices in science." *Social Studies of Science* 35:581–621.

Rounseville, Cheryl. 1992. "Phantom limb pain: The ghost that haunts the amputee." *Orthopaedic Nursing* 11:67–71.

Rubin, Herbert J., and Irene S. Rubin. 2005. *Qualitative interviewing: The art of hearing data.* 2nd edition. Thousand Oaks, CA: Sage.

Russell, W. R. 1949. "Painful amputation stump and phantom limbs: Treatment by repeated percussion to stump neuromata." *British Medical Journal* 1:1024–26.

Rybarczyk, Bruce, Robert Edwards, and Jay Behel. 2004. "Diversity in adjustment to a leg amputation: Case illustrations of common themes." *Disability and Rehabilitation* 26:944–53.

Saadah, E. S., and R. Melzack. 1994. "Phantom limb experiences in congenital limb-deficient adults." *Cortex* 30:479–85.

Sacks, Oliver W. 1987. *The man who mistook his wife for a hat and other clinical tales.* New York: Perennial Library.

Sakagami, Y., T. Murai, and H. Sugiyama. 2002. "A third arm on the chest: Implications for the cortical reorganization theory of phantom limbs." *Journal of Neuropsychiatry and Clinical Neurosciences* 14:90–91.

Sargent, Michael G. 2005. *Biomedicine and the human condition: Challenges, risks, and rewards.* Cambridge: Cambridge University Press.

Satchithananda, D. K., J. Parameshwar, I. Hardy, and S. R. Large. 1998. "Phantom-limb lengthening after heart transplant." *Lancet* 352:292.

Scarry, Elaine. 1985. *The body in pain: The making and unmaking of the world.* New York: Oxford University Press.

Scatena, P. 1990. "Phantom representations of congenitally absent limbs." *Perceptual and Motor Skills* 70:1227–32.

Scheper-Hughes, Nancy. 1994. "Embodied knowledge: Thinking with the body in critical medical anthropology," in *Assessing cultural anthropology*, edited by R. Borofsky. New York: McGraw Hill.

———. 2001. "Bodies for sale: Whole or in parts." *Body and Society* 7:1–8.

———. 2005. "The last commodity: Post-human ethics and the global traffic in 'fresh' organs," in *Global assemblages: Technology, politics, and ethics as anthropological problems*, edited by A. Ong and S. J. Collier. Malden, MA: Blackwell.

———. 2006. "Organ trafficking: The real, the unreal, and the uncanny." *Annals of Transplantation* 11:16–30.

———. 2011. "The body in tatters: Dismemberment, dissection, and the return of the repressed," in *A companion to the anthropology of the body and embodiment*, edited by F. E. Mascia-Lees. Malden, MA: Wiley-Blackwell.

Scheper-Hughes, Nancy, and Margaret M. Lock. 1987. "The mindful body: A prolegomenon to future work in medical anthropology." *Medical Anthropology Quarterly* 1:6–41.

———. 1991. "Message in the bottle: Illness and the micropolitics of resistance." *Journal of Psychohistory* 18:409–32.

Schilder, P. F. 1935. *The image and appearance of the human body: Studies in the constructive energies of the psyche.* London: Routledge.

Schuch, Michael C., and Charles H. Pritham. 2002. "International standards organization terminology: Application to prosthetics and orthotics." *Journal of Prosthetics and Orthotics* 6:29–33.

Schwartz, Hillel. 1992. "Torque: The new kinaesthetic of the twentieth century," in *Incorporations*, edited by J. Crary and S. Kwinter. New York: Zone Books.

———. 1996. *The culture of the copy: Striking likenesses, unreasonable facsimiles.* New York: Zone Books.

Schwartz, Jeffrey M., and Sharon Begley. 2002. *The mind and the brain: Neuroplasticity and the power of mental force.* New York: HarperCollins.

Schwarz, Berthold E. 1964. "Phantom embolism." *Psychosomatics* 5:52–54.

Schwenkreis, Peter, K. Witscher, Frank Janssen, Burkhard Pleger, Roman Dertwinkel, Michael Zenz, J. P. Malin, and Martin Tegenthoff. 2001. "Assessment of reorganization in the sensorimotor cortex after upper limb amputation." *Clinical Neurophysiology* 112:627–35.

Scott, W. C. M. 1948. "Some embryological, neurological, psychiatric, and psychoanalytic implications of the body scheme." *International Journal of Psychoanalysis* 29:141–55.

Sem-Jacobsen, C. W. 1968. *Depth-electrographic stimulation of the human brain and behavior.* Springfield, IL: Charles C. Thomas.

Serlin, David. 2002. "Engineering masculinity: Veterans and prosthetics after World War Two," in *Artificial parts, practical lives: Modern histories of prosthetics*, edited by K. Ott, D. Serlin, and S. Mihm. New York: New York University Press.

———. 2004. *Replaceable you: Engineering the body in postwar America.* Chicago: University of Chicago Press.

———. 2006. "The other arms race," in *The disabilities studies reader*, edited by L. Davis. New York: Routledge.

Sherman, Richard A. 1989. "Stump and phantom limb pain." *Neurologic Clinics* 7:249–64.

———. 1994. "Phantom limb pain: Mechanism-based management." *Clinics in Podiatric Medicine and Surgery* 11:85–106.

———. 1997. "History of treatment attempts," in *Phantom pain*, edited by R. A. Sherman, M. Devor, and K. Heermann-Do. New York: Plenum Press.

———. 1999. "Utilization of prostheses among US veterans with traumatic amputation: A pilot survey." *Journal of Rehabilitation Research and Development* 36:100–108.

Sherman, Richard A., J. G. Arena, C. J. Sherman, and J. L. Ernst. 1989. "The mystery of phantom pain: Growing evidence for psychophysiological mechanisms." *Biofeedback and Self Regulation* 14:267–80.

Sherman, Richard A., and G. M. Bruno. 1987. "Concurrent variation of burning phantom limb and stump pain with near surface blood flow in the stump." *Orthopedics* 10:1395–1402.

Sherman, Richard A., J. L. Ernst, R. H. Barja, and G. M. Bruno. 1988. "Phantom pain: A lesson in the necessity for careful clinical research on chronic pain problems." *Journal of Rehabilitation Research and Development* 25:vii–x.

Sherman, Richard A., J. Katz, Joseph J. Marbach, and Kim Heermann-Do. 1997. "Locations, characteristics, and descriptions." *Phantom pain*, edited by R. A. Sherman, M. Devor, and K. Heermann-Do. New York: Plenum.

Sherman, Richard A., and C. J. Sherman. 1983. "Prevalence and characteristics of chronic phantom limb pain among American veterans: Results of a trial survey." *American Journal of Physical Medicine* 62:227–38.

———. 1985. "A comparison of phantom sensations among amputees whose amputations were of civilian and military origins." *Pain* 21:91–97.

Sherman, Richard A., C. J. Sherman, and G. M. Bruno. 1987. "Psychological factors influencing chronic phantom limb pain: An analysis of the literature." *Pain* 28:285–95.

Sherman, Richard A., C. J. Sherman, and N. G. Gall. 1980. "A survey of current phantom limb pain treatment in the United States." *Pain* 8:85–99.

Sherman, Richard A., C. J. Sherman, and L. Parker. 1984. "Chronic phantom and stump pain among American veterans: Results of a survey." *Pain* 18:83–95.

Shildrick, Margrit. 1997. *Leaky bodies and boundaries.* London: Routledge.

———. 1999. "The body which is not one: Dealing with difference." *Body and Society* 5:77–92.

———. 2008. "Corporeal cuts: Surgery and the psycho-social." *Body and Society* 14:31–46

———. 2010. "Some reflections on the socio-cultural and bioscientific limits of bodily integrity." *Body and Society* 16:11–22.

Shilling, Chris. 2003. *The body and social theory.* London: Sage.

———. 2005. *The body in culture, technology and society.* Thousand Oaks, CA: Sage.

Shorter, Edward. 1992. *From paralysis to fatigue: A history of psychosomatic illness in the modern era.* New York: Free Press.

Shreeve, James. 1993. "Touching the phantom." *Discover* 14:1–6.

Shukla, G. D., S. C. Sahu, R. P. Tripathi, and D. K. Gupta. 1982. "Phantom limb: A phenomenological study." *British Journal of Psychiatry* 141:54–58.

Shurr, Donald G., and Thomas M. Cook. 1990. *Prosthetics and orthotics.* Norwalk, CT: Appleton & Lange.

Sideris, Lisa, Charles McCarthy, and David H. Smith. 1999. "Roots of concern with nonhuman animals in biomedical ethics." *ILAR* 40:1–10.

Siebers, Tobin. 2008. *Disability theory.* Ann Arbor: University of Michigan Press.

———. 2010. "In the name of pain," in *Against health: How health became the new morality,* edited by J. M. Metzl and A. Kirkland. New York: New York University Press.

Silber, Jerome, and Sydelle Silverman. 1958. "Studies in the upper limb amputee." *Artificial Limbs* 5:88–116.

Simmel, Marianne L. 1956. "On phantom limbs." *Archives of Neurology and Psychiatry* 75:637–47.

———. 1959. "Phantoms, phantom pain, and 'denial.'" *American Journal of Psychotherapy* 13:603–13.

———. 1961. "The absence of phantoms for congenitally missing limbs." *American Journal of Psychology* 74:467–70.

———. 1962. "Phantom experiences following amputation in childhood." *Journal of Neurology, Neurosurgery, and Psychiatry* 25:69–78.

———. 1966a. "Developmental aspects of the body scheme." *Child Development* 37:83–95.

———. 1966b. "A study of phantoms after amputation of the breast." *Neuropsychologia* 4:331–50.

———. 1967. "The body percept in physical medicine and rehabilitation." *Journal of Health and Social Behavior* 8:60–64.

Slocum, D. 1949. *An atlas of amputations.* Philadelphia: Mosby.

Smith, Doug. 2001. "Notes from the medical director: Limb loss is difficult for patient and surgeon." *InMotion* 11:1.

Smith, Stephen. 1871. "Analysis of four hundred and thirty-nine recorded amputations in the contiguity of the lower extremity," in *Surgical memoirs of the war of the rebellion,* edited by F. Hamilton. Cambridge, MA: Riverside.

Sobchack, Vivian. 2010. "Living a 'phantom limb': On the phenomenology of bodily integrity." *Body and Society* 16:51–67.

Solomon, George F., and Michael K. Schmidt. 1978. "A burning issue: Phantom limb pain and psychological preparation of the patient for amputation." *Archives of Surgery* 113:185–86.

Spitzer, M., P. Bohler, M. Weisbrod, and U. Kischka. 1995. "A neural network model of phantom limbs." *Biological Cybernetics* 72:197–206.

Stannard, Catherine F. 1993. "Phantom limb pain." *British Journal of Hospital Medicine* 50:583–84, 586–87.

Star, Susan Leigh. 1989. *Regions of the mind: Brain research and the quest for scientific certainty.* Stanford, CA: Stanford University Press.

Star, Susan Leigh, and Elihu M. Gerson. 1987. "The management and dynamics of anomalies in scientific work." *Sociological Quarterly* 28:147–69.

Stattel, Florence M. 1954. "The painful phantom limb." *American Journal of Occupational Therapy* 8:156–57.

Stein, J. M., and C. A. Warfield. 1982. "Phantom limb pain." *Hospital Practice* 17:166–67, 171.

Stiker, Henri-Jacques. 1997. *A history of disability.* Translated by W. Sayers. Ann Arbor: University of Michigan Press.

Stone, T. T. 1950. "Phantom limb pain and central pain: Relief by ablation of a portion of posterior central cerebral convolution." *Archives of Neurology and Psychiatry* 63:739–48.

Strauss, Anselm C. 1987. *Qualitative analysis for social scientists*. Cambridge: Cambridge University Press.

Strauss, Anselm C., and Juliet M. Corbin. 1998. *The basics of qualitative research: Techniques and procedures for developing grounded theory*. 2nd edition. Newbury Park, CA: Sage.

Suchman, Lucy. 2005. "Affiliative objects." *Organization* 12:379–99.

Suchman, Lucy, Jeanetee Blomberg, Julian E. Orr, and Randall Trigg. 1999. "Reconstructing technologies as social practice." *American Behavioral Scientist* 43:392–408.

Sumitani, Masahiko, Satoru Miyauchi, Arito Yozu, Yuko Otake, Youichi Saitoh, and Yoshitsugu Yamanda. 2010. "Phantom limb pain in the primary motor cortex: Topical review." *Journal of Anesthesiology* 24:337–41.

Sweetman, Paul. 1999. "Anchoring the (postmodern) self? Body modification, fashion, and identity." *Body and Society* 5:51–76.

Synnott, A. 1993. *The body social: Symbolism, self, and society*. New York: Routledge.

Szasz, Thomas S. 1974. *The myth of mental illness*. New York: Harper & Row.

Taub, Edward. 2005. Phone interview by author. July 26.

Tessler, M. J., M. Angle, and S. Kleiman. 1992. "Is phantom limb pain induced by spinal anaesthesia in lower limb amputees?" *Canadian Journal of Anaesthesia* 39:A78.

Thomas, Atha, and Chester C. Haddan. 1945. *Amputation prosthesis: Anatomic and physiologic considerations, with principles of alignment and fitting designed for the surgeon and limb manufacturer*. Philadelphia: Lippincott.

Thomson, Rosemarie Garland. 1996. "From wonder to error: A genealogy of freak discourse in modernity," in *Freakery: Cultural spectacles of the extraordinary body*, edited by R. G. Thomson. New York: New York University Press.

———. 2001. *Seeing the disabled: Visual rhetorics of disability in popular photography*. New York: New York University Press.

Titchkosky, Tanya. 2000. "Disability studies: The old and the new." *Canadian Journal of Sociology* 25:197–24.

———. 2007. *Reading and writing disability differently: The textured life of embodiment*. Toronto: University of Toronto Press.

Toepter, Susan. 1999. "Aimee Mullins: Athlete/model." *People Weekly Magazine* 51:144.

Tofts, Darren. 2002. "On mutability," in *Prefiguring cyberculture: An intellectual history*, edited by D. Tofts. Cambridge, MA: MIT Press.

Turner, Bryan S. 1987. *Medical power and social knowledge*. London: Sage.

———. 1991. "Recent developments in the theory of the body," in *The body: Social processes and cultural theory*, edited by M. Featherstone, M. Hapworth, and B. Turner. London: Sage.

———. 1996. *The body and society: Explorations in social theory*. Thousand Oaks, CA: Sage.

Ulger, Ozlem, Semra Topuz, Kezban Bayramlar, Gul Sener, and Fatih Erbahceci. 2009. "Effectiveness of phantom exercises for phantom limb pain: A pilot study." *Journal of Rehabilitation Medicine* 41:582–84.

Uncles, D. R., C. J. Glynn, and L. E. Carrie. 1996. "Regional anaesthesia for repeat Cae-sarean section in a patient with phantom limb pain." *Anaesthesia* 51:69–70.

VA. 2002a. "About VA." *Department of Veterans Affairs*: www.va.gov.

———. 2002b. "Veterans' Health Administration." *Department of Veterans Affairs*: http://www.va.gov/health/default.asp.

———. 2010. "VA history." *Department of Veterans Affairs*: www.va.gov.

van der Schans, Cees P., and Jan H. B. Geertzen. 2002. "Phantom pain and health-related quality of life in lower limb amputees." *Journal of Pain and Symptom Management* 24:429–36.

Van Dijck, José. 2005. *The transparent body: A cultural analysis of medical imaging.* Seattle: University of Washington Press.

Van Loon, Joost. 2002. "A contagious living fluid: Objectification and assemblage in the history of virology." *Theory, Culture, and Society* 19:107–24.

Van Wirdum, P. 1965. "A new explanation of phantom symptoms." *Psychiatria Neurologia Neurochirurgia* 68:306–13.

Varma, S. K., S. K. Lal, and A. Mukherjee. 1972. "A study of phantom experience in amputees." *Indian Journal of Medical Sciences* 26:185–88.

Vidal, F. 2009. "Brainhood, anthropological figure of modernity." *History of the Human Sciences* 22:5–36.

Vitali, Miroslaw. 1978. *Amputations and prostheses.* London: Bailliáere Tindall.

Vrancken, M. 1989. "Schools of thought on pain." *Social Science and Medicine* 29:435–44.

Wade, Nicholas. J. 2003. "The legacy of phantom limbs." *Perception* 32:517–24.

Wade, Nicholas J., and Stanley Finger. 2003. "William Porterfield and his phantom limb." *Neurosurgery* 52:1196–98.

———. 2010. "Phantom penis: Historical dimensions." *Journal of the History of the Neurosciences* 19:299–312.

Walby, Catherine. 2000. "Fragmented bodies, incoherent medicine." *Social Science and Medicine* 30:465–74.

Wangensteen, Owen H., Jacqueline Smith, and Sarah D. Wangensteen. 1967. "Some highlights in the history of amputation: Reflecting lesions in wound healing." *Bulletin of the History of Medicine* 41:97–131.

Wartan, S. W., W. Hamann, J. R. Wedley, and I. McColl. 1997. "Phantom pain and sensation among British veteran amputees." *British Journal of Anaesthesia* 78:652–59.

Watson, Nick. 2002. "Well, I know this is going to sound very strange to you, but I don't see myself as a disabled person: Identity and disability." *Disability and Society* 17:509–27.

Webster, Andrew. 2002. "Innovative health technologies and the social: Redefining health, medicine, and the body." *Current Sociology* 50:443–57.

Weeks, Sharon R., Victoria C. Anderson-Barnes, and Jack W. Tsao. 2010. "Phantom limb pain: Theories and therapies." *Neurologist* 16:277–86.

Weeks, Sharon R., and Jack W. Tsao. 2010. "Incorporation of another person's limb into body image relieves phantom limb pain: A case study." *Neurocase* 16:461–65.

Wegenstein, Bernadette. 2002. "Getting under the skin." *Configurations* 10:221–59.

Weinstein, S., and E. A. Sersen. 1961. "Phantoms in cases of congenital absence of limbs." *Neurology* 11:905–11.

Weinstein, Sidney, E. A. Sersen, and R. J. Vetter. 1964. "Phantoms and somatic sensation in cases of congenital aplasia." *Cortex* 1:276–90.

Weinstein, S., R. J. Vetter, and E. A. Sersen. 1970. "Phantoms following breast amputation." *Neuropsychologia* 8:185–97.

Weinstein, S., R. J. Vetter, G. Shapiro, and E. A. Sersen. 1969. "The effects of brain damage on the phantom limb." *Cortex* 5:91–103.

Weiss, Andor A. 1956. "The phantom limb." *Annals of Internal Medicine* 44:668–77.

Weiss, S. A., and B. Lindell. 1996. "Phantom limb pain and etiology of amputation in unilateral lower extremity amputees." *Journal of Pain and Symptom Management* 11:3–17.

Weiss, Samuel A. 1958. "The body image as related to phantom sensation: A hypothetical conceptualization of seemingly isolated findings." *Annals of the New York Academy of Sciences* 74:25–29.

Weiss, Samuel A., and S. Fishman. 1963. "Extended and telescoped phantom limbs in unilateral amputees." *Journal of Abnormal Social Psychology* 66:489–97.

Weiss, T., W. H. Miltner, T. Adler, L. Bruckner, and E. Taub. 1999. "Decrease in phantom limb pain associated with prosthesis-induced increased use of an amputation stump in humans." *Neuroscience Letters* 272:131–34.

Weitz, Rose. 1996. *The sociology of health, illness, and health care: A critical approach.* Belmont, CA: Wadsworth.

Whelan, Emma. 2003. "Putting pain to paper: Endometriosis and the documentation of suffering." *Health* 7:463–82.

Whitaker, H. A. 1979. "An historical note on the phantom limb." *Neurology* 29:273.

Whyte, A. S., and L. J. Carroll. 2002. "A preliminary examination of the relationship between employment, pain, and disability in an amputee population." *Disability and Rehabilitation* 24:462–70.

Whyte, A., and C. A. Niven. 2004. "The illusive phantom: Does primary care meet patient need following limb loss?" *Disability and Rehabilitation* 26:894–900.

Wiley, Bell Irvin. 2002. "Heroes and cowards," in *The Civil War soldier: A historical reader*, edited by M. Barton and L. M. Logue. New York: New York University Press.

Williams, Anne, and Susan B. Deaton. 1997. "Phantom limb pain: Elusive, yet real." *Rehabilitation Nursing* 22:73–77.

Williams, Simon J. 1997. "Modern medicine and the 'uncertain body': From corporeality to hyperreality?" *Social Science and Medicine* 45:1041–49.

———. 1998. "Health as moral performance: Ritual, transgression, and taboo." *Health* 16:435–57.

Williams, Simon J., and Gillian Bendelow. 1998. *The lived body: Sociological themes, embodied issues.* New York: Routledge.

———. 2000. "'Recalcitrant bodies'? Children, cancer, and the transgression of corporeal boundaries." *Health* 4:51–71.

Williams, Simon J., Stephan Katz, and Paul Martin. 2011. "Beyond medicalization? Memory, medicine, and the brain," in *Sociological reflections on the neurosciences*, edited by M. D. Pickersgill and I. V. Keulen. Bingley, UK: Emerald.

Williamson, V. C. 1992. "Amputation of the lower extremity: An overview." *Orthopaedic Nursing* 11:55–65.

Willoch, F., G. Rosen, T. R. Tolle, I. Oye, H. J. Wester, N. Berner, M. Schwaiger, and P. Bartenstein. 2000. "Phantom limb pain in the human brain: Unraveling neural circuitries of phantom limb sensations using positron emission tomography." *Annals of Neurology* 48:842–49.

Wilson, A. Bennett. 1998. *A primer on limb prosthetics*. Springfield, IL: Charles C. Thomas.

Wilson, P. R., J. R. Person, D. W. Su, and J. K. Wang. 1978. "Herpes zoster reactivation of phantom limb pain." *Mayo Clinic Proceedings* 53:336–38.

Winchell, E. 1995. *Coping with limb loss*. New York: Avery.

Winston, Burton J. 1950. "The use of tetraethylammonium chloride in treatment of phantom pain." *Circulation* 1:299–301.

Wood, Gaby. 2002. *Living dolls: A magical history of the quest for mechanical life*. London: Faber and Faber.

Woolgar, Steve. 1991. "Configuring the user: The case of usability trials," in *A sociology of monsters: Essays on power, technology, and domination*, edited by J. Law. New York: Routledge.

Wyer, Mary, Mary Barbercheck, Donna Giesman, Hatice Orun Ozturk, and Marta Wayne. 2001. *Women, science, and technology: A reader in feminist science studies*. New York: Routledge.

Young, Allan. 1995. *The harmony of illusions: Inventing post-traumatic stress disorder*. Princeton, NJ: Princeton University Press.

Young-Bruehl, Elisabeth. 1988. *Anna Freud: A biography*. New York: Summit.

Yuh, W. T., D. J. Fisher, R. K. Shields, J. C. Ehrhardt, and F. G. Shellock. 1992. "Phantom limb pain induced in amputee by strong magnetic fields." *Journal of Magnetic Resonance Imaging* 2:221–23.

Zeher, Michael J., Robert S. Armiger, James M. Burck, Courtney Moran, Janid Blanco Kiely, Sharon R. Weeks, Jack W. Tsao, Paul F. Pasquina, R. Davoodi, and G. Loeb. 2011. "Using a virtual integration environment in treating phantom limb pain." *Studies in Health Technology and Informatics* 163:730–36.

Zola, Irving Kenneth. 1972. "Medicine as an institution of social control." *Sociological Review* 20:487–504.

Zuk, Gerald H. 1956. "The phantom limb: A proposed theory of unconscious origins." *Journal of Nervous and Mental Disease* 124:510–13.

ableism, 3, 203, 240, 146, 220, 240, 246, 248, 253n7, 265n19

absolute synchronicity, 22, 24, 216–217, 249; phantom fusion, 22, 216

actant, 149, 151–152, 231

Advisory Council on Artificial Limbs (ACAL), 202

"affiliative objects," 191, 192, 193–194, 249

American Board for the Certification in Orthotics, Prosthetics and Pedorthics (ABC), 261n10

American Civil War, 109–111, 195, 197–198, 260n3, 261n9

American Orthopedic Limb Manufacturers Association (AOLMA), 200

American Orthotic and Prosthetic Association (AOPA), 202

American Taylorism, 25, 43

amputation surgery, 9, 20, 28, 194, 198, 201, 204–208, 213, 244, 255n1, 260n4; collaboration with prosthetic science, 204–205

amputee/ation: ambiguous figure, 197–148; authentic, 29, 224; children, 129, 144, 256n8; conduit, 28, 148, 158; congenital, 6, 44, 62, 67, 115–116, 128–130, 141, 143, 144–145, 188, 233–235, 244, 256n8, 265n21, 266n24; degradation of the self, 196; elective (see also apotemnophilia), 6, 181, 220, 235–241, 241, 244, 262n3; emasculation/feminization, 9, 12, 29, 107, 111, 124, 132, 139, 146, 199, 205–207, 230, 248, 261n12; guilt, 4; hybridization, 17, 129, 194, 207, 239; hysteria, 111; icon, 194, 195, 198, 206, 213, 225, 247–248; imagery, 14, 15, 203–204, 206–208, 246; in/dependence, 9, 197, 199, 248, 250; investment, 184, 209, 241; malleability, 10–11, 214, 221; pioneer, 28, 158;

productivity, 9, 10, 12, 18, 111, 132, 195, 197, 199, 203, 205–206, 209, 229; prosthetized, 12, 14, 17, 197, 213, 247–248; reduplication, 176; restorative(tion), 184, 241; survival, 139

Amputee Coalition of America (ACA), 1–3, 17, 215, 251n1

"anatomical atlas," 191

"anatomo-politics," 5, 30

apotemnophilia(philes)/wannabe(s), 29, 220, 224, 235–241, 249, 262n4, 262n7, 263n8, 263n11, 263n13, 264n15, 264n16; acrotomophilia(philes)/devotee(s), 237, 262n3, 263n11; alien, 237–238; pretender(s), 263n11; pruning, 238, 239; self-actualization, 238

Artificial Limb Program (ALP), 202

biomedical commodification, 99, 105, 229, 241

biomedical gaze, 30, 95, 138, 256n9

biomedical legitimation, 4, 19, 24, 30, 31, 74, 89, 105, 108, 140, 155, 202, 224, 225, 229, 230, 237, 239, 244, 249, 252n4, 256n9; phantom penis, 225–229; visualization, 156, 169, 191, 232

biomedical rationalization/management, 20, 25, 33, 67, 70, 106, 138, 150, 151, 160, 176, 192, 223, 229, 230, 245

biomedical resistance, 19–20, 150–152, 192, 230; body scheme/image, 125–126; pain, 82–83

biomedical territorialization, 74, 158, 162, 177, 191, 229

bio-monitoring, 135, 191, 208

biopolitical order, 4, 71, 84, 99, 100, 107, 150, 157, 158, 160, 185, 191, 193, 223, 232, 233, 250, 253n5

biopower, 71, 74, 152, 250

body, 27, 30–31, 37, 44, 59, 196–197, 214, 219, 227, 231, 245, 253n5; absence, 19–20, 75–76; agential, 19; augmented, 221, 229, 244, 247, 253n6, 253n7; (bio)medical(ized), 138, 150, 223; birthed, 115, 128, 239, 264n13; in-the-brain/brain-based, 28, 29, 147, 150, 156–158, 160, 162–164, 167, 176, 179, 186, 191, 208, 223–224, 230–235, 241, 250; character, 196; docile, 5, 30, 246; in dreams, 134–135, 250; economy of motion, 25, 43–44, 45–49; emancipated, 245; epiphenomenal, 27, 29, 148, 150, 159–160, 224, 230–232; "fractioned," 106, 107, 111, 159, 179, 191, 229, 230, 250; healthy, 48, 244; homuncular, 163, 230, 258n15; hybridized, 150; idealized, 134; inadequacies, 15, 245; male, 146, 163, 164, 165, 199, 203, 208, 229, 230; mechanistic, 25, 37–38, 256n9; mind-body, 28, 157, 159, 219, 223, 231, 253n5, 256n9; normal/natural, 3–4, 30, 150, 217; optimization, 5, 213; pained, 76, 95; as phantom, 159, 160; phenomenology, 117, 134, 228; postmodern, 214, 244–245; recalcitrant, 19, 71, 150–152, 192; reorganized, 162; as self, 8–9, 12, 13, 14, 19, 28, 42, 45, 49, 59–60, 69, 110–112, 117, 118–119, 125, 147, 157, 159–160, 196–197, 208, 210, 214, 223, 231, 238–239; 245, 264n13, 264n14; sleep, 135; social, 29, 108, 150, 185, 244, 248; superfluous, 55, 150, 160, 231, 232; wholeness, 29, 110–111, 125–126, 127, 128, 131, 134, 135, 166, 215, 224, 239–240, 248, 250
Body Dismorphic Disorder (BDD), 236, 262n7
"body love," 136–137
body part: atrophied, 183; deep connection, 136–138, 241; homuncular parts/areas, 172, 179, 183, 186, 208, 218, 229, 241, 258n15; interactional effects, 151; proper handling, 114, 133–138, 241; scheme-ed, 229; value, 31, 114, 118–119, 122, 123, 131, 136, 165–166, 241, 264n17; virtual, 219, 220, 229, 250
body scheme/image, 26, 134, 147, 165, 167, 233, 235, 239, 241, 255n5, 264n16; archetypal engram, 116, 130, 241; child amputee(s), 129–130, 243; coinciding, 210; complete, 126, 131, 133, 240; congenital amputee(s), 128–130, 145; denial, 130–131, 134, 141, 166; exposure, 122–124; gender, 234–235; gestalt, 125–129, 131, 166; Head and Holmes, 114–116, 118, 130, 143, 145, 146; ness, 243; malleable/plastic, 243; mimesis,

126; neuroprosthetic, 189; theory, 113–116; the psychological organ, 116–122, 130, 143
brain/cortex: captivation, 156; cartography, 157, 160, 168, 169, 192; conflation with the mind, 156, 231; deafferentation, 142, 180, 182, 186, 258n8, 259n20; dysfunction, 160, 182, 183; experience/sensation, 159, 231; functionality, 28, 115, 146, 157, 160, 164, 167, 176, 180–183, 185, 186, 188, 189, 191, 222; hard-wired paradigm, 13, 28, 29, 160, 169, 180, 224, 233, 241, 258n11; of interest, 158, 224, 232; male, 162–163, 208, 230, 224; motor cortex/motor homunculi(us), 160–165, 166, 170, 176, 180, 183, 185, 189, 218, 241, 254n3, 257n14, 258n6, 259n17, 259n19; somatosensory cortex/sensory homunculi(us), 147, 160–165, 166, 168, 169, 170, 172, 176, 180, 183, 185, 189, 218, 230, 241, 254n3, 257n14, 258n6, 259n17, 259n19

Campbell, Kelly, 142, 153, 213
castration, 131–132, 139
Civil War, 109–111, 195–198, 260n3, 261n9; postbellum, 10, 139, 195, 207
Committee on Prosthetic Devices (CPD), 202, 203, 261n7
content analysis, 252n3
corporeal(ity), 4, 8, 11, 110, 126, 160, 166, 177, 191, 210, 215, 229, 231, 264n13; activity, 135; aesthetics, 17; biographies, 5, 149; enhancement, 3, 225, 248; futures, 114; ghosts, 122, 229; histories, 27, 42, 136; ideologies, 24, 27, 30–31, 37, 71, 150, 229, 240; technologies, 5; transcendence, 2; transformations, 5, 29, 244–246; transgressions, 150, 152, 249
cortical reorganization/remapping, 13, 170, 171, 172–175, 176, 177–178, 180–187, 221, 223, 233–234 (see also neuronal sprouting/arborization; neuronal unmasking); dead zones/islands of allegiance, 183–184, 189, 242, 259n20; decreased, 189; dramatic/massive, 169, 170, 180, 182, 241; dynamic, 179; encroachment, 169, 218; functional, 182–183, 217; injury-related, 181; invasion, 172, 175, 177, 180, 182, 184, 218; maladaptive, 160, 182–183; masking, 186–187; permanent, 180; phantom pain, 182–184, 189, 259n18, 259n19; pain memories, 183; plasticity, 13, 28, 160, 174, 180–186, 189, 218–222, 233–234, 243; prevention, 13, 180, 184–185, 189–190; reversal/reoccupation, 188, 189, 212, 218, 222, 234; stable, 179, 180,

184; telescoping, 183; use-dependent, 181, 190, 218, 241, 259n18

Crittenden, Chad, 2

cyborg, 4, 5, 10–11, 15, 17, 37, 206–208, 244, 246–248, 261n14

Czerniecki, Joseph M., 32–33, 77–78, 94, 104, 147

Dedlow, George, 109–111, 132, 206; "fraction of a man," 109–111

deeply embodied technologies, 7–8, 9, 11, 213, 219, 221, 222, 242

denial, 125, 130–138, 139, 140, 142, 159, 179; egoistic, 131–138, 140; secure, 131, 133

"diffusionist localizationism," 152, 167

disability, 2, 29, 31, 71, 138, 140, 167, 196, 197, 204, 223, 224, 240–241, 244, 246–248, 256n9, 261n12, 263n11, 265n19

disturbances of continuity, 24, 58–65

embodiment, 4–5, 8–9, 11, 13, 59, 155, 191, 199, 208, 209, 210, 213, 215, 222, 223, 240, 242, 246, 253n5; fraudulence, 29, 107, 111, 224, 230; of-the-body, 8, 11, 117, 216; perfection/ing, 7, 18, 25, 56, 69, 128, 198, 232

epidemiology, 112, 150

experimental phantoms, 142, 145–146

"explicit localizationism," 152, 167, 183, 185

flesh(y), 5, 8, 11, 14, 33, 66, 80, 160, 176, 186, 191, 214, 215, 217, 220, 224, 225, 229, 231, 262n14; limbs, 6, 7, 10, 24, 25, 27, 33, 45, 47, 66, 75

Freud, Anna, 125, 130

Freud, Sigmund, 117, 131, 135, 157

gangrene, 42, 54, 101, 109, 143, 144, 195, 236

gate-control theory, 85, 97–99

grounded theory, 3, 251n2, 252n3

Head, Sir Henry, and Holmes, Gordon Morgan, 114–116, 117, 118, 130, 143, 145, 146, 165

Holy Grail, 19, 27, 149–152, 157–160, 223, 250

human kinesthetic, 45–46

homunculus, 146, 166–167, 173, 186, 208, 218, 230, 233, 235, 257n14, 257n4, 257n5; amputation, 238, 241; appendages, 186; body scheme/image, 165, 166, 234, 239; breast, 163; ear, 163, 172; face, 168, 175; feet, 163, 258n14; gapping, 164; genitalia/penis, 163, 172, 208, 230; geography, 176, 184, 189,

221, 241, 149, 152, 158, 176, 177, 179, 180, 184, 189, 241; hand/arm, 163, 168, 172, 175; invasion, 177; motor, 160–165, 180, 218, 241; Penfield, 160–165, 166, 173, 176, 258n6; sensory, 160–165, 180, 218, 241; telescoping, 164, 166

imaging technologies, 13, 17, 149, 155, 156, 158, 185–186, 191–192, 230, 232, 257n1, 258n7

Jensen, Mark, 217

Katz, Joel, 32, 39, 42, 47–78, 60, 69, 92–93, 100, 158, 170, 183, 192, 218, 234, 254n9, 259; pain memories, 102–103

kinesthetic legacy, 146, 230

Korean War, 122, 205, 209, 262n15

language of pain, 73, 82–85, 86, 89

leprosy, 116, 143, 144,

lobotomy, 96–97

masculinity, 12, 111, 132, 146, 197, 199, 224, 229, 230, 261n12; hegemonic masculinity, 163, 200, 207–208

McGill Pain Questionnaire (MPQ), 73, 74, 85–89; pain quality, 89–95

medicalization, 12, 26, 108, 138–139, 142

Melzack, Ronald, 42, 46, 47, 48, 52, 53, 54, 56, 58, 59–60, 64–65, 67, 70, 76, 81, 87, 128, 142, 153–154, 159, 231, 254n1; archetypal engram, 143–146; gate-control theory, 98–99; the McGill Pain Questionnaire, 85–92; the neuromatrix, 147–148, 208, 224, 230, 233, 235, 249, 257n15; pain memory, 102–103; pain memory, correlation with, 212–214

Merleau-Ponty, Maurice, 116, 117–118

Merzenich, Michael, 258n7

mirror neurons, 224, 242–243, 249

mislocation phenomenon, 23, 170–179, 192; "dual percepts," 170, 172; modality-specific, 174–179; orgasm, 172–173; referred sensation, 32, 170–175, 177–178, 179, 184; referred to the breast, 172, 173–174, 176; referred to the foot/feet, 172, 173, 176; referred to genitalia, 172, 258n14; referred to the hand(s), 171, 174–175, 176, 179; "remote trigger zone(s)"/far-removed, 171–177; topographically-precise, 174–179; trigger zone(s), 170, 174–176, 258n13

Mitchell, Silas Weir, 12, 20–21, 22, 34, 35, 48, 49, 75, 101, 108–112, 197, 226, 255n2, 256n6
modernization of amputation, 6, 28, 142, 163, 194, 195–200, 223, 244
modernization of combat, 198–199
Mullins, Aimee, 15–17

National Association of Prosthetic-Orthotic Educators (NAPOE), 261n10
National Commission on Orthotic and Prosthetic Education (NCOPE), 261n10
natural phantom, 23, 43, 62, 69, 72, 74, 106, 201
nerve irritation theory, 112–113, 121, 152–154, 171
neural interfacing, 10, 253n6
neuroimaging, 149, 156, 158, 186, 191–192, 258n7
neuroma, 97, 113, 153–154
neuronal sprouting/arborization, 152, 169–170, 184, 186, 241, 259n20
neuronal unmasking, 152, 186, 241, 259n20
neuroscientific, 13, 19, 27, 29, 71, 108, 139–140, 148, 149, 152, 157, 160, 167, 178, 180, 223, 230, 232, 235; neuroscientist(s), 148, 158, 160, 168, 176, 181, 188, 191, 194, 231, 249, 250, 258n7
nosology, 82, 112, 150

object relations, 49–52, 71, 89, 192, 193–194, 249; body scheme/image, 117; "object centered socialities," 18–19; pain, 75–76, 77, 83; penetrating, 7, 27, 127–128, 178; utility, 115; "work object," 149–151
Office of War Information (OWI), 203, 261n11
ontology, 7, 10, 19, 25, 30, 62, 150, 159, 223, 240, 246, 159

pain medicine, 26, 73, 74, 82, 83, 89, 92, 94–95, 105, 244
pain memory, 23, 72, 102, 100–105, 178, 179, 183
pained subject, 74, 95
Paré, Ambrose, 108, 255n1, 255n2, 256n6
Penfield, Wilder, 161–165, 166, 167, 168, 169, 172, 173, 176, 257n3, 258n6
phantom animation, 22, 24, 48, 149, 184, 188, 190, 191, 192, 209, 211, 215–217, 222, 249, 250; inhabit, 11, 22, 24, 149, 194, 209
phantom awareness, 7, 22, 23, 32, 56, 75–76, 81, 104, 154, 187, 200, 235

phantom breast, 76–77, 114, 119–121, 172–173, 176, 227–228, 235, 256n6
"the phantom complex," 32
phantom distortion, 23–24, 25–26, 33–34, 55, 68–72, 105, 107, 114, 141, 147, 149, 179, 192, 201, 212, 223, 229, 233; pain, 103; proliferation, 20, 22, 28, 31, 35, 176; supernumerary phantoms, 24, 65–69, 147, 233
phantom exercise, 48, 49, 55, 72, 184–185, 189, 209, 218–219, 222, 228, 242
phantom disappearance, 20, 23–24, 52, 54–55, 62, 70, 114, 127, 133–134, 141, 154, 166, 179, 187, 192, 200–201, 211, 216–217, 222, 254n3, 259n16
phantom fading, 23, 53, 54, 55, 56, 59, 62, 114, 166, 188, 200–201, 216, 254n3
phantom floating, 56–60, 70, 91, 166
phantom forgetting, 20, 22, 23, 42–45, 55, 72
phantom gaps/holes, 7, 22, 24, 36, 47, 58–59, 60, 164
phantom jactitation/spasming, 21, 22, 23, 46, 48–49, 212
phantom limb: alienation, 20, 42, 107; cleaved, 141–142; congenital, 27, 53, 126, 141, 144, 233; dream morphology, 13, 134–135; experimental objects, 148, 157; extinction/displacement, 24, 29, 194, 221–222, 223, 235, 225, 235, 248–250; healthy, 49, 55, 185, 190, 209, 218; idiosyncratic, 52, 71, 229, 232–233; indispensable, 160, 190, 210, 214–215, 235; intercourse, 172, 173, 258n16; mental compromise/insanity, 79, 95, 111, 112, 139–142, 223, 230; more real than real, 14, 160, 232, 242, 254n1; morphology, 25, 33, 70, 110, 149, 154, 164, 176, 187, 229; penetration, 22, 50, 127–128, 178; prevalence rate, 222, 226, 254n4; provoking, 28, 53–54, 154, 197, 200, 216; socially/materially substantive, 9, 19, 52, 70, 105, 107, 127, 149, 151, 160, 223; transgressive, 70, 77, 152, 176, 192, 235; treatment, 20, 26, 72, 74, 78, 89, 93, 95–101, 106, 114, 133, 153–154, 181, 184–185, 224, 254n8, 257n11; universal, 81, 120, 122, 140, 222, 227; vulnerable/at risk populations, 27, 108, 114, 121, 142–144, 230; willed, 23, 46–49, 72, 185, 186, 218; window, 13, 158, 159, 191, 235, 250
phantom mimesis, 6–7, 31, 35, 68–69, 70, 71–72, 75, 107, 114, 125, 160, 176, 179, 224; body scheme/image, 119; forgetting, 42–44; movement, 36–38, 45–49; pain,

102–103; posture, 35–36; sensation, 34–35, 38–39; unconscious, 110; utility, 55
phantom morphology, 70, 154, 164, 176, 187
phantom occupation, 22, 24, 52
phantom pain, 125, 154, 190; cortical reorganization, 188, 189, 190; epidemic, 25, 72, 103, 106, 212, 230; exposure, 23, 27, 114, 122–124, 243; intersubjective understanding, 82–85, 89; mental compromise/insanity, 79–80, 95, 104, 109, 124; narcissism, 131–132, 139, 140; neurosis, 95–96; peak of pain, 74, 100, 103, 212; prevent(ion), 74, 103, 106, 155, 184–185, 188, 189–190, 211–212, 217; provoking, 54, 123; prevalence rate, 25, 26, 74, 80–82, 99, 100, 104–106, 119, 132, 217; treatment, 95–100, 154, 184–185, 187–188, 242, 243
phantom paralysis, 7, 22, 23, 27, 49–52, 55, 101, 126–128, 142, 144, 178, 187–188, 224, 229; learned paralysis, 49–50, 55, 114, 242
phantom parts, 23–24, 113–114, 118–121, 227, 228: proliferation, 108, 121, 176, 230; brain-based, 157, 176, 243
phantom penis, 29, 119, 121, 224, 225–229, 234, 255n2
phantom peripheralism, 154–155
phantom pleasure, 7, 23, 26, 70, 74, 75–80, 94, 105, 106, 212, 224, 228, 231
phantom proliferation, 20–24, 27, 108, 118–122, 168, 176, 192, 230, 235; and pain, 22, 26, 74, 77, 89, 94
phantom reawakening, 23, 54, 185, 187, 188, 189, 192, 200, 211, 224, 249, 250, 253n1
phantom regrowth, 23, 64, 197, 201
phantom shape-shifting/protean nature, 20, 34, 69, 70, 71, 168, 176, 180, 192, 221, 250
phantom shrinking, 24, 58, 60, 66, 127, 178
phantom shunning, 24, 52, 128
phantom taming/domestication, 28, 108, 210–214, 216, 229
phantom telescoping, 58–59, 61–65, 70, 140, 164–166, 178, 183, 187, 197, 200, 212, 259n18, phantom utility, 24, 28–29, 44–45, 49, 55, 63, 72, 188, 189–194, 209–210, 216, 217–221, 222, 223; cortical organization, 217–222
phantom window, 13, 28, 158, 159, 191, 235, 250
phantom-prosthetic relations, 9, 17–20, 22, 24, 28–29, 155, 190–192, 193–194, 200, 210–211, 221–225, 230, 248
phylogenetic recapitulation, 63, 119
Pons, Timothy, 167, 168–170, 176, 177, 186, 258n7, 259n20

preemptive analgesia, 103–104, 106
prostheses/artificial limbs, 229, 232, 247; coaxing/fooling the phantom, 65, 190, 197; cortical reorganization, 189, 192, 213; cosmetic, 190, 200–201, 213, 218; coupling/ investment, 2, 7–8, 10, 184, 208–209, 211, 216, 247, 249, 261n14; curative, 14, 28, 98, 190–191, 200–204, 211–214, 216, 217; facility, 18, 24, 28, 48, 76, 181, 184, 189–190, 209, 215, 217; functional, 190, 201, 213, 217, 219, 221; hiding disfigurement, 6, 197, 196, 206; incorporation, 184, 215, 221; masculinization, 197, 199, 208; mobility, 10, 18, 196, 204; myoelectric, 190, 213; normalization, 205; pain, 192, 218; pity, 195; productivity, 195; quickening, 3, 5, 11, 211, 250; taming, 28, 210–214, 216, 229; therapeutic, 8, 12, 28, 212, 216
prosthetic animation, 8, 18, 22, 24, 48, 149, 184, 190, 192, 209–212, 215–217, 222, 249; coinciding, 208–210, 216
prosthetic design, 7, 9–10, 11–12, 15, 195, 205–206, 245, 262n16; militarization, 12, 140, 205–208, 247
prosthetic imaginary, 9, 13–17, 29, 214, 225, 247, 248
prosthetic manufacturers, 1–3, 15, 251n1
prosthetic science, 3, 140, 194, 199–202, 204, 206, 222, 244–245
prosthetic taken-for-grantedness, 11, 210
prosthetization, 6, 10, 12, 17, 150, 191, 196, 197, 210, 212, 213, 215, 222; absolution, 196; cortical reorganization/remapping, 182, 190, 212, 213, 217; cyborg warrior, 206, 207–208; disability, 2, 204, 246, 248, 253n6; embodiment, 208–209, 213, 222, 243; esthetics, 15, 17; interface, 246; militarized, 206; miracle of, 196, 198, 201, 206; mobility, 10, 18, 196, 204, 206; normalization, 205; of phantoms, 28, 194, 210; pain, 212; rebirth, 1, 3–6, 9, 13–15, 29; soldier, 206–207; salvation, 196–197; surveillance, 208; therapeutic, 18; tolerable deviance, 196; transcendent/transformative, 6, 194, 198, 201, 205–207, 215, 224–225, 229, 245, 248, 249; prosthetic imaginary, 13, 247
provoking the phantom, 28, 53–54, 123, 154, 197, 200–204, 216, 257n13

qualitative, semi-structure interviewing, 3, 251n1, 252n4, 259n20

Ramachandran, Vilayanur, 39, 45, 48, 65, 99, 102, 144, 160, 162, 168–169, 180, 220, 229, 232, 235, 238, 257n2, 258n14, 259n18; Holy Grail, 157–159; invasion, 172; learned paralysis, 49; mirror box, 187, 188, 192, 250; "overcomplete" body, 239–240; referred sensation, 177–179; transsexuals, 232–235; "trigger zones," 174–175; unmasking hypothesis, 186–188
Reinertsen, Sarah, 2
relational materialism, 151
relationality, 6, 18, 75, 117, 150–151, 192, 193

Schilder, Paul, 116–117, 118, 125, 165
Sherman, Richard, 39, 77, 79, 80, 92, 147, 154–155, 260n4; disability, 265n19; phantom pain treatment, 93, 100, 106, 181, 254n8; psychopathology, 132–133, 257n11; Sherman's typology, 92–93, 94–95, 148, 154–155
Simmel, Marianne, 6, 7, 34, 36,50, 56, 59, 76, 79, 81, 91, 115, 128–129, 140–141, 165–166, 227–228
situational analysis, 251n2
specificity theory, 97–98, 254n6
superadded features, 23, 39–42, 72
supernumerary limbs, 24, 65–69, 147, 233
symptomatology, 105, 112, 150, 230

Taub, Edward, 148, 168, 177–178, 181–182, 184, 221, 234, 258n9, 259n20

techno-corporeality, 2, 3–6, 11, 17, 18, 29, 191, 207, 214, 224, 245, 247–248, 249
techno-induced liberation, 140, 194, 204–208, 225, 247
technologic conjoin-ment, 4, 15, 18, 192, 224, 248
technologic fetishism, 6, 15, 38, 223; cyborg, 208
technological liberation, 140,
technology(ies)-of-the-body, 7- 9, 11, 18, 216
transsexual(ity), 29, 224,232–235, 238, 249, 263n13,

Veterans Administration (VA), 32, 124, 200, 202, 261n7, 261n8, 262n16
Vietnam War, 205, 209, 262n15
virtual reality, 185, 186, 188, 190, 218–219, 224, 242, 250; artificial, 190; augmented, 188, 242; immersive, 188
vulnerable populations, 27, 108, 114, 142–144, 230

wish-fulfillment theory, 43, 131, 134–136, 139–140, 142, 159, 166
work object, 149–150
Wright, Alexa, 40, 51, 57, 60, 62, 64
WWI (World War I), 122, 198–200, 201, 207, 262n15
WWII (World War II), 12, 37, 78, 114, 122, 123 124, 140, 192, 201, 205–207, 209, 216, 243, 262n15

Cassandra S. Crawford was born and raised in California, where she received her Ph.D. in Sociology from the University of California–San Francisco. She is Assistant Professor at Northern Illinois University and Faculty Associate in Women's Studies and in Lesbian, Gay, Bisexual, and Transgender Studies.